Man-Tak Leung · Lee-Ming Tan
Editors

Applied Psychology Readings

Selected Papers from Singapore Conference on Applied Psychology, 2016

Springer

Editors
Man-Tak Leung
Department of Counselling
and Psychology
Hong Kong Shue Yan University
North Point
Hong Kong

Lee-Ming Tan
East Asia Research Pte. Ltd.
Singapore
Singapore

ISBN 978-981-10-2795-6 ISBN 978-981-10-2796-3 (eBook)
DOI 10.1007/978-981-10-2796-3

Library of Congress Control Number: 2016953326

Printed on acid-free paper

This Springer imprint is published by Springer Nature
The registered company is Springer Nature Singapore Pte Ltd.
The registered company address is: 152 Beach Road, #22-06/08 Gateway East, Singapore 189721, Singapore

Preface

2016 Singapore Conference on Applied Psychology (SCAP 2016), organised by East Asia Research (EAR) and supported by the Hong Kong Shue Yan University, Singapore University of Technology and Design and Association of Psychotherapists and Counsellors (Singapore), was held during June 14–15, 2016 at Holiday Inn Singapore Atrium.

The special theme for SCAP 2016 was 'Towards Education Cohesiveness—A Psychological Perspective'. The annual SCAP conference series organised by EAR are major international events aimed at supporting the Applied Psychology and HR communities in Asia. Psychologists, healthcare professionals, academicians and researchers from all fields of applications get to meet, network and learn here.

The programme consisted of an opening speech by the conference chair, Dr. Man-Tak Leung, Hong Kong Shue Yan University and three half-hour plenary lectures by Dr. Jaclyn Lee, Dr. Po Gim Tee Jeffrey and Abigail Lee. There are also two parallel sessions of 27 oral presentations (20 min each). A total of 55 registered delegates from the following countries participated in SCAP 2016: Australia, Austria, France, Hong Kong, India, Indonesia, Macao, Malaysia, Philippines, Singapore, Taiwan, Thailand, UK and USA. Participants were invited to submit papers to the present volume. We wish to thank Dr. Man-Tak Leung from Hong Kong Shue Yan University, SCAP 2016 Conference Chair, for coordinating the reviewing of the submitted papers.

East Asia Research (EAR)

Established in Singapore in 2015, EAR envisions to be the gateway to improving lives and enhancing productivity in Asia through promoting cross-geographical exchange of ideas and knowledge in various faculties. This will be achieved through the dissemination of knowledge from the Asia-focused research conferences and publications by EAR.

EAR academic conferences provide a meaningful platform for researchers, postgraduates, academicians, and industry practitioners to share unique insights and drive innovation. This is a great opportunity for expanding contact networks beyond a singular field and kick-starting a strategic collaboration. Such partnership can bridge the resources and expertise of multiple disciplines to spearhead pioneer movements, giving rise to breakthroughs in long-standing issues.

The present volume embraces various research topics in applied psychology such as psychometrics, educational psychology, cognitive psychology, psychoanalysis, sport psychology, social psychology, cyber psychology, emotion and motivation, structural equation modelling, item response theory, and their crossovers. These papers will serve as supplementary readings and references for applied psychologists in doing their research.

North Point, Hong Kong — Man-Tak Leung
Singapore, Singapore — Lee-Ming Tan

Acknowledgments

The editors would like to express gratitude to Dr. Jane Montague, Discipline Lead for Psychology; Assistant Head of Department of Life Sciences, University of Derby, for her professional advice on preparing this book. Dr. Montague had recently published a paper: 'Worlds within worlds: A strategy for using interpretative phenomenological analysis with focus groups. Qualitative Research in Psychology.' which can be reached at: http://www.tandfonline.com/eprint/8UJ8gjpiwuArpwUghDnS/full.

Contents

About the Editors

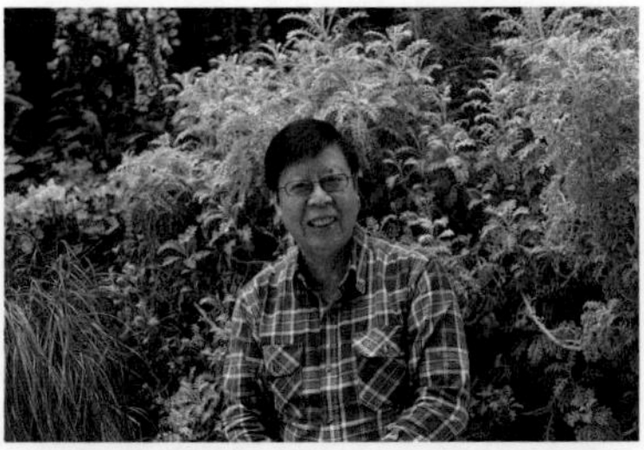

Dr. Man-Tak Leung is currently Assistant Professor of Counselling and Psychology at the Hong Kong Shue Yan University. Dr. Leung obtained his Ph.D. in Educational Psychology from the Chinese University of Hong Kong, three Master Degrees from Hong Kong University in Educational Assessment (M.Ed.), Applied Statistics (M.Soc.Sc), and Information Technology in Education (M.Sc.) respectively. His research embraced undergraduates and high school students' achievement emotions, achievement goals, social achievement goals, achievement motives related with their study processes, learning strategies and self-regulated learning with various antecedents such as personality traits, enneagram, attachment styles, sense of school belonging, cyber-informatics addictive behaviour, classroom climate, action and control belief, eastern and western parenting styles, Chinese values, motivational beliefs, epistemological belief in ability, implicit belief in intelligence, self-construal, self-efficacy, and academic self-concepts leading to subsequent achievement outcomes. He had presented not less than 50 conference papers in various international conferences as well as local conferences held in Australia, New Zealand, Hawaii, Singapore, Japan, Malaysia, Mainland China and Hong Kong. Dr. Leung has published academic papers in international peer-reviewed journals, book chapters, conference proceedings, theses, dissertations and consulting reports and they were awarded Distinguished Paper Award in ISEP 2013, Best Paper Award in ACAP 2014, ACAP 2015 and SCAP 2016, respectively. He adores Jack Russell terriers, enjoys travelling and taking photos, listens to music and enjoys doing research and supervising students' research projects.

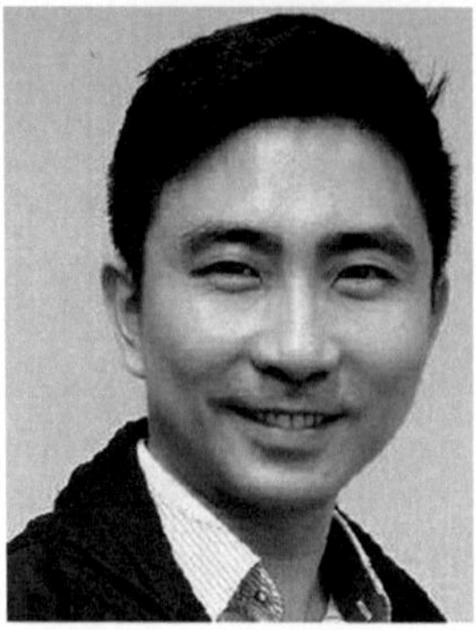

Mr. Lee-Ming Tan is the founder of East Asia Research and he obtained his Master of Applied Finance from the University of Adelaide. He is deeply interested in how humans function and react with each other. An insight into how people's minds think and how they work together is invaluable in just about every field. Outside of work, Anthony Tan enjoys outdoor activities and occasional computer games.

Scap Advisory Board

Conference Chair

Dr. Man-Tak Leung, Department of Counselling and Psychology, Hong Kong Shue Yan University

Committee Members

Dr. W. Quin Yow, Ph.D., Director, Language and Social Cognition Lab, Assistant Professor (Psychology), Singapore University of Technology and Design
Dr. Zhou, Dehui Ruth, Department of Counselling and Psychology, Hong Kong Shue Yan University
Dr. Ho, Sin-Wan Bianca, Department of Counselling and Psychology, Hong Kong Shue Yan University
Dr. Tan Jing Hee, Executive Director and Chairman of its Academic Board of East Asia Institute of Management
Dr. Po Gim Tee Jeffrey, Ph.D., Former President of the Association of Psychotherapists and Counsellors (Singapore)
Ms. Abigail Lee, President of the Association of Psychotherapists and Counsellors (Singapore)

Conference Organiser

East Asia Research

Conference Sponsors

Qatar Airways

Routledge Taylor and Francis Group

Chapter 1
The Phenomenology and Ontology of the Oedipus Complex

Matthew Gildersleeve

Abstract This paper will continue my earlier work that provided a phenomenological and ontological explanation of Jung's complex theory (Gildersleeve in Procedia Soc Behav Sci 217:967–976, 2016). This paper will contribute to that earlier work by providing a phenomenological explanation of Freud's writing on the Oedipus complex and this phenomenological description will also allow the ontological meaning of the Oedipus complex to be understood. This work reveals the convergent ideas between Martin Heidegger's philosophy and Sigmund Freud's psychoanalysis and this provides support to defend the existence of Freud's arguments on the Oedipus complex by explaining it through the lived experience vocabulary of phenomenology. This article also demonstrates that Jung's and Freud's writing on complexes possess the same phenomenological and ontological structure and this shows that their respective theories can be integrated to develop psychoanalytic theory and practice in new ways. Finally, this work contributes to the writing of Medard Boss and the Daseinsanalysis literature that has yet to provide a Daseinsanalytic interpretation of the Oedipus complex.

Keywords Jung · Heidegger · Freud · Phenomenology · Complexes

1.1 Introduction

Askay and Farquhar (2013) have demonstrated how psychoanalysis can benefit from using Heidegger's philosophy by highlighting similarities between Freud and Heidegger that include developing a comprehensive and unified explanation of the human being. Consequently Askay and Farquhar (2013) argue that there is

M. Gildersleeve (✉)
School of Social and Behavioural Sciences, University of Queensland,
Brisbane, QLD, Australia
e-mail: m.gildersleeve@uq.edu.au

M.-T. Leung and L.-M. Tan (eds.), *Applied Psychology Readings*,
DOI 10.1007/978-981-10-2796-3_1

an “intimate belonging together” (Askay and Farquhar 2013, p. 1228) of Being and the unconscious. These authors emphasize this has been supported by a number of philosophers and psychologists including Needleman, Richardson, Binswanger, Boss, Loewald, Chessick, Frie, Mills and Thompson. Accordingly, Askay and Farquhar (2013) argue that a merger of Heidegger’s work with Freud’s will provide an enhanced and more comprehensive explanation of the human being (Askay and Farquhar 2006).

1.2 Phenomenology, Lived Experience and the Human Sciences

Heidegger (2001) explicitly engaged with psychoanalysis in the Zollikon seminars organized by psychiatrist Medard Boss from 1959 to 1969. As a result of this engagement, Boss developed psychoanalysis with Heidegger’s phenomenology and ontology to establish a new psychotherapeutic method named Daseinsanalysis (Boss 1963). Boss and Heidegger felt the Zollikon seminars were required. Instead of building his explanation of the human mind on Heidegger’s fundamental ontology, Freud uncritically adopted the assumptions of the metaphysical tradition of Cartesianism. This involves conceptualizing the mind from the third person point of view and as a mechanical object. This resulted in concealing the lived experience and ontological meaning of a human. In contrast, phenomenology is understood as a human science compared to psychoanalysis that is understood as a natural science and “The distinction of “Human” Science versus “Natural” Science is often attributed to Wilhelm Dilthey” (Van Manen 1990, p. 3). Storolow explains “According to Dilthey, the human sciences are to be distinguished from the sciences of nature because of a fundamental difference in attitude toward their respective objects of investigation: the natural sciences investigate objects from the outside whereas the human sciences rely on a view from the inside” (Stolorow and Atwood 1984, p. 88).

Since Freud adhered to the natural scientific tradition he assumed that the human can be completely explained by inferring the meaning of behaviour and “the continuity of causal connections” (Askay and Farquhar 2006, p. 216). Heidegger highlights the problem of inferring the meaning of behaviour that lays outside of the lived experience as Freud’s creation of the unconscious postulated a hidden entity to explain the mind that was not found in everyday experience and could not be perceived. This distinction between the natural scientific view of human behaviour in psychoanalysis and the phenomenological view in Daseinsanalysis is evident when Freud says: “We do not seek merely to describe and classify phenomena but to comprehend them as indications of a play of forces in the mind, as expressions of tendencies striving towards a goal, which work together or against one another. In this conception, the trends we merely infer are more prominent than the phenomena we perceive”. (Freud 1920, p. 60)

Consequently, it appears Freud constructed hypothetical explanations for human behaviour because he followed the common mode of scientific thinking where "human beings reject the importance of things experienced directly. They do not count. Meanwhile, most proofs rest on mere hypotheses" (Heidegger 2001, p. 215). In contrast, Heidegger's philosophy describes and explains human behaviour using direct evidence found in the phenomena of lived experience and Boss highlights this tenet by saying "what Heidegger's teaching has taught me" is "only to open my eyes" (Boss 1988, p. 41).

Medard Boss adhered to Heidegger's fundamental ontology of Dasein and articulated an appropriate response to natural scientific method of psychoanalysis (Heidegger 2001, p. 269). Boss's work aimed to develop an ontologically suitable psychoanalysis. Boss acknowledged the importance of Freud's psychoanalytic techniques to help a person achieve mental health but Boss rejected Freud's theory to explain human behaviour. Therefore, Boss's writing aimed to explain and re-interpret Freud's theoretical writing through the light of Heidegger's phenomenology. Boss avoided applying the natural science method to human behaviour which distorts the knowledge built in this area because "psychology, anthropology, and psychopathology have considered the human being as an object in a broad sense, as something present-at-hand, as a domain of beings" (Heidegger 2001, p. 153). By conceiving humans as an object, the lived experience dimension of that human is not included in knowledge construction.

Richardson (2003), who recognized that psychoanalytic theories that adhere to natural science are unnecessary since phenomenology can explain behaviour through direct lived experience, also supports the phenomenological method applied to psychoanalysis. With the use of natural scientific method, psychoanalysis has distorted and obstructed human behaviour to be explained correctly, because this explanation is not verified by lived experience. Alternatively, Daseinsanalysis avoids the construction of unverifiable concepts to explain human behaviour by building explanations from direct lived experience through the method of phenomenology.

Loparic (1999) says when Heidegger critiques psychoanalysis he accepts Freud's observations but these observations need to be translated into a "language of description of phenomena" (Heidegger 2001, p. 345). Heidegger recognizes that Freud has discovered many 'ontic' experiences such as projection, identification, regression and repression, however for these behaviours to be adequately explained, these discoveries need to be re-interpreted in the light of Heidegger phenomenological ontology of Dasein. Thus, Loparic declares all behaviour encountered in psychoanalysis must be understood as "particular modes of being in the world, which make them possible" (Loparic 1999, p. 14). Spinelli also provides an explanation of the essential features of Daseinsanalysis that include rejecting the idea of a human being as "a psychic apparatus" which is determined by "unseen psychic structures and forces" (Spinelli 1996, p. 32).

Daseinsanalysis attempts to acquire a more accurate understanding of human behavior using Heidegger's "analysis of Dasein" (Boss 1963, p. 4). Boss emphasizes that Daseinsanalysis urges theories in psychology to be constructed by remaining with what is immediately perceived and to "not get lost in "scientific" abstractions, derivations, explanations, and calculations estranged from the immediate reality of the given phenomena" (Boss 1963, p. 30). Daseinsanalysis avoids the "dangerous scientific tendency to flee from the immediately given phenomena" (Boss 1963, p. 59) and unverified assumptions which construct abstractions "behind" direct experience. Consequently, Boss states that Daseinsanalysis's criticism towards psychoanalysis "is positive" (Boss, 1963, p. 59) because it is capable of explaining human behaviour through lived experience rather than from "distant and abstract positions" (Boss 1963, p. 59). Daseinsanalysis demonstrates the inadequacy of the secondary, "speculative superstructure" of psychoanalytic theory, because Daseinsanalysis can elucidate "on the basis of immediate experience, all those psychic phenomena that forced Freud to invent the unconscious" (Boss 1963, p. 94).

With all the success that has been achieved through the natural scientific method in psychology "the natural scientific approach repeatedly finds itself confronting a realm to which it cannot gain access" (Boss 1977). Thus, the role of Daseinsanalysis is to gain access to the lived first person experience and explain behaviour from the areas of life which natural science cannot reach. Boss says Freud uncritically thought that the natural scientific path was the only way to truth. Unfortunately, by adhering to this method, psychoanalysis constructs "conclusions that are alien to the actual appearance of our objects of study, with abstractions that depart from what can actually be seen" (Boss 1977, p. 84).

Finally, in "Daseinsanalysis: A Quest for Essentials", Craig (1988) also calls for all psychoanalytic theories to re-interpreted with Heidegger's fundamental ontology. Craig explains Boss has lead the way in this task by explaining a variety of psychoanalytic concepts such as "transference", "countertransference", "resistance", "repetition compulsion" and "acting out", "in the philosophically "purified" light of phenomenological reflection" (Craig 1988, p. 15). However, Boss nor any other Daseinsanalysts are yet to apply this purified light to the Oedipus complex and this article focuses on this task since the Oedipus complex "is probably the most important segment in Freud's developmental explanatory scheme" (Kupfersmid 1995, p. 536). Furthermore, it is important to provide phenomenological support to the Oedipus complex since "its recognition has become the shibboleth that distinguishes the adherents of psycho-analysis from its opponents" (Freud 2001b, p. 226) and the phenomenological explanation presented in this article may assist in turning opponents into adherents for the benefit of unifying the dispersed psychotherapeutic community. Consequently, this article fills this "knowledge gap" left by Boss by re-interpreting Freud's writing on the Oedipus complex in the "purified" light of phenomenology. This article continues the work of Boss who aimed to cure therapists "of what he refers to as "a new neurosis best called 'psychoanalytis'" (Craig 1988, p. 15) which means to explain the findings in psychoanalysis through the precise and appropriate method of phenomenology.

1.3 The Oedipus Complex

The significance of this article is further highlighted by the phenomenological support it provides to the theory of the Oedipus complex and this is important since its introduction "has provoked the most violent opposition among adults" (Freud 2001d, p. 207). Dimas et al. (2008, p. 1343), also highlight "The theory of the oedipus complex has its opponents, who often question its validity due to the lack of sufficient empirical investigation" and "the term is based on anecdotal evidence that is subject to personal biases". It is no surprise there has been violent disapproval by opponents who question the validity of the Oedipus complex since it has been described with "conclusions that are alien to the actual appearance of our objects of study, with abstractions that depart from what can actually be seen" (Boss 1977, p. 84).

In contrast to the natural scientific method, this article describes the Oedipus complex using the human scientific method of phenomenology. Phenomenology is capable of turning violent opposition into adherents of the Oedipus complex when this phenomenon can be presented by remaining with what is immediately perceived and to "not get lost in "scientific" abstractions, derivations, explanations, and calculations estranged from the immediate reality of the given phenomena" (Boss 1963, p. 30). As a result, this article recognizes and addresses Poland's concern with the Oedipus complex "The controversy is centrally a problem of definition having to do with levels of abstraction, with the difference between unique phenomenological experiences and the theorizing generalizations drawn from and about them. Human experience is always specific, singular, particular, unique" (Poland 2007, p. 561).

Before starting this work, I will end this introduction with a brief prelude to the terminology used in this article. Throughout this article the word 'Oedipus' will be placed in parentheses to emphasize that the arguments being made are applicable to both Freud and Jung's writings on complexes. The parentheses have been inserted to accommodate the Freudian reference to complexes (Freud writes 'Oedipus complex') and the Jungian reference to complexes (Jung only writes 'complex'). The final note on terminology used in this article concerns the word 'Dasein'. Dasein will be used to refer to the specific ontology of human existence that Heidegger explains in his book *Being and Time* (Heidegger 2000).

1.4 The Phenomenology and Ontology of a (Oedipus) Complex

By the end of this paper, this article will demonstrate that the ontological meaning of a (Oedipus) complex is phenomenologically disclosed when Dasein's world is conspicuously experienced as unready to hand and "not—being-at-home". In the experience of a (Oedipus) complex, angst, conscience and guilt are saliently disclosed in a moment of conspicuous obstructiveness and obstinacy, which results in the ready to-hand losing its readiness-to-hand in a certain way. The inauthentic and authentic understanding of the meaning of the (Oedipus) complex because of this moment will also be described. Finally, this article also integrates Jung's writing on complexes with Freud's to demonstrate both possess the same ontological structure and this highlights the potential for both Freud's and Jung's theory to be combined together with Heidegger's phenomenological ontology to advance psychoanalytic theory in the future.

In *Being and Time*, Heidegger explains that to the everydayness of Being-in-the-world there belong certain modes of concern. This permits the entities with which Dasein concerns itself to be encountered in such a way that the worldly character of what is within the world comes to be faced. When Dasein is concerned with something, entities that are ready-to-hand may be met as something unusable and not appropriately modified for the use that has been chosen. As a result, when unusability is discovered, equipment becomes conspicuous and "This conspicuousness presents the ready-to-hand equipment as in a certain un-readiness-to hand" (Heidegger 1962, p. 103). This explanation of Dasein's being in the world is very informative to both Freud and Jung's concept of a complex. Both Jung and Freud implicitly recognize the similar disturbance and conspicuousness of "un-readiness-to hand" a complex has on a person. For example, Jung, commenting on his word association experiment results says, "At the very simplest words there appear obstructions and other disturbances which can be explained only by the fact that the stimulus word has excited a complex" (Jung 1907, p. 43). On the other hand, Freud says, "In the very earliest years of childhood (approximately between the ages of two and five) a convergence of the sexual impulses occurs of which, in the case of boys, the object is the mother. This choice of an object, in conjunction with a corresponding attitude of rivalry and hostility towards the father, provides the content of what is known as the Oedipus complex" (Freud 1925, p. 120).

This comparison shows both Freud and Jung converge with Heidegger here as they all place emphasis on highlighting a conspicuous experience that disturbs and obstructs a person's life. The similarity between Jung's descriptions from his experiments on the experience of a complex on a person's consciousness and Freud's description of the experience of hostility towards the father is very much the same as Heidegger's description of Dasein encountering the world as conspicuous and unready to hand. This combination initially suggests a defining feature of a complex appears to be the experience of what Heidegger calls 'unreadiness to hand', where the disruption may be caused by a word (Jung) or the father (Freud). Due to this initial connection between Jung's, Freud's and Heidegger's work, the psychoanalytic concept of the complex will now be phenomenologically and ontologically developed and clarified.

The phenomenological and ontological meaning of the experience of a complex can be further understood by recognizing that "In our concernful dealings, however, we not only come up against unusable things within what is ready-to-hand already: we also find things which are missing which not only are not 'handy' but are not 'to hand' at all" (Heidegger 1962, p. 103). When Dasein notices the un-ready-to-hand, the world of entities ready-to-hand becomes obstructive, which means the world "cannot be budged without the thing that is missing" (Heidegger 1962, p. 103). Consequently, anything that is un-ready-to-hand is disturbing to Dasein, and enables Dasein to see the obstinacy of that with which Dasein must concern itself (the (Oedipal) complex). "With this obstinacy, the world makes itself known in a new way as the Being of that which still lies before us and calls for our attending to it" (Heidegger 1962, p. 104). In other words, the ontological meaning of the experience of the (Oedipus) complex calls for Dasein's attending to its obstinate obstructiveness to being in the world.

Now as both Freud's and Jung's writing highlighted before, the experience of a (Oedipus) complex disturbs and hinders daily life just in the same way Heidegger phenomenologically describes the world as unready to hand. As a result, what should now be apparent from the introduction of Heidegger's writing is that the experience of a disturbing (Oedipus) complex is an important moment to Dasein. It not only indicates that the current way of existing is unsuitable because of conspicuous obstructiveness of the world but it also indicates its obstinacy and need for attention to remove this obstructiveness from being in the world. This can be further understood when Heidegger says that the "structure of the Being of what is ready-to-hand as equipment is determined by references or assignments" (Heidegger 1962, p. 105). As a result, when the world of Dasein becomes conspicuously unready to hand from the experience of a (Oedipus) complex, the reference or assignment has become explicit and the obstructive environment has been disclosed which means it has been opened or unconcealed. This opening of the obstructiveness of the world is a fundamental step in the process of making the unconscious (Oedipus) complex, conscious in the process of individuation (Jung) or the formation of the super-ego (Freud). A phenomenological explanation of the process of authentically understanding the (Oedipus) complex and overcoming the obstructiveness it presents will be presented in the last third of this article, under the heading "Authentic Understanding of the Experience of a (Oedipus) Complex".

From both Freud's and Jung's writing on (Oedipus) complexes displays the characteristics of individualizing a person from other beings and in the same moment there appears to produce a feeling of "not-being-at-home" in the world. The uncanniness of this individualized "not being at home" event of the experience of a complex reflects the writing of Heidegger's description of Dasein's experience of angst. For example, Jung says that the feeling of a complex disrupts consciousness in the same way Heidegger explains angst disrupts Dasein's being in the world. This similarity of emotion linking the complex with angst is evident when Jung suggests the "The emotional inhibition must be cited as the main hindering cause" (Jung 1907, p. 43) to consciousness. Similarly, Freud says, "The ego reacts with feelings of anxiety (conscience anxiety) to the perception that it has not come up to the demands made by its ideal, the super-ego" (Freud 2001g, p. 167). In other words, the ego experiences anxiety when there is an obstruction (e.g. the father) in the way of the desired mother (demands from the super-ego) and this produces a phenomenological experience of "not-being-at-home" in the world.

To add to this, Heidegger says, "that in the face of which one has anxiety is Being-in-the world" (Heidegger 1962, p. 231) however, that in the face of which one has anxiety is not an entity within the world. To understand the ontology and phenomenology of a (Oedipus) complex it is also important to note that Heidegger says that in the face of which one is anxious is completely indefinite and this tells Dasein that entities within-the-world are not relevant. Thus, when something threatening brings itself close, the experience of the anxiety of a (Oedipus) complex "does not 'see' any definite 'here' or 'yonder' from which it comes" (Heidegger 1962, p. 231). The (Oedipus) complex is unconscious and therefore "that in the face of which one has anxiety is characterized by the fact that what threatens is nowhere" (Heidegger 1962, p. 231).

This is relevant to understanding the phenomenology and ontology of the (Oedipus) complex because it highlights that angst reveals that the (Oedipus) complex is unconscious to Dasein. As long as it is unconscious, Dasein will be "tenderly attached to the parent of the opposite sex, while its relation to the parent of its own sex is predominantly hostile" (Freud 2001h, p. 225). When Dasein is "tenderly attached to the parent of the opposite sex, while its relation to the parent of its own sex is predominantly hostile" Dasein encounters angst. Dasein is unconscious to the task of renouncing "the intense object-cathexes which he has deposited with his parents" and to compensate for this loss with "a strong intensification of the identifications with his parents" (Freud et al. 2005, p. 490).

In addition to this attunement to anxiety in the experience of an unconscious (Oedipus) complex, Heidegger's phenomenology of existence suggests that conscience would also take part in this experience. The experience of angst can also be understood to reveal the call of conscience as an appeal to Dasein. Heidegger says the call of conscience calls Dasein back to be called forth to an authentic understanding in the face of anxiety from "not being home in the world". Conscience calls conspicuously to disclose that the world cannot be understood in the current familiar everydayness mode of being. Conscience calls Dasein forth to understand the truth of the meaning of the world that it is anxious about. Therefore, the experience a (Oedipus) complex can also be ontologically understood as a call to Dasein to reveal Dasein's inauthenticity to itself. Conscience calls Dasein inauthentic because the experience of a (Oedipus) complex reveals, "the child has psychically to accommodate the reality of a 'creative relationship of which he is the product and from which he is excluded'" (Waddell 2003, p. 53). Dasein has been inauthentic and experiences "not being home in the world", angst and the call of conscience because the (Oedipus) complex has not been destroyed where "The object-cathexes are given up and replaced by identifications. The authority of the father or the parents is introjected into the ego, and there it forms the nucleus of the super-ego, which takes over the severity of the father and perpetuates his prohibition against incest, and so secures the ego from the return of the libidinal object-cathexis" (Freud et al. 2005, p. 398).

Finally, the last component of providing a phenomenological and ontological explanation of the meaning of the experience of a (Oedipus) complex involves Heidegger's work on guilt. Heidegger says that the 'voice' of conscience speaks of Dasein's 'guilt'. The call of guilty by conscience means "'having responsibility for'-that is, as Being-the basis for…" or "Being the-basis of a nullity" (Heidegger 1962, p. 331). Thus, the experience of a (Oedipus) complex can now be appropriately phenomenologically elucidated with Heidegger's ontology of guilt. The experience of a (Oedipus) complex results in conscience calling Dasein guilty for being the basis for its unfamiliar and obstructive "not being at home in the world" (Heidegger 1962, p. 233). In addition, conscience calls Dasein guilty for the "special affection for his mother, whom he regards as belonging to him" and "to feel his father as a rival who disputes his sole possession" (Freud 2001d, p. 207). As a result, the phenomenological experience of the (Oedipus) complex is argued to consist of anxiety, conscience and guilt that is authentically understood as a call of care from Dasein to itself.

Understanding that Dasein has been called guilty by itself in the experience of a (Oedipus) complex constitutes Dasein's care for its authentic being in the world. In the experience of a (Oedipus) complex, Dasein stands together with the truth of its primordial Being. Conscience calls to Dasein to understand that it is not at home so to call Dasein forth to the possibility of authentically finding its home within the truth of Being by removing the (Oedipus) complex from Dasein's world. When conscience calls, it keeps silent to summon Dasein into the stillness of itself, and Dasein is called "back as something that is to become still" (Heidegger 1962, p. 343). When Dasein encounters a (Oedipus) complex, the world is disclosed in a conspicuous, obstructive and obstinate character, which shows the world to Dasein as insignificant and in need of attention and care. This phenomenological explanation is highlighted in Freud's generic description of the (Oedipus) complex where he says, the child "begins to desire his mother herself in the sense with which he has recently become acquainted, and to hate his father anew as a rival who stands in the way of this wish" (Freud and Gay 1995, p. 392). The father is a rival who stands in the way (conspicuous, obstructive and obstinate) of the child's wish (the child's wish is in need of attention and the care of reflection due to this experience).

Consequently, the experience of a (Oedipus) complex is an important moment for Dasein's being in the world because it has the potential to liberate Dasein to turn towards its authentic meaning for Being by renouncing the "incestuous wish toward the mother and internalizes the paternal authority that demands this renunciation" (Benjamin 1987, p. 213). If Dasein understands itself authentically in the experience of a (Oedipus) complex, this allows Dasein to critically interpret its being-in-the-world to determine those obstructive elements that have been neglected and so threaten its care while being in the world. By falling prey to a (Oedipus) complex, Dasein encounters an obstinate and obstructive existence which calls Dasein forth to individuate "to its ownmost being-in-the-world, which as understanding, projects itself essentially upon possibilities" (Heidegger 1996, p. 176) so the desire for the mother can be "sublimated into more civilized filial feelings" (Benjamin 1987, p. 213). Importantly, the positive nature of the experience of a (Oedipus) complex can bring Dasein face to face with concealed authentic possibilities of existence that have the potential to appropriate the unready to hand and obstructive world in the act of individuation (Jung) or identification (Freud). This will be discussed in part three of this paper.

1.5 Inauthentic Understanding of the Experience of a (Oedipus) Complex

This section of this paper outlines the phenomenology and ontology of an inauthentic understanding of a (Oedipus) complex. Freud "frequently affirmed the importance of the Oedipus complex. Several times he stated that it is the genesis of all neurosis" (Kupfersmid 1995, p. 536) and this section will ontologically explain how an inauthentic understanding of the experience of a (Oedipus) complex is the origin of neurosis.

This section will demonstrate how an inauthentic understanding of the experience of a (Oedipus) complex occurs. This occurs when Dasein has not tolerated "the impossibility of claiming and winning one parent at the expense of the other, but also to endure the position of observer of a relationship in which he or she does not belong—of being at the lonely point of the triangle and of having to acknowledge the existence of a different kind of relationship from that available with either parent" (Waddell 2003, p. 54). Sophocles, King Oedipus is the archetypal example of a neurotic and inauthentic understanding of the experience of a (Oedipus) complex and this is in agreement with Freud who says, "King Oedipus, who slew his father Laïus and married his mother Jocasta, merely shows us the fulfilment of our own childhood wishes. But, more fortunate than he, we have meanwhile succeeded, in so far as we have not become psychoneurotics, in detaching our sexual impulses from our mothers and in forgetting our jealousy of our fathers" (Freud 2001a, p. 262). Jung's work can also contribute to explain how an inauthentic understanding of the experience of a (Oedipus) complex occurs and is the origin of neurosis and this is where this section begins.

Jung states that complexes are psychic contents that are outside the control of the conscious mind because "They have been split off from consciousness and lead a separate existence in the unconscious" (Jung 2001, p. 81). Therefore, it is now important to provide a phenomenological description as to how it is ontologically possible for complexes to be split off from consciousness and to exist unconsciously as this will help to understand how Dasein can understand a (Oedipus) complex inauthentically. First, it is essential to recognize that by its ontological nature, Dasein is always projecting possibilities for its existence as long as it is and therefore can flee the possibility of choosing to exist authentically. If Dasein follows an familiar average everydayness which turns away from authentically understanding a (Oedipus) complex, the care for its being in the world project goes astray which Heidegger calls "the entanglement of Da-sein" (Heidegger 1996, p. 164). Heidegger says entanglement leads to Dasein "Falling prey to the "world", its absorption in being-with-one-another guided by idle talk, curiosity, and ambiguity" (Heidegger 1996, p. 164) instead of an authentic understanding of the experience of a (Oedipus) complex. Falling prey is the constitution of inauthentically turning away from understanding the meaning of the experience of a (Oedipus) complex and falling prey to familiar average everydayness "tears understanding away from projecting authentic possibilities" (Heidegger 1996, p. 167) which leaves a (Oedipus) complex covered and active within the unconscious.

To further explain how neurosis can arise from an inauthentic understanding of a (Oedipus) complex, it is important to note that Heidegger says "The absorption of Da-sein in the 'they' and in the world taken care of reveals something like a flight of Da-sein from itself as an authentic potentiality for being itself" (Heidegger 1996, p. 172). In this flight, Dasein avoids a confrontation with its authentic existence that involves facing the obstructiveness and obstinacy of a (Oedipus) complex that is disclosed through guilt, angst and conscience. This flight can be understood by relating it to Freud's writing on the role of wishful phantasies in the Oedipus complex. Freud says "The deeper you penetrate into the pathogenesis of nervous illness"; "You will be taught that we humans, with the high standards of our civilization and under the pressure of our internal repressions, find reality unsatisfying quite generally, and for that reason entertain a life of phantasy in which we like to make up for the insufficiencies of reality by the production of wish fulfilments" (Freud 2001c, p. 50). When Dasein encounters the experience of a (Oedipus) complex, Dasein can turn away from authentically understanding the meaning of the complex through "the production of wish fufilments". By producing phantasies and wish fulfilments, Dasein has inauthentically understood the meaning of the experience of a (Oedipus) complex and with this; Dasein flees the truth of its authentic self and the ability to remove a (Oedipus) complex remains unconscious to Dasein.

As a result, when Dasein flees the truth of its authentic self though the phantasy of inauthentic understanding, Dasein has not mastered a (Oedipus complex) and "It has been found to be characteristic of a normal individual that he learns to master his Oedipus complex, whereas the neurotic subject remains involved in it" (Freud 1955, p. 245). This allows the creation of neurosis out of the experience of a (Oedipus) complex to be phenomenologically understood because of Dasein covering over its authentic possibilities for care that remain undiscovered. Dasein's essence as being-in-the-world is care, but if the phantasy of an inauthentic understanding of its being is present, Dasein can fall prey to neurosis when Dasein is "fleeing from it and of forgetting" (Heidegger 1996, p. 41) it's authentic understanding of the meaning of a (Oedipus) complex. Consequently "We see that human beings fall ill when, as a result of external obstacles or of an internal lack of adaptation, the satisfaction of their erotic needs in reality is frustrated" (Freud 2001c, p. 49). This frustration can be understood to occur when Dasein covers over its authentic possibilities for care through the phantasy of an inauthentic understanding of a (Oedipus) complex, where “no solution at all is arrived at: the son remains all his life bowed beneath his father’s authority and he is unable to transfer his libido to an outside sexual object. In this sense the Oedipus complex may justly be regarded as the nucleus of the neuroses” (Freud 1963, p. 337).

To add to this, Jung explains that complexes originate and always contain something like a “conflict-they are either the cause or the effect of a conflict” (Jung 1969, p. 98). This conflict is clearly an illustration of an inauthentic understanding of a (Oedipus) complex. For example, Freud explains, “Hans really was a little Oedipus who wanted to have his father ‘out of the way’, to get rid of him, so that he might be alone with his beautiful mother and sleep with her” (Freud 1962, p. 111). This explanation highlights the conflictual nature of a (Oedipus) complex where Hans is in conflict with his father who is “in the way” of Hans “beautiful mother”. Freud also says, “It is the fate of all of us, perhaps, to direct our first sexual impulse towards our mother and our first hatred and our first murderous wish against our father” (Freud, 2001a, p. 262) and this highlights examples of the conflictual nature of a (Oedipus) complex.

Consequently, if Dasein has not developed an authentic understanding of the meaning of a (Oedipus) complex, the conflict is experienced as “““vulnerable points” which we do not like to remember and still less to be reminded of by others, but which frequently come back to mind unbidden and in the most unwelcome fashion” (Jung 2001, p. 81). Furthermore, Heidegger’s phenomenological description of uncanniness also highlights what Jung is saying, which is that the truth of Being (which is experienced as a conflict) that has been attempted to be escaped, can only be escaped inauthentically and “This uncanniness pursues Dasein constantly, and is a threat to its everyday lostness, though not explicitly” (Heidegger 1962, p. 234). Therefore, the obstructiveness and conflict of a (Oedipus) complex will continue to be encountered if Dasein has a neurotic (inauthentic) understanding of the meaning of a (Oedipus) complex and “The detachment of the child from his parents is thus a task that cannot be evaded if the young individual’s social fitness is not to be endangered” (Freud 2001c, p. 48).

Therefore, for Dasein to exist authentically without neurosis, Dasein requires a discovery of the authentic meaning of a (Oedipus) complex. The experience of a (Oedipus) complex ontologically represents the truth of Dasein’s Being which Dasein does not want to face. However, inauthentically fleeing is ineffective as the truth continues to exist even if Daseininauthentically flees the truth of Being and this explains how neurosis develops from the conflict of a (Oedipus) complex. Since the truth of Being persists although Daseininauthentically prefers otherwise, a (Oedipus) complex “always contain memories, wishes, fears, duties, needs, or views, with which we have never really come to terms, and for this reason they constantly interfere with our conscious life in a disturbing and usually a harmful way” (Jung 2001, p. 81). Thus, as long as Dasein has an inauthentic understanding of a (Oedipus) complex, Dasein has yet to “really come to terms” with the need to be “able to bear relinquishment” (Waddell 2003, p. 54) of the desire for the mother and to remove the father.

Without an authentic understanding of the meaning of a (Oedipus) complex, Dasein's Being is constantly threatened by its conflict with the father because Dasein is in the obstructive untruth of Being and therefore cannot appropriately or realistically care for its being in the world. The experience of a (Oedipus) complex contains the truth of Dasein's undiscovered possibilities for being authentic and although "Complexes represent a kind of inferior consciousness" (Jung 2001, p. 82) they contain "an opening to new possibilities of achievement" (Jung 2001, p. 82) and "Complexes are therefore, in this sense, focal or nodal points of psychic life which we would not wish to do without" (Jung 2001, p. 82).

Jung further explains that the genesis of a complex "arises from the clash between a requirement of adaptation and the individual's constitutional inability to meet the challenge" (Jung 2001, p. 82). Jung suggests, "Naturally, in these circumstances there is the greatest temptation simply to follow the power Instinct and to identify the ego with the self outright, in order to keep up the illusion of the ego's mastery" (Jung 1969, p. 224). When this aspect of Jung's writing is analysed phenomenologically, it can be appreciated that identifying with the ego means Dasein has fled from an authentic understanding of the experience of a (Oedipus) complex to identify with an inauthentic understanding. Identifying with the ego and the inability to adapt to life's challenges can be explained as fleeing from authentically understanding "the reality of a 'creative relationship of which he is the product and from which he is excluded' (Rusbridger 1999, p. 488)" (Grier 2005, p. 74). He or she has not only to tolerate the impossibility of claiming and winning one parent at the expense of the other, but also to endure the position of observer of a relationship in which he or she does not belong—of being at the lonely point of the triangle and of having to acknowledge the existence of a different kind of relationship" (Waddell 2003, p. 54).

This illustrates that neurosis as created out of a (Oedipus) complex can be explained to arise when Daseininauthentically understands the experience of a (Oedipus) complex. Dasein "does so by turning away from it in falling; in this turning-away, the "not-at-home" gets 'dimmed down'" (Heidegger 1962, p. 234). Dasein does not authentically accept the need "to devote himself to the great task of detaching himself from his parents, and not until that task is achieved can he cease to be a child and become a member of the social community" (Freud 1977, p. 418). This is also reflected in Jung's own words when he says the complex can be "fled from with an effort of will, but not argued out of existence, and at the first suitable opportunity it reappears in all its original strength" (Jung 1969, p. 96). The antithesis to fleeing an authentic understanding is to accept that "his libido should not remain fixated to these first objects; later on, it should merely take them as a model, and should make a gradual transition from them on to extraneous people" (Freud 2001c, p. 48). The next section of this chapter will explain how this occurs through authentically wanting to have a conscience. In wanting to have a conscience lies "the choosing to choose a kind of Being-one's-Self which, in accordance with its existential structure, we call "resoluteness"" (Heidegger 1962, p. 314). Resoluteness allows Dasein to relinquish the object cathexes toward the mother and are "replaced by identifications, and the authority of the father is introjected into the ego, thereby forming the nucleus of the superego. This protects the child from the dangerous Oedipal wishes, and the libidinal trends become "desexualized and sublimated" and transformed into impulses of affection" (Freud et al. 2005, p. 398). Resoluteness will be examined in more detail in the last section of this chapter.

1.6 Authentic Understanding of the Experience of a (Oedipus) Complex

This final section of this article outlines the phenomenology and ontology of an authentic understanding of the experience of an (Oedipus) complex which allows neurosis to be surpassed and this will also highlight how "the beginnings of religion, morals, society and art converge in the" (Freud 1950, p. 156) destruction of a (Oedipus) complex. To recap, when Dasein encounters a (Oedipus) complex, the world becomes obstructive and obtrusive and Dasein feels "not at home" from an experience of angst, guilt and conscience. Dasein experiences angst, guilt and the call of conscience because Dasein's understanding is inauthentic when there is a "special affection for his mother, whom he regards as belonging to him" and "to feel his father as a rival who disputes his sole possession" (Freud 2001d, p. 207).

Dasein experiences angst and is called guilty by conscience in the experience of a (Oedipus) complex and this constitutes Dasein's care for its authentic being in the world. Dasein is anxious because the "special affection for his mother" is obstructed by the father and this results in Dasein experiencing the world as "not being at home" due to the obstruction. As a result of this, conscience calls Dasein forth to its authentic understanding of a (Oedipus) complex which it has fallen prey to. The call of conscience discloses Dasein as being the basis or being guilty for the obstructiveness of "not being at home in the world". Alternatively, Dasein's understanding of a (Oedipus) complex is authentic when Dasein understands it has not discovered possibilities missing from being in the world. Dasein has left possibilities undiscovered and missing from its world and thus the world falls into unreadiness to hand that is experienced as a (Oedipus) complex. The importance of the task of mastering a (Oedipus) complex by discovering the possibilities missing from the readiness to hand is explained by Freud: "Every new arrival on this planet is faced by the task of mastering the Oedipus complex; anyone who fails to do so falls a victim to neurosis" (Freud 2001b, p. 226).

To discover the possibilities that are missing that brings Dasein to experience obstructiveness of a (Oedipus) complex means to let them be involved in the readiness to hand. The possibilities that have not been discovered "consists in detaching his libidinal wishes from his mother and employing them for the choice of a real outside love-object" (Freud 1963, p. 337). As long as Daseininauthentically understands the meaning of the experience of a (Oedipus) complex, these possibilities that are missing from Dasein's world cannot be involved in the readiness to hand and thus remain undiscovered and unconscious.

Heidegger says the readiness-to-hand of the world belongs to any region that has been discovered and "has the character of inconspicuous familiarity" (Heidegger 1962, p. 137). Heidegger also explains that "Dasein, in its very Being, has this Being as an issue" (Heidegger 1962, p. 67) and Dasein discovers some regions of being and leaves others undiscovered. Importantly for the arguments, concerning the phenomenology of a (Oedipus) complex presented in this paper he also says "The region itself becomes visible in a conspicuous manner only when one discovers the ready-to-hand circumspectively and does so in the deficient modes of concern". (Heidegger 1962, p. 138) and "Often the region of a place does not become accessible explicitly as such a region until one fails to find something in its place" (Heidegger 1962, p. 138). Therefore, it can be phenomenologically explained from this that when Dasein has an inauthentic understanding of the meaning of a (Oedipus) complex, the region where the (Oedipus) complex is experienced is left undiscovered and thus remains conspicuously obstructive to being in the world. Alternatively, when Dasein has an authentic understanding of the meaning of the (Oedipus) complex, Dasein has the possibility of discovering the unconscious possibilities required for Dasein to unconceal the truth of its authentic home in the world.

As Dasein discloses possibilities in a factical world to itself understandingly, Dasein not only discloses its own possibilities for care but other beings are also disclosed and "freed for their own possibilities" (Heidegger 1996, p. 135). This is important because for Dasein to understand a (Oedipus) complex authentically also means to free other beings for their own authentic possibilities by letting them be involved in the readiness to hand. This now needs to be understood in relation to Freud's writing on identification in the process of the dissolution of the Oedipus complex. To authentically free other beings for their authentic possibilities "consists in detaching his libidinal wishes from his mother and employing them for the choice of a real outside love-object" (Freud 1963, p. 337). In addition, Freud explains, "the boy's object-cathexis of his mother must be given up. Its place may be filled by one of two things: either an identification with his mother or an intensification of his identification with his father" (Freud et al. 2005, p. 455). What this quote tells us is that identification allows Dasein to discover and free other beings for their own authentic possibilities and for Dasein to abandon the object-cathexis of the (Oedipus) complex.

In "The Dissolution of the Oedipus Complex" Freud also says "The libidinal trends belonging to the Oedipus complex are in part desexualized and sublimated (a thing which probably happens with every transformation into an identification) and in part inhibited in their aim and changed into impulses of affection". In addition, "the ego is formed to a great extent out of identifications which take the place of abandoned cathexes" (Freud et al. 2005, p. 398). As a result, this suggests that Dasein can remove the angst, guilt and call of conscience of the obstructive (Oedipus) complex by freeing other beings for their authentic possibilities through discovering the possibilities of abandoning the object-cathexis and identification. This also explains that when "libidinal cathexes are abandoned, desexualized and in part sublimated; its objects are incorporated into the ego, where they form the nucleus of the super-ego and give that new structure its characteristic qualities. In normal, or, it is better to say, in ideal cases, the Oedipus complex exists no longer, even in the unconscious; the super-ego has become its heir" (Freud et al. 2005, p. 410).

This means the super-ego, which retains "essential features of the introjected persons" (Freud 2001g, p. 167) is "established after that complex has been disposed of" (Freud 1949, p. 121), when Dasein has freed other beings for their own authentic possibilities. This is achieved by discovering possibilities through identification, this allows Dasein to make space, and room for the authentic possibilities of other beings and this removes Dasein's inauthentic understanding and the obstructiveness of a (Oedipus) complex. Furthermore, the super ego is "the inheritor of the parental influence" (Freud 1997, p. 242) and "becomes a representative of the real external world as well and thus also becomes a model for the endeavours of the ego" (Freud 2001g, p. 167). Phenomenologically this means, the super-ego discloses beings to Dasein in their possibilities. When the super-ego becomes a representative of the real external world through identification "innerworldly beings are discovered, that is, have come to be understood, we say that they have meaning" (Heidegger 1996, p. 142). When Dasein understands and frees other beings for their authentic possibilities through identification, the super-ego removes the obstructiveness of a (Oedipus) complex. As a result, it is clear then that overcoming a (Oedipus) complex by freeing other beings for their authentic possibilities through identification is also "the source of our individual ethical sense, our morality" and "Conscience and morality have arisen through the overcoming, the desexualization, of the Oedipus complex" (Freud 2001g, p. 169).

This can be understood further when Heidegger says Being-true "means to-be-discovering" (Heidegger 1996, p. 201) and being true means to let beings be seen in their unconcealment (discoveredness). Therefore, the process of freeing other beings for their authentic possibilities and understanding the unconscious, obstructive (Oedipus) complex can be understood in Heideggerian terms as taking being out of concealment. This unconcealment of possibilities through identification by the super-ego is in contrast to the untruth of falling prey that misunderstands the experience of the (Oedipus) complex. Furthermore, the truth of discovering the authentic possibilities of other beings "must always first be wrested from beings. Beings are torn from concealment" (Heidegger 1996, p. 204). This distinctive and authentic understanding "is attested in Dasein itself by its conscience-this reticent self-projection up on one's ownmost Being-guilty, in which one is ready for anxiety-we call "resoluteness"" (Heidegger 1962, p. 343). This authentic disclosedness through resoluteness modifies the experience of a (Oedipus) complex in "both the way in which the 'world' is discovered and the way in which the Dasein-with of Others is disclosed" Heidegger (1962, p. 344) and Dasein is resolute when Dasein "identifies with the father and internalizes his power to form the superego; in so doing, he relinquishes his Oedipal attachment to the mother and takes the father as his ego ideal" (Jones 1999, p. 455).

As a result, "The 'world' which is ready-to-hand does not become another one 'in its content', nor does the circle of Others get exchanged for a new one;

but both one's Being towards the ready-to-hand understandingly and concernfully, and one's solicitous Being with Others, are now given a definite character in terms of their ownmost potentiality-for-Beingtheir-Selves" (Heidegger 1962, p. 344). Consequently, when Dasein has authentically understood the experience of a (Oedipus) complex and Dasein has been resolute to unconceal the truth of Being, Dasein let's possibilities be free for their involvement in the ready to hand which removes the obstructiveness of the (Oedipus) complex from being in the world. Dasein can remove the (Oedipus) complex by discovering the authentic possibilities of other beings through the super-ego by identification. This allows Dasein to understand "'You ought to be like this (like your father)'" and also "the prohibition: 'You may not be like this (like your father)—that is, you may not do all that he does; some things are his prerogative'" (Freud et al. 2005, p. 457).

By understanding the authentic possibilities of other beings that were an "obstacle to a realization of his Oedipus wishes"; the "infantile ego fortified itself for the carrying out of the repression by erecting this same obstacle within itself" (Freud et al. 2005, p. 458). In addition, by understanding the authentic meaning of a (Oedipus) complex in this way, Dasein "makes it possible to let the Others who are with it 'be' through solicitude which leaps forth and liberates" (Heidegger 1962, p. 344). Thus, when Dasein understands the truth of Being instead of neurotically and inauthentically understanding the experience of a (Oedipus) complex, Dasein's world is no longer experienced as obstructive and unready to hand and by overcoming a (Oedipus) complex through identification "the superego sets the stage for child socialization" (Kupfersmid 1995, p. 536). The importance of removing the obstruction of the (Oedipus) complex "is central to psychoanalytic thinking on (a) the nature of child development, (b) the cause of human neurosis, (c) the development of an individual's values/morality, and (d) the focus of clinical treatment".

Finally, it is important to summarize and reiterate that a (Oedipus) complex can temporally remain unconscious "in a dormant condition, it seems as if there were absolutely nothing in this hidden region" (Jung 1981, p. 279). However, the truth of Being remains even though Dasein can neurotically and inauthentically understands the experience of a (Oedipus) complex. By ignoring the truth of Dasein's authenticity disclosed by angst, guilt and conscience though phantasy and wish fulfilment, a (Oedipus) complex cannot be understood as real and "Hence we are continually surprised when something unknown suddenly appears "from nowhere"" (Jung 1981, p. 279). Alternatively, an authentic resoluteness which understands that angst, guilt and conscience reveal Dasein's primordial truth to itself allows Dasein to understand that "possibilities of future development may also come to light in this way, perhaps in just such an outburst of affect which sometimes radically alters the whole situation" (Jung 1981, p. 279). Therefore, by being authentically resolute, a (Oedipus) complex can be surpassed when Dasein does not become absorbed in only one of its possibilities for being and has instead interpreted new possibilities for being in the world. This is achieved when the "superego will perform the paternal function within his own psyche, proclaiming autonomy at the price of sexual renunciation and former dependency"

(Benjamin 1987, p. 213). Lastly, resoluteness allows “a differentiation within the psyche, the development of the superego through identification” (Benjamin 1987, p. 213). When Dasein discovers the authentic possibilities of other beings (e.g. mother and father) to remove the obstructiveness of a (Oedipus) complex, there is also a “transition from fear of external authority to self-regulation; authority is replaced by independent conscience, prohibition by self-control, need for approval by autonomy” (Benjamin 1987, p. 213).

1.7 Conclusion

To close, it is important to note that overcoming complexes “are not limited to the infantile years (in Kleinian theory) nor to early childhood (in Freudian theory). They are life-long. Struggles of this kind have to be ‘reworked in each new life situation, at each stage of development, and with each major addition to experience or knowledge’ (Britton 1989, p. 38)” (Waddell 2003, p. 54). This article has explained the phenomenological experience of a (Oedipus) complex as well as the inauthentic and authentic understanding of this experience and overcoming complexes should be understood as “a process of constant recasting and assimilation, involving repeated reorganization through new identifications and altered object relations. It is to do with the capacity to allow for this continuous evolution of the personality, for the transitions from one state to another” (Waddell 2003, p. 56) By overcoming complexes “In the course of development the super-ego also takes on the influences of those who have stepped into the place of parents-educators, teachers, people chosen as ideal models. Normally it departs more and more from the original parental figures; it becomes, so to say, more impersonal” (Freud 2001e, p. 64). Thus identifications which “come about with these later parents as well”; “make important contributions to the formation of character” (Freud 2001e, p. 64) for Dasein to authentically care for the meaning of its Being by removing obstructive complexes from being in the world.

In conclusion, this chapter has built on the work of my previous paper (Gildersleeve 2016) by illustrating the further congruency between Heidegger and psychoanalysis. Specifically, this chapter provided a phenomenological description of Freud’s Oedipus complex theory with the use of Heidegger’s phenomenological ontology. Finally, this chapter has highlighted the compatibility of Jung’s and Freud’s writing on complexes. Casement comments that Jung’s word association experiments on complexes brought “Jung and Freud into collaboration with each other” (Casement 2001, p. 13). This collaboration advanced both Jung’s and Freud’s work on complexes where “From Jung’s point of view, the tests confirmed the latter’s theory of repression, one of the cornerstones of psychoanalysis, which threw light on how complexes worked. For Freud, on the other hand, the association tests conducted by Jung provided a scientific underpinning to important parts of his work” (Casement 2001, p. 13). This paper has contributed to understanding how this collaboration was possible by demonstrating Freud’s and Jung’s theories possess the same ontological meaning and phenomenological experience of a complex. It is important this has been established because it highlights the potential for both Freud's and Jung's theory to be further combined in the future with Heidegger's phenomenological ontology to advance psychoanalytic philosophy.

References

Askay, R., & Farquhar, J. (2006). *Apprehending the inaccessible: Freudian psychoanalysis and existential phenomenology*. Evanston: Northwestern University Press.

Askay, R., & Farquhar, J. (2013). *Being Unconscious: Heidegger and Freud*. Oxford Handbooks Online.

Benjamin, J. (1987). The decline of the Oedipus complex. In J. M. Broughton (Ed.), *Critical theories of psychological development*. New York: Plenum

Boss, M. (1963). *Psychoanalysis and daseinsanalysis*. New York: Basic Books.

Boss, M. (1977). *Existential foundations of medicine and psychology*. Northvale, NJ: Jason Aronson.

Boss, M. (1988). Recent considerations in daseinsanalysis. *The Humanistic Psychologist, 16*(1), 58–74.

Britton, R. (1989). The missing link: parental sexuality in the Oedipus complex. *The Oedipus complex today: Clinical implications*, 83-101.

Casement, A. (2001). *Carl Gustav Jung* (Vol. 11). London: Sage.

Craig, E. (1988). Introduction: daseinsanalysis: A quest for essentials. *The Humanistic Psychologist, 16*(1), 1.

Dimas, C., Reiss, D., & Neiderhiser, J. (2008). Triangular relationships in adolescence predict adult psychopathology: An empirical validation of the Oedipus Complex? *Journal of the American Psychoanalytic Association, 56*(4), 1342–1348.

Freud, S. (1920). *A general introduction to psychoanalysis*. New York: Boni and Liveright.

Freud, S. (1925). *Collected papers. Vol. 5, Miscellaneous papers, 1888–1938*. London: Hogarth Press.

Freud, S. (1949). *An outline of psychoanalysis* (J. Strachey, Trans.). Norton.

Freud, S. (1950). *Totem and taboo: Some points of agreement between the mental lives of savages and neurotics* (Vol. 94, p. 124) (J. Strachey, Trans.). New York: Routledge.

Freud, S. (1955). *The standard edition of the complete psychological works of Sigmund Freud* (Vol. 18). London: Hogarth Press.

Freud, S. (1962). *The Standard Edition of the Complete Psychological Works of Sigmund Freud: (1909) Two case histories ('Little Hans' and the 'Rat Man')*. London: Hogarth Press

Freud, S. (1963). *1916–1917 Introductory lectures on psycho-analysis Standard Edition 15 and 16*. London: Hogarth Press.

Freud, S. (1977). *Introductory lectures on psychoanalysis of Sigmund Freud*. New York: Norton.

Freud, S. (1997). *Writings on art and literature*. Stanford: Stanford University Press.

Freud, S. (2001a). *Complete psychological works of Sigmund Freud* (Vol. 4). New York: Random House.

Freud, S. (2001b). *Complete psychological works of Sigmund Freud* (Vol. 7). New York: Random House.

Freud, S. (2001c). *Complete psychological works of Sigmund Freud* (Vol. 11). New York: Random House.

Freud, S. (2001d). *Complete psychological works of Sigmund Freud* (Vol. 15). New York: Random House.

Freud, S. (2001e). *Complete psychological works of Sigmund Freud* (Vol. 16). New York: Random House.

Freud, S. (2001g). *Complete psychological works of Sigmund Freud* (Vol. 19). New York: Random House.
Freud, S. (2001h). *Complete psychological works of Sigmund Freud* (Vol. 21). New York: Random House.
Freud, S., Freud, A., & Strachey, J. (2005). *The essentials of psycho-analysis*. New York: Random House.
Freud, S., & Gay, P. (1995). *The Freud Reader*. New York: WW Norton & Company.
Gildersleeve, M. (2016). The phenomenology and ontology of complexes. *Procedia-Social and Behavioral Sciences, 217*, 967–976.
Grier, F. (2005). *Oedipus and the Couple*. Karnac Books.
Heidegger, M. (1962). *Being and time*, trans. J. Macquarrie and E. Robinson.
Heidegger, M. (1996). *Being and time* (J. Stambaugh, Trans.). SUNY series in contemporary continental philosophy.
Heidegger, M. (2000). *Being and time* (J. Macquarrie, & E. Robinson, Trans.). Harper Collins.
Heidegger, M. (2001). *Zollikon seminars: Protocols, conversations, letters*. Evanston: Northwestern University Press.
Jones, G. Y. (1999). 'Beyond the oedipal complex': Freud and lacan revisited. *Psychodynamic Counselling, 5*(4), 453–463.
Jung, C. G. (1907). *The psychology of dementia praecox* (F. Peterson, Trans.). New York: Nervous and Mental Disease Publ. Co.
Jung, C. G. (1969). *The structure and dynamics of the psyche* (R. Hull, Trans.). The collected works of CG Jung, 8.
Jung, C. G. (1981). *The archetypes and the collective unconscious* (G. Adler, & R. Hull, Trans.). Princeton University Press.
Jung, C. G. (2001). *Modern man in search of a soul* (W. Dell, Trans.). Psychology Press.
Kupfersmid, J. (1995). Does the Oedipus complex exist? Psychotherapy: Theory. *Research, Practice, Training, 32*(4), 535.
Loparic, Z. (1999). Heidegger and Winnicott. *Naturezahumana, 1*(1), 103–135.
Poland, W. S. (2007). Oedipal complexes, Oedipal schemas. *American Imago, 64*(4), 561–565.
Richardson, W. J. (2003). Heidegger and Psychoanalysis? *Naturezahumana, 5*(1), 9–38.
Spinelli, E. (1996). *Martin Heidegger and psychotherapy*. Brussels: Society for Existential Analysis, International Federation of Daseinsanalysis.
Stolorow, R. D., & Atwood, G. E. (1984). Psychoanalytic phenomenology: Toward a science of human experience. *Psychoanalytic Inquiry, 4*(1), 87–105.
Van Manen, M. (1990). *Researching lived experience: Human science for an action sensitive pedagogy*. New York: Suny Press.
Waddell, M. (2003). Coming into one's own: The Oedipus complex and the couple in late adolescence. *Journal of Child Psychotherapy, 29*(1), 53–73.

Chapter 2
The Behavioral-Related Conditioned Sound in Cross Modal Stroop Task

Hau Lam Agnes Chan and De-Hui Ruth Zhou

Abstract This study examined the effect of conditioned sound as stimuli in an audiovisual Stroop task. It is know that the conditioned sound is induced under the pairing of a sound stimulus with conditioned behaviors in our daily life. For example, the sound of pedestrian traffic light is conditioned with the meaning of crossing the road or not crossing the road. In this study, a cross modal audiovisual Stroop task was used to test the effect of conditioned sound, since it is always presented with other visual cues in our daily life. It was hypothesized that conditioned sound would produce interference effect in the Stroop task. A 2 (audio stimuli: conditioned sound/voiced representation) × 2 (visual stimuli: pictorial representation/text representation) × 2 (congruence: audio stimuli and visual stimuli are congruent in meaning/audio stimuli and visual stimuli are incongruent in meaning) × 2 (tasks: answer corresponding to visual stimuli/answer corresponding to audio stimuli) factorial design was constructed. Sixty Hong Kong college students with permanent Hong Kong resident status participated in this study. ANOVA tests had been employed to explore and analyze the data, aiming to show that both audio stimuli (conditioned sound and voiced representation) might induce interference effect; while voiced representation created greater interference than conditioned sound. The results were in congruence with the previous literature on the induction of behavioral interference under the Stroop task. The study showed that conditioned sound resulted from our daily conditioned behavior affected human perception in the multimodal Stroop effect. The study also supported the attenuation model in selective attention. As conditioned sound may give slower and more inaccurate responses than spoken word, it is suggested that the use of conditioned sound as indicators in different instruments and tools used in our daily life can be

H.L.A. Chan (✉) · D.-H.R. Zhou
Department of Counselling and Psychology, Hong Kong Shue Yan University, North Point, Hong Kong, China
e-mail: agnes_chl@yahoo.com.hk

D.-H.R. Zhou
e-mail: dhzhou@hksyu.edu

M.-T. Leung and L.-M. Tan (eds.), *Applied Psychology Readings*,
DOI 10.1007/978-981-10-2796-3_2

replaced by spoken word to enhance their effectiveness by facilitating quicker and more accurate responses.

Keywords Audiovisual Stroop test · Cross modal · Automaticity · Conditioned sound

2.1 Introduction

There are many signals consisting of sound signal and other signals for human perception in our daily life, for example, the sound signal of the pedestrian traffic light to help the blind people, the sound signal produced by the computer when an USB is inserted or removed to indicate the completion of the process, etc. After familiarizing to these sound signals, which had no meaning attached to them originally, people used to perceive these sounds with their particular meanings. By pairing these sounds with particular behavioral meaning, this kind of linkage formation between a sound and a behavioral-related meaning is called behavioral conditioning (Settlage and Harlow 1936). This study used the term conditioned sound to relate these sounds with a specific conditioned behavioral meaning. As it is questionable that the process of meaning retrieval by conditioned sound is the same as spoken word; this study is going to compare these two sounds in a Stroop test.

2.1.1 The Stroop Effect and Its Variations

There are a number of studies on the Stroop effect and its variations in the past 80 years (e.g., Acosta and Simon 1976; Dalrymple-Alford 1968; Jensen and Rohwer 1966; Simon et al. 1975; Stroop 1935). The standard Stroop test is an effect of color word interference (Stroop 1935), which involved a set of color words printed with different color-ink. Under the congruent condition, the color ink of the word had the same meaning as the word did (e.g., the word "blue" was printed with blue-ink; the word "crimson" was printed with red-ink). Under the incongruent condition, the color ink of the word was different from the meaning of the word (e.g., the word "blue" was printed with yellow-ink; the word "crimson" was printed with purple-ink). Reaction time was measured when the participants were asked to read the words or name the color-ink of the words separately. The results showed that the response time under the congruent condition was shorter than that under the incongruent condition; and under the incongruent condition, the response time for reading the words was shorter than that of naming the color-ink.

Interference is the main process leading to the result of the Stroop effect. Interference effect occurs when there is conflict between two or more perceptual or cognitive processes, where additional time is needed to solve the conflict, causing negative performance impact (Lidwell et al. 2010). Several studies suggested that interference effect was not involved in the encoding stage (Acosta and Simon 1976; Simon 1982; Simon and Berbaum 1990; Simon and Pouraghabagher 1978), but in the response selection stage (Acosta and Simon 1976; Simon 1982; Simon et al. 1975; Van der Molen and Keuss 1981). Simon and Berbaum (1988) suggested that interference occurred between the process of perceptual encoding and response activation, during the process of decoding and information retrieval from short-term memory, which Seymour (1977) mentioned these stages as the conceptual encoding process. In the standard Stroop test, the incongruence of the target (the color-ink of the printed word) and the distractor (the meaning of the printed word) caused conflict between their information retrieval processes which led to interference. Therefore, having shorter response time under the congruent condition than that under the incongruent condition was due to the interference effect.

In addition, automaticity is also observed in the Stroop effect. Automaticity in the Stroop tests refers to the forming of automatic process for reading (i.e., the printed word), brought by long practice and does not need controlled attention (consciously paid attention) to occur (Stirling 1979). Although no controlled attention was needed in the automatic reading process, it still used up part of the attentional resources, thus reduced the resources available to process and name the target (i.e., the color-ink of the printed word; Stirling 1979).

As both the color word and the color-ink in the standard Stroop test required visual sensation to perceive, this kind of Stroop tests are called the visual Stroop tests. Similar visual Stroop effect studies had also shown similar results (e.g., Dalrymple-Alford 1968; Jensen and Rohwer 1966).

Auditory Stroop tests are a kind of variation from the standard Stroop test. The difference between visual Stroop tests and auditory Stroop tests is that the stimuli of visual Stroop tests were visual stimuli (words, pictures, etc.), whereas that of auditory Stroop tests were audio stimuli (sounds, spoken words, etc.). Auditory Stroop tests also got similar results with standard Stroop test (e.g., Green and Barber 1981; Gregg and Purdy 2007; Jerger et al. 1988).

Another kind of variation form of the standard Stroop test is the cross modal audiovisual Stroop tests. It involved both auditory and visual stimuli in the test. Limited studies had investigated this cross modal audiovisual Stroop effects, and Peng and Prime (2014) was the only study that investigated it in both directions (i.e., having both visual distractor and auditory distractor) by a color-naming task. The test involved a set of color words (visual stimulus), a set of color patches (visual stimulus), and a set of sound tract with spoken color words (audio stimulus). Reaction time was measured when participants were asked to read the words (with auditory distractor), named the color patches (with auditory distractor) and read the color word they heard (with visual distractor) separately. The response time under the congruent condition (i.e., the spoken word was congruent with the presented color word or color patches) was shorter than that under the incongruent condition (i.e., the spoken word was different with the presented color word or color patches) due to the interference effect. In addition, under the incongruent conditions, the response time for the participants to read out the color word they heard (with visual distractor) was slower than that of reading out the words or naming the color patches they saw (with auditory distractor). This showed that visual distraction might exert greater cross modal Stroop interference than audio distraction. To sum up, their study showed that Stroop effects between visual and audio stimuli were multidirectional and visual distractors exerts stronger cross modal Stroop interference (Peng and Prime 2014).

2.1.2 Audiovisual Interference

Apart from those audiovisual studies for the Stroop effects, the audiovisual word interference task was also quite common in the multimodal studies of audiovisual interaction (Calvert et al. 2000; Laurienti et al. 2004; McGurk and MacDonald 1976; Molholm et al. 2002; Soto-Faraco et al. 2004; Van Atteveldt et al. 2004). For instance, McGurk and MacDonald (1976) had reported that visual distraction created by observing the speaker's lip movement might affect the perception of the auditory phonemes. This showed that the audiovisual interaction do really interact with each other, and may then affect the perception of information. On the other hand, the behavioral studies showed that the congruency effect of audiovisual cues might affect behaviors, that is, under the congruent condition (i.e., with the cue of listening to "red" while watching a red circle), the behavioral response would be made faster than normal (i.e., without any cues), whereas under the incongruent condition, the behavior would be slower than normal (Laurienti et al. 2004). This further supported the congruency effect in the audiovisual multimodality (Schriefers and Meyer 1990).

2.1.3 Sound Stimuli: The Conditioned Sound Versus Spoken Word

Auditory Stroop tests which involved audio stimuli (e.g., Cohen and Martin 1975; Green and Barber 1981; Gregg and Purdy 2007; Hamers and Lambert 1972; Jerger et al. 1988), had never used conditioned sound as a stimulus before. A conditioned sound refers to a tone which is conditioned with a meaning. For examples, different traffic light sounds are conditioned with the meaning of "crossing" or "not crossing"; ringing of doorbell is conditioned with the meaning of someone's arrival. Conditioned sound was usually used in the studies of behavioral conditioning (e.g., Imani et al. 2012; Settlage and Harlow 1936). Studies of audio Stroop effects, however, only focused on gender, pitch and color, and did not investigate the effect of conditioned sound before.

The conditioned sound, when compared with a spoken word as a stimulus that is well-studied, has a great difference in the format of meaning.

Listening to spoken words, in the nature of speech, could be a type of variation of reading automaticity as they are comparable in nature. They are both the only way of perceiving semantic information but different towards the type of sensation as reading perceives visual semantic information, whereas listening perceives auditory information. This study assumed that automaticity effect could occur in both reading and listening.

The conditioned sound is not the same as a spoken word, which is originally a meaningful sound, but a meaningless sound paired with a specific meaning over a long time of exposure. Hence, it is hypothesized that the perception process could be different between perceiving spoken word, which is assumed to be automatically listened and its meaning is directly perceived without requiring controlled attention, and perceiving conditioned sound, which involves controlled attention.

2.1.4 Visual Stimuli: Picture Versus Written Words

Several studies had been carried out on the effect of pictures, instead of colors, combined with an embedded written word, as the visual stimuli in visual Stroop tests (e.g., Cattell 1886; Dyer 1973; Fraisse 1969; Golinkoff and Rosinski 1976; Rosinski 1977; Rosinski et al. 1975). The result of the incongruent condition (i.e., meaning of the picture and the embedded word is different) showed that the distraction of written word greatly interfered with the meaning of the picture, but there was only little distraction brought by the picture to the written word when perceived (e.g., Golinkoff and Rosinski 1976; Rosinski 1977; Rosinski et al. 1975).

As a stimulus, picture is similar to the conditioned sound. It does not involve the automaticity effect as written word does, and is paired with a meaning. This study used picture as one of the independent visual stimulus in order to investigate the effect of automaticity.

2.1.5 Key Press Response in Stroop Tests

The standard Stroop test and many of its variations had used oral response for measurement (e.g., Green and Barber 1981; Gregg and Purdy 2007; Jerger et al. 1988; Stroop 1935); but Simon (1969) and some others had studied a variation of visual Stroop effects with the key press response (e.g., Simon 1969, 1982).

Key press response was introduced to study the interference of direction in Simon effect as the action of key pressing in different hands would be interfered by directional cue (Simon 1969). The success of Simon's study (1969) had raised the use of key press response into wide application for Stroop experiments. Benefits from the advantages of key press response in comparing to the oral response can then be brought into the Stroop studies. As key press response can be collected and measured by electronic devices, the measurement of key press response would be more accurate than the manual measurement (MacLeod 2005). In addition, by using electronic measurement, the experiment can exclude the presence of the experimenter (MacLeod 2005). The concrete key pressing action may also avoid faked oral response (i.e., uncertainty delayed in oral response, such as: um, uh-hah, I think, etc.) (MacLeod 2005). Using key press response can maximize the accuracy of data collection.

2.2 Purpose of Study and Research Question

Although researches in Stroop effects were common, there were only limited numbers of audiovisual Stroop studies (e.g., Cowan and Barron 1987; Peng and Prime 2014), and most of them were studying the unidirectional model of how auditory distraction interfered with visual stimulus (e.g., Cowan and Barron 1987). As such, this study intended to be an audiovisual Stroop study examining the two-directional modal of how the audio and visual components distract and interfere with each other.

Conditioned sound is an unstudied audio stimulus especially in the field of Stroop effect. As it is paired with meaning, it could be used to study the Stroop effect. Yet, until now, no examination was made on the conditioned sound. This study did used conditioned sound to study the Stroop effect.

The research question for this study is asking whether the perception process of pictures and conditioned sounds may differ from that of words in the Stroop effect based on the theory of automaticity.

There are four research hypotheses in the present study as follows:

H1 The incongruent condition would exert greater interference than the congruent condition;

H2 Visual distractor would exert greater interference than auditory distractor;

H3 Vocal sound would exert greater interference than conditioned sound; and

H4 Words would exert greater interference than pictures.

2.3 Method

2.3.1 Design

This experiment has a between-subject and within-subjects design. The experiment used 2 test conditions (congruent/incongruent) $\times$ 2 audio stimuli (spoken word/conditioned sound) $\times$ 2 visual stimuli (written word/picture) within-subjects design. In addition, the between-subject design involves two task conditions

Table 2.1 The eight combinations of condition variables, audio variables, and visual variables

Condition	Auditory stimuli	Visual stimuli	
		Word	Picture
Congruent	Word	Congruent	Congruent
		Spoken word	Spoken word
		Written word	Picture
	Conditioned sound	Congruent	Congruent
		Conditioned sound	Conditioned sound
		Written word	Picture
Incongruent	Word	Incongruent	Incongruent
		Spoken word	Spoken word
		Written word	Picture
	Conditioned sound	Incongruent	Incongruent
		Conditioned sound	Conditioned sound
		Written word	Picture

(choose answers according to the visual stimuli/choose answer according to the audio stimuli) in counterbalanced task design. In the experiment, task A referred to participants choosing answers corresponding to the audio stimuli, and task V referred to participants choosing answers corresponding to the visual stimuli. Table 2.1 shows the combinations of the above variables.

2.3.2 Participants

Sixty participants (30 male and 30 female participants) were recruited in this study. The recruited participants were physically healthy without any auditory, visual, or finger motion defects. They were college students aged between 17 and 24 and continuously lived in Hong Kong in the past 10 years.

2.4 Materials

The research materials used in task A and task V were identical. It were presented on a computer device (screen size: 27 cm high × 34 cm wide; resolution: 1280 wide × 1024 high; orientation: landscape; brightness: 100 %) with the E-PRIME software (Schneider et al. 2001). It included eight combinations of stimuli as listed in Table 2.1 above. Each combination had included eight task items. Hence, each task contained 64 task items and the whole experiment contained totally 128 task items.

Each of the 128 task items first showed a fixation page with a "+" (in the middle of the page; bolded; font: Courier New; size: 50) for 250 ms, then it would automatically change to the question page until a response was received, and finally changed to a blank page for 100 ms after the response was given in the question page. Afterwards, it would automatically change to another fixation page to start another task item. Each question page consisted of an audio stimulus (either a conditioned sound or a spoken word in a specific theme, e.g., USB insertion, pedestrian traffic light, etc.; volume: 25 in window 7; presented in 90 ± 1 Hz) which started to present together in joint presentation with the visual stimulus in white background (either a picture or a written word; in a specific theme corresponding to the audio stimuli; picture presented in the middle of the screen, resolution: 1280 wide × 1024 high; written words presented in font "新細明體," size: 50, bolded) circled by a red circle (used to highlight the visual image) and the answer choices (either a picture or a written word as same as the visual stimulus; in a specific theme corresponding to the visual stimulus presented above; picture presented in the two sides at the bottom of the screen, resolution: 1280 wide × 1024 high; written word presented in font "新細明體," size: 40, bolded) presented on the same screen at the same time. A letter "A" or "L" (in capital letter; bolded; font: Calibri; size: 50) was placed right above the answer choice to indicate that participant might press either the letter key "A" or "L" in the keyboard provided for answering each task item. Participants should answer as soon as possible after the answer choices were presented in each task item, which then ended the task item. The 128 task items were continuously carried out in this sequence until the whole task had been completed. The above would be repeated for every task item.

The time to complete all of these 128 task items by one participant was approximately 8 min, whereas the whole process including the training task was approximately 15 min.

2.4.1 Procedures

The experiment was divided into two parts, mainly to separate the two tasks (task A and task V) by a break so as to minimize the mixing up of the two tasks.

Before the start of the experiment, the experimental content and task instruction was first explained to the participants, then followed by a trial exercise consisted of 16 task items. Feedback showing their accuracy and response time under the trial exercise was provided after each task item for 1000 ms to increase their understanding to the operation of the experiment.

A recognition training was then presented to ensure the participants could recognize the images and conditioned sound used in the experiment later on.

After that, the experiment was started and participants were required to answer the 64 task items in the first task (either task A or task V). A 2-min break was then given, followed by the second part of the experiment.

In the second part of the experiment, the instruction for the required task (either task A or task V opposite to the first part) was first provided and then followed by a trial exercise, as those carried out in the first part. After making sure they got the correct way to do the task, the second task started.

Participants were required to finish all of the 128 task items in both parts of the experiment. The response time and accuracy of each task item were recorded immediately by the E-Prime software during the test.

2.4.2 *The Control of the Extraneous Factors*

Several controlling measurements used to minimize the extraneous factors were implemented in the study.

The recognition training was used to identify and train-up the less familiar stimuli (especially conditioned sound) to limit the individualized differences of conditioning effect. The restriction in participant recruitment on those continuously living in Hong Kong for the past 10 years might ensure the accessibility of the local stimuli used in the experiment.

A big red circle placed surrounding the visual stimuli was to enhance the participants both to look at the visual stimuli and listen the audio stimuli before giving their responses with a view to reduce the possibility of the attentional bias that the participants might choose not to look at the visual distractor in the audio task; while it was assumed that the participants should be distracted equally by the visual and audio distractor in both tasks in the experiment.

2.5 Results

A $2 \times 2 \times 2 \times 2$ four-way repeated-measure ANOVA was conducted with average reaction time of corrected response and sum of accuracy as the dependent variables, and tasks (visual task, audio task); congruence conditions (congruence, incongruence); visual stimuli (picture, word); together with the audio stimuli (conditioned sound, voice) as the independent variables. Table 2.2 and Table 2.3 showed the mean and standard deviation of the average reaction time and sum of accuracy, respectively, for each independent variable.

2.5.1 *Average Reaction Time*

There was a significant main effect for tasks [$F(1,944) = 146.39$, $p < .001$, partial $\eta^2 = .13$], with those doing the visual task ($M = 863.69$, SD $= 273.47$) reporting

Table 2.2 Means, standard deviations, and AVOVA for average reaction time

	M (SD)	ANOVA
Task		
Visual task	863.69 (273.47)	146.39***
Audio task	1105.55 (357.69)	
Congruence condition		
Congruent condition	951.31 (322.71)	11.11**
Incongruent condition	1017.94 (354.50)	
Visual stimuli		
Picture	1012.93 (368.11)	8.02**
Word	956.31 (308.09)	
Audio stimuli		
Conditioned sound	1026.71 (380.63)	17.74***
Spoken word	942.53 (289.14)	

** $p < .01$; *** $p < .001$

Table 2.3 Means, standard deviations, and ANOVA for sum of accuracy

	M (SD)	ANOVA
Task		
Visual task	6.78 (1.09)	9.78**
Audio task	6.58 (1.22)	
Congruence condition		
Congruent condition	7.11 (1.07)	183.63***
Incongruent condition	6.24 (1.09)	
Visual stimuli		
Picture	7.08 (1.13)	158.10***
Word	6.27 (1.05)	
Audio stimuli		
Conditioned sound	6.60 (1.21)	6.13*
Spoken word	6.75 (1.11)	

* $p < .05$; ** $p < .01$; *** $p < .001$

significantly shorter average reaction time than those doing the audio task ($M = 1105.55$, SD = 357.69). Hypothesis 2 was confirmed.

There was a main effect for congruence conditions [$F(1,944) = 11.11$, $p < .01$, partial $\eta^2 = .01$], with those under congruent condition ($M = 951.31$, SD = 322.71) reporting significantly shorter reaction time than those under incongruent condition ($M = 1017.94$, SD = 354.50). Hypothesis 1 was confirmed.

There was a main effect for different visual stimuli [$F(1,944) = 8.02$, $p < .01$, partial $\eta^2 = .01$], with those using words as visual stimulus ($M = 956.31$, SD = 308.09) reporting significantly shorter reaction time than those using pictures as visual stimulus ($M = 1012.93$, SD = 368.11). Hypothesis 4 was confirmed.

There was also a main effect for different audio stimuli [$F(1{,}944) = 17.74$, $p < .001$, partial $\eta^2 = .02$], with those using voice as audio stimulus ($M = 942.53$, SD = 289.14) reporting significantly shorter reaction time than those using conditioned sound ($M = 1026.71$, SD = 380.63). Hypothesis 3 was confirmed.

Apart from the main effects, there was a significant task and audio stimuli interaction with average reaction time [$F(1{,}944) = 21.49$, $p < .001$, partial $\eta^2 = .02$]. In the visual task, the responses with spoken word as distractor ($M = 867.94$, SD = 262.58) would have longer reaction time and that with conditioned sound as distractor ($M = 859.45$, SD = 284.42) would have shorter reaction time. On the other hand, in the audio task, responses toward spoken word ($M = 1017.12$, SD = 295.68) would have shorter reaction time and responses toward conditioned sounds ($M = 1193.98$, SD = 391.51) would have longer reaction time.

It was also found that there was a significant tasks × congruence conditions × audio stimuli interaction [$F(1{,}944) = 4.38$, $p < .05$, partial $\eta^2 = .01$].

2.5.2 *Sum of Accuracy*

The result showed a significant main effect for tasks [$F(1{,}944) = 9.78$, $p < .01$, partial $\eta^2 = .01$], with those doing the visual task ($M = 6.78$, SD = 1.09) reporting significantly higher accuracy than those doing the audio task ($M = 6.58$, SD = 1.22). Hypothesis 2 was confirmed.

There was also a significant main effect for congruence conditions [$F(1{,}944) = 183.63$, $p < .001$, partial $\eta^2 = .16$], with those having congruent condition ($M = 7.11$, SD = 1.07) reporting significantly higher accuracy than those having incongruent condition ($M = 6.24$, SD = 1.09). Hypothesis 1 was confirmed.

In addition, there was a significant main effect for different visual stimuli [$F(1{,}944) = 158.10$, $p < .001$, partial $\eta^2 = .14$], with those using pictures as visual stimulus ($M = 7.08$, SD = 1.13) reporting significantly higher accuracy than those using words as visual stimulus ($M = 6.27$, SD = 1.05). Hypothesis 4 was rejected as the result showed a reversed pattern.

There was also a main effect for different audio stimuli [$F(1{,}944) = 6.13$, $p < .05$, partial $\eta^2 = .01$], with those using voice as audio stimulus ($M = 6.75$, SD = 1.11) reporting significantly higher accuracy than those using conditioned sound as audio stimulus ($M = 6.60$, SD = 1.21). Hypothesis 3 was confirmed.

There was a significant task and audio stimuli interaction with sum of accuracy [$F(1{,}944) = 12.38$, $p < .001$, partial $\eta^2 = .01$]. In the responses in visual task, spoken word as distractor ($M = 6.74$, SD = 1.11) would have a lower accuracy and those with conditioned sound as distractor ($M = 6.81$, SD = 1.08) would have a higher accuracy; meanwhile in the audio task, responses toward spoken word ($M = 6.75$, SD = 1.11) would have a higher accuracy and responses toward conditioned sounds ($M = 6.60$, SD = 1.21) would have a lower accuracy.

2.6 Discussion

Three out of four hypotheses in the study were confirmed by the results, except hypothesis 4 which was rejected due to the showing of an opposite pattern of result for sum of accuracy.

According to the attention network model, the three sub-functions of attention, namely alerting, orienting, and executive attention have their specific function (Posner and Rothbart 2007). In this research, alerting and orienting had been kept constant in all situations, and only executive attention had been measured as conflicts brought by the different sensory information arisen in the task. Selective attention might also present in the experiment as the experimental design had instructed the participants to answer only toward one sensory stimulus, and participants might choose to focus on the attended information and ignore the unattended information.

As a cross modal Stroop task, the major discussion would be whether the visual or audio channel have exerted greater distraction on the other. The experiment had replicated the result of Peng and Prime (2014), showing that visual stimuli would exert greater distraction to the task than audio stimuli. Therefore, when participants were required to complete the audio task (to response towards what they heard), as having been distracted largely by the visual stimuli, the responses would become slower and more inaccurate.

2.6.1 Audiovisual Interaction in a Cross Modal Task

The significant main effects in congruence condition aspect had confirmed that the Stroop tasks had triggered interference effect in the experiment. The results had supported other studies under incongruent condition, which concluded that the responses would have longer average reaction time and lower sum of accuracy (e.g., McGurk and MacDonald 1976; Peng and Prime 2014; Schriefers and Meyer 1990).

It showed that the audiovisual cross modal interaction effect was present with the incongruent condition. As there was only one distractor in each condition, and that distractor was another sensory stimuli (i.e., if visual stimulus is the target stimuli, audio stimuli would be the distractor, and vice versa), the Stroop effects shown under the incongruent condition must be due to the interference brought by the interaction between the two different sensory stimuli, resulting in a longer reaction time and lower accuracy. Therefore, this study supported the results of other cross modal studies that the audiovisual interaction would affect the perception of information and result in altering the response as showed under the incongruent condition of the task (e.g., Laurienti et al. 2004; McGurk and MacDonald 1976; Schriefers and Meyer 1990).

2.6.2 Meaning and the Automaticity Effect

The research question of this study was whether the perception process of picture and conditioned sound were the same as word. With the assumed presence of automaticity effect on word, this study hypothesized that the perception process of picture and conditioned sound was different with that of word. The results showed that both written and spoken word would trigger faster response than picture or conditioned sound. According to automaticity effect, word required less attention and resources to be perceived as it was well-practiced (Stirling 1979). The result thus supported that the presence of automaticity effect had taken role in the perception of word, thus shortened the time needed to perceive the word.

One of the evidence of the experiment was the significant main effect showed under different audio stimuli with slower reaction time and lower sum of accuracy for response with conditioned sound when compared with spoken word. This might be explained by the automaticity effect of listening to word (Stirling 1979) as hypothesized at the beginning of this study. As spoken word was automatically perceived with its meaning, while conditioned sound would require more effort to perceive its meaning, the reaction time for answers with spoken word was faster. Thus, this study had supported the presence of automaticity effect on spoken word.

It was interesting to note that for the responses towards visual stimuli, written words may trigger faster response, while picture might have higher accuracy. This result had rejected the findings of similar researches that picture would give slower reaction time and lower accuracy (e.g., Cattell 1886; Fraisse 1969). This could be explained by the data-driven error of automaticity effect. Data-driven error takes place when the incoming sensory information has overridden the intended variables in an automatic action sequence (Reason 1990). Thus, the responses toward automatic processed written word may more easily be affected by the audio distractor in comparing with picture which requires more attention to be perceived. Another possible explanation is that the picture used in this study and other studies (e.g., Cattell 1886; Fraisse 1969) are different in nature. The pictures used in this study are highly accessible in our daily life and these pictures could be well-conditioned with its meaning. In opposite to the conditioned sound, people usually make judgement based on visual aid, including those picture used in this study. Therefore, participants could give very accurate response when they saw these familiar pictures. The pictures used in other visual Stroop studies are normal line drawings (e.g., Geng et al. 2014; Lupker 1979), and therefore do not show higher accuracy than written word in their studies.

By comparing visual and audio stimuli, the results showed that both picture and conditioned sound would produce longer reaction time for response, while picture would trigger higher accuracy but conditioned sound would lead to a lower accuracy when comparing with written and spoken word, respectively. This confirmed that both picture and conditioned sound were perceived differently from word, hence required different time to be processed in the perception processes. Thus, the results in this study supported that picture and conditioned sound were having different modes of perception from that of word. Further studies can focus on the difference between picture and conditioned sound in perception and interpretation process as to compare with words.

2.6.3 Selective Attention

There are multiple different attentional models proposed to explain the mechanism of selective attention, such as the Broadbent's model, the selective filter model, and the late-filter model. All these selective attention models had proposed that the filter of blocking most irrelevant information (only personal information can pass through the filter) was placed before the short-term memory stage, and would not affect the response making (Broadbent 1958; Deutsch and Deutsch 1963; Moray 1959; Norman 1968; Wood and Cowan 1995). However, this study did not support these models but showed that even though information were coming from different sensory organs and were interpreted as different sensory information, they did interact with each other to alter the response even participants had tried to eliminate the distraction of one of them.

In fact, this research supported the attenuation model proposed by Treisman (1960) for selective attention. Please refer to Fig. 2.1 for the Treisman's attenuation model. The attenuation model proposes that all stimuli inputs, including both attended and unattended information are equally passed through the sensory register (equally received by the sensory organs). When they pass through the attenuation control, the capacity of the unattended information would be limited, while the attended information would not be limited. Finally, with the different capacity of various information they would pass through the perceptual processes and get into the short-term memory before responses were given. In this way, as the unattended information has limited capacity, the response would be more affected by the attended information (the target stimuli in this study), even though the unattended information (the distractors in this study) still has the capacity to interact with the attended information in order to alter the response. Therefore, even the executive attention is working to eliminate the irrelevant information, the conflict brought by the incongruent condition (conflict between the meaning of visual

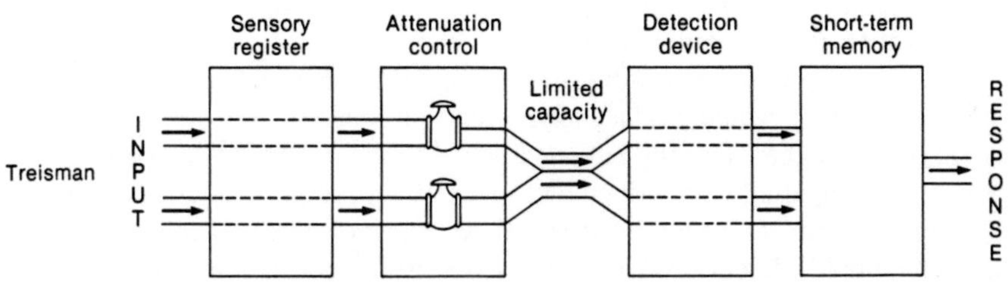

Fig. 2.1 Treisman's attenuation model

and audio stimuli) may still lead to poorer performance (longer reaction time and lower accuracy).

Therefore, this research supported the attenuation model with evidence that the capacity of unattended information had been reduced by selective attention but it still had the capacity to alter the responses triggered by the attended stimuli.

2.7 Implications

This study has addressed the interaction effect of picture and conditioned sound as comparing with written and spoken words. The results showed that spoken word would have shorter response time and higher accuracy than conditioned sound. This implies that usage of conditioned sounds as indicators in most daily instruments and tools (such as the pedestrian traffic lights in transportation system, the payment devices in public transports and stores, etc.) could be considered to be replaced by spoken words in order to increase the effectiveness of the instruments and tools to the users. This might be particularly useful for those instructions requiring high compliance or quick response. For example using spoken words in the pedestrian traffic lights can insert greater interaction effect on pedestrians and the chance of traffic accident could be greatly reduced.

Apart from using spoken word to replace conditioned sound as the automaticity effect of spoken word could provide greater interaction effect, the implication in visual aspect might be different. The results in this study showed that in the perceptual process, picture might give higher accuracy and written word might give faster response. To maximize the effectiveness of the instruments and tools, it is suggested that picture and written word can be used together as indicators to replace using only written word or picture sign separately in our daily applications. The use of combining picture and written word in instruments to improve the effectiveness of it is in fact similar to the use of spoken word (instead of conditioned sound) as mentioned in the above paragraph.

To sum up, refining instruments and tools for different aspect, such as the transportation system, medical devices, or banking transaction tools, etc., by using spoken instructions and combining picture with written word would be useful suggestion from the results of this study in order to increase the compliancy of users.

2.8 Limitations

Although every effort was employed to minimize the drawbacks of this study, there are two major limitations on this study as mentioned below.

The facilitation effect brought by the congruence of two stimuli as mentioned in some literature (e.g., Hamers and Lambert 1972; McLeod 1998; Stirling 1979) was not included in this study as limited accessible stimuli with conditioned sound could be used to construct a neutral condition. Further study could focus on the facilitation and interference with conditioned sound to verify whether facilitation also takes place with the presence of conditioned sound.

The individualized conditioning effect may affect the current results. However, it is also the nature of conditioned sound that people seldom really pay much attention or be very familiar with the conditioned sound. Thus, this research still reflected the actual circumstances of cross modal interaction effect with conditioned sound. Further study can investigate the interaction effect with different extent of conditioning and whether conditioned sound with greater conditioning effect may override the automaticity effect of spoken word.

2.9 Conclusion

This study had introduced the cross modal interaction effect given by picture, conditioned sound and word. The findings had demonstrated that all of the stimuli, including the conditioned sound, would create interference under incongruence of visual and audio stimuli. The results proved that the automaticity effect of spoken word may trigger faster and more accurate responses than that of conditioned sound, while picture may trigger higher accuracy and written word may give faster response. Therefore, it is suggested that the daily use of conditioned sound could be replaced by spoken word and those visual signs could be modified by combining both picture and written word in our daily instruments and tools employed by various disciplines so as to increase their effectiveness.

Acknowledgments This study has obtained the ethical approval from the Research Committee of the Hong Kong Shue Yan University.

References

Acosta, E., Jr., & Simon, J. R. (1976). The effect of irrelevant information on the stages of processing. *Journal of Motor Behavior, 8*, 181–487.

Broadbent, D. E. (1958). *Perception and communication*. Oxford: Pergamon.

Calvert, G. A., Campbell, R., & Brammer, M. J. (2000). Evidence from functional magnetic resonance imaging of crossmodal binding in the human heteromodal cortex. *Current Biology, 10*, 649–657.

Cattell, J. M. (1886). The time it takes to see and name objects. *Mind, 11*, 63–65.

Cohen, G., & Martin, M. (1975). Hemisphere differences in an auditory Stroop test. *Perception and Psychophysics, 17*, 79–83.

Cowan, N., & Barron, A. (1987). Cross-modal, auditory-visual Stroop interference and possible implications for speech memory. *Perception and Psychophysics, 41*(5), 393–401.

Dalrymple-Alford, E. C. (1968). Interlingual interference in a colornaming task. *Psychonomic Science, 10*, 215–216.

Deutsch, J. A., & Deutsch, D. (1963). Attention: Some theoretical considerations. *Psychological Review, 70*, 80–90.

Dyer, F. N. (1973). The Stroop phenomenon and its use in the study of perceptual, cognitive, and response processes. *Memory and Cognition, 1*, 106–120.

Fraisse, P. (1969). Why is naming longer than reading? *Acta Psychologica, 30*, 96–103.

Geng, J., Schnur, T. T., & Janssen, N. (2014). Relative speed of processing affects interference in Stroop and picture-word interference paradigms: evidence from the distractor frequency effect. *Language, Cognitive and Neuroscience, 29*(9), 1100–1114.

Golinkoff, R. M., & Rosinski, R. R. (1976). Decoding, semantic processing, and reading comprehension skill. *Child Development, 47*, 252–258.

Green, E. J., & Barber, P. B. (1981). An auditory stroop effect with judgements of speaker gender. *Perception and Psychophysics, 30*(5), 459–466.

Gregg, M. K., & Purdy, K. A. (2007). Graded auditory stroop effects generated by gender words. *Perceptual and Motor Skills, 105*, 549–555.

Hamers, J. F., & Lambert, W. E. (1972). Bilingual interdependencies in auditory perception. *Journal of Verbal Learning and Verbal Behavior, 11*, 303–310.

Imani, A., Pourbakht, A., Akbari, M., & Kashani, M. M. (2012). Effect of sound conditioning on click auditory brainstem response threshold shifts in guinea pigs. *Audiology, 21*(3), 77.

Jensen, A. R., & Rohwer, W. D., Jr. (1966). The Stroop color-word test: A review. *Acta Psychologica, 25*, 36–93.

Jerger, S., Martin, R. C., & Pirozzol, F. J. (1988). A developmental study of the auditory Stroop effect. *Brain and Language, 35*, 84–104.

Laurienti, P. J., Kraft, R. A., Maldjian, J. A., Burdette, J. H., & Wallace, M. T. (2004). Semantic congruence is a critical factor in multisensory behavioral performance. *Experimental Brain Research, 158*, 405–414.

Lidwell, W., Holden, K., & Butler, J. (2010). *Universal principles of design, revised and updated: 115 Ways to enhance usability, influence perception, increase appeal, make better design decisions, and teach through design*. Beverly, MA: Rockport Publishers.

Lupker, S. J. (1979). The semantic nature of response competition in the picture-word interference task. *Memory and Cognition, 7*(6), 485–495.

MacLeod, C. M. (2005). The Stroop task in cognitive research. In A. Wenzel & D. C. Rubin (Eds.), *Cognitive methods and their application to clinical research* (pp. 17–40). Washington, DC: American Psychological Association.

McGurk, H., & MacDonald, J. (1976). Hearing lips and seeing voices. *Nature, 264*, 746–748.

McLeod, C. M. (1998). Training on integrated versus separated Stroop task: The progression of interference and facilitation. *Memory and Cognition, 26*, 201–211.

Molholm, S., Ritter, W., Javitt, D. C., & Foxe, J. J. (2002). Multisensory visual-auditory object recognition in humans: A high density electrical mapping study. *Cerebral Cortex, 14*, 452–465.

Moray, N. (1959). Attention in dichotic listening: Affective cues and the influence of instructinos. *Quarterly Journal of Experimental Psychology, 11*, 56–60.

Norman, D. A. (1968). Toward a theory of memory and attention. *Psychological Review, 75*, 522–536.

Peng, D. C., & Prime, S. L. (2014). Clarifying the crossmodal stroop effect in an auditory-visual colour naming task with words and non-words stimuli. *Journal of Vision, 14*(10), 446.

Posner, M. I., & Rothbart, M. K. (2007). Research on attention networks as a model for the integration of psychological science. *Annual Review of Psychology, 58*, 1–23.

Reason, J. (1990). *Human error*. New York: Cambridge University Press.

Rosinski, R. R. (1977). Picture-word interference is semantically based. *Child Development, 48*, 643–647.

Rosinski, R. R., Golinkoff, R. M., & Kukish, K. S. (1975). Automatic semantic processing in a picture-word interference task. *Child Development, 46*, 247–253.

Schneider, W., Eschman, A., & Zuccolotto, A. (2001). *E-Prime user's guide*. Pittsburgh: Psychology Software Tools Inc.

Schriefers, H., & Meyer, A. S. (1990). Experimental note: Cross-modal, visual-auditory picture-word interference. *Bulletin of the Psychonomic Society, 28*(5), 418–420.

Settlage, P., & Harlow, H. F. (1936). Concerning the sensory pathway in the conditioned reflex. *Journal of Comparative Psychology, 22*(2), 279–282.

Seymour, P. H. K. (1977). Conceptual encoding and locus of the Stroop effect. *Quarterly Journal of Experimental Psychology, 29*, 245–265.

Simon, J. R. (1969). Reactions toward the source et stimulation. *Journal of Experimental Psychology, 81*, 174–176.

Simon, J. R. (1982). Effect of an audio stimulus on the processing of a visual stimulus under single-and dual-tasks conditions. *Acta Psychologica, 51*, 61–73.

Simon, J. R., Acosta, E., Jr., & Mewaldt, S. P. (1975). Effect of locus of warning tone on auditory choice reaction time. *Memory and Cognition, 3*, 167–170.

Simon, J. R., & Berbaum, K. (1988). Effect of irrelevant information on retrieval time for relevant information. *Acta Psychologica, 67*, 33–57.

Simon, J. R., & Berbaum, K. (1990). Effect of conflicting cues on information processing: The 'Stroop effect' vs. the 'Simon effect'. *Acta Psychologica, 73*, 159–170.

Simon, J. R., & Pouraghabagher, A. R. (1978). The effect of aging on the stages of processing in a choice reaction time task. *Journal of Gerontology, 33*, 553–561.

Soto-Faraco, S., Navarra, J., & Alsius, A. (2004). Assessing automaticity in audio-visual speech integration: Evidence from the speeded classification task. *Cognition, 92*, B13–B23.

Stirling, N. (1979). Stroop interference: An input and an output phenomenon. *Quarterly Journal of Experimental Psychology, 31*, 121–132.

Stroop, J. R. (1935). Studies of interference in serial verbal reactions. *Journal of Experimental Psychology, 18*, 643–662.

Treisman, A. M. (1960). Contextual cues in selective listening. *Quarterly Journal of Experimental Psychology, 12*, 242–248.

Van Atteveldt, N. M., Formisano, E., Goebel, R., & Blomert, L. (2004). Integration of letters and speech in the human brain. *Neuron, 43*, 271–282.

Van der Molen, M. W., & Keuss, P. J. G. (1981). Response selection and the processing of auditory intensity. *Quarterly Journal of Experimental Psychology, 33A*, 177–184.

Wood, N., & Cowan, N. (1995). The cocktail party phenomenon revisited: How frequent are attention shifts to one's name in an irrelevant auditory channel? *Journal of Experimental Psychology. Learning, Memory, and Cognition, 21*, 255–260.

Chapter 3
Media Multitaskers and Attentional Bias Toward Emotional Stimuli

Shanu Shukla

Abstract Individuals with high propensity toward media multitasking have been found to be vulnerable toward attention problems and mind wandering behavior. Their "breadth-biased" behavior style inclines them to pay attention to a large set of stimuli. As a result, they become susceptible to interferences. However in the environment, the nature of stimuli can be emotional—positive, negative, or neutral. In the realistic scenario, one may ask whether the media multitaskers follow the breadth-biased focused style or are they biased toward any one of the positive, negative, or neutral stimuli on the basis of their recurrent thoughts. The present study attempts to explore the nature of attentional bias among the high- and low media multitaskers (HMM and LMM) through the "facial dot probe task" paradigm.

Keywords Attentional bias · High media multitaskers · Low media multitaskers · Facial dot probe task

3.1 Introduction

Media multitasking, a simultaneous consumption of two or more media, has become a popular behavioral choice among the adolescents and the young adults (Carriera et al. 2009; Anderson and Rainie 2013). Several studies (Rideout et al. 2010; Voorveld et al. 2014) have suggested that the consumption of multiple media has increased from average 6.3 to 7.6 h a day (for US users aged between 8 and 18 years). This leads to an emerging need to understand the effect of excessive media multitasking on the users' behavior. One such area of concern is selective attention. Researchers suggested that the HMM employ breadth-biased style of processing information (Ophir et al. 2009; Lin 2009; Minear et al. 2013; Uncapher et al. 2016).

S. Shukla (✉)
Human Factors and Applied Cognition Lab, Department of Psychology,
Indian Institute of Technology Indore, Simrol, Madhya Pradesh 453552, India
e-mail: shanu.shukla11@gmail.com

M.-T. Leung and L.-M. Tan (eds.), *Applied Psychology Readings*,
DOI 10.1007/978-981-10-2796-3_3

This implies that the HMM pays attention to all the stimuli in a similar manner and thus are easily susceptible to interferences. However, these results emerged from the laboratory based studies where the experimental stimuli were designed to be neutral in nature. But in the real scenario the nature of stimuli can be emotional—positive, negative, or neutral. Thus, the present study makes an attempt to understand the effect of excessive media multitasking behavior on selective attention toward emotional stimuli (for example, facial expressions of emotions) using the facial dot probe paradigm (MacLeod et al. 1986).

The cognitive theory behind the dot probe task paradigm entails that the individual will selectively attend those stimuli in the environment (in facial dot probe task it is the facial expressions of emotion) which will reflect its own internal mental state or mood (Bullock and Bonanno 2013). Therefore, if a person is positively biased, he (or she) will selectively focus his (or her) attention toward the positive stimuli in the environment and if he (or she) is negatively biased he (or she) will orient his (or her) attention toward the negative stimuli (Bar-Haim et al. 2007; Becker and Leinenger 2011).

From the affective and well-being related studies, it has been noted that the HMM display a positive relationship with the symptoms of anxiety, depression, and stress disorders (Becker et al. 2013; Mark et al. 2014). According to Felix Economakis (http://www.bps.org.uk/news/media-multitasking-anxiety-and-depression), this occurs because media multitasking produces multiple demands on the brain which results in releasing stress hormones and anxiety. However, there are other studies which suggested that the excessive media multitasking has no effect on the emotions or well-being of an individual (Shih 2013; Xu et al. 2016). Some argue that it is not the media multitasking that influence the emotional states of an individual but those are other moderators such as time management that influence an individual emotional well-being (Yang et al. 2015). There is another study which revealed that the participants had displayed positive emotions during media multitasking situation (Laine-Hernandez et al. 2013). Collectively, on the basis of these researches it can be said that there is no clear relationship between the emotional state and HMM.

Hence through the facial dot probe task one aim to know two things: First, whether the HMM focus upon all the stimuli in a similar way or will they show preferences toward emotional stimuli. Second, which kind of attentional bias will they display (which can be an indirect reflection of their internal mood/mental states) toward facial emotional stimuli.

3.2 Experiment

3.2.1 Methods

3.2.1.1 Participants

A total of 30 participants [mean $(M) = 19.3$ years; standard deviation $(\mathrm{SD}) = 1.25$; within the age range 16–22 years] pursuing Bachelor of Technology programme at an institute of technology voluntarily participated in the experiment.

There were 18 males and 12 females in the sample. Each participant was tested individually. The data of two participants were discarded due to their failing to complete media multitasking questionnaire. Thus, in total data of 28 participants were included in the subsequent analyses.

3.2.1.2 Material

A media multitasking questionnaire identical to that of Ophir et al. (2009) was used to assess the media multitasking habits among the participants. The questionnaire is divided into two parts. Part one inquires about the number of hours one spends in a week using the given media (it has in total 12 media options such as print media, television, computer based video, etc.). Part two assesses one's media multitasking habit and frequency to be engaged with other media while using primary medium through a four-point rating scale. A formula was used to calculate Media Multitasking Index (MMI) for each participant as mentioned in Ophir et al. (2009) study.

Facial Dot Probe Task is a modified form of the original dot probe task (MacLeod et al. 1986). This was designed in the *OpenSesame* (Mathôt et al. 2012) software and was run on a Windows 8 Laptop. It consists of photographs from two databases; Amsterdam Dynamic facial expression Set (Van der Schalk et al. 2011) and Indian Movie Face Database (Setty et al. 2013). The rationale behind using two different databases was to provide exposure to cross-cultural facial emotional stimuli to the participants. The facial stimuli pairs display an emotional face (high and low intensity of positive and negative images from the databases) and a neutral face of the same actor. Twenty emotions-neutral pairs were used in a practice trial and 192 trials were used for the experimental task.

An "informed consent form" briefly detailing the structure of the study was provided to the participant to get their written consent. They were also provided with "Demographic Questionnaire" where their personal details, educational qualification, and other factual data were recorded.

3.2.1.3 Procedure

Upon arrival the participants were given the briefing of the experiment and subsequently the "consent form" was filled. The experiment was divided into two sessions. In session one, participants were required to fill the Demographic Questionnaire and media multitasking questionnaire. After this session, participants were introduced to "Facial dot probe task". They were seated approximately 75 cm away from the Laptop screen and were given 20 practice trials so as to familiarize themselves with the task.

Each trial began with a fixation dot that lasted for 500 ms followed by a pair of pictures (emotional and a neutral facial expression) for 1000 ms. After the stipulated time the pictures disappeared and either of them was replaced by a small dot. The dot was visible till the participants press one of the two response keys ("*p*" if the dot is on right side and "*q*" if it is on left side). There were in total 192 trials presented in the experimental task and each task lasted for 14 min (average time taken by participants). The response time and accuracy for each response was recorded. Besides, errors in identifying target dot probe or response time of more than 2000 ms were not included in the data analysis.

3.3 Results

3.3.1 Media Multitasking Index (MMI)

Media Multitasking Index (MMI) refers to the average number of media that an individual can be engaged in simultaneously. For each participant, it was calculated using the Ophir et al. (2009) criteria. The following formula was employed:

$$\mathrm{MMI} = \sum_{i=1}^{n} \frac{m_i h_i}{h_{\mathrm{total}}},$$

where m_i was the number of media typically used while using primary medium i, h_i was the total number of hours spent on an average day using primary medium i, and h_{total} was the total number of hours spent on an average day with all primary media.

Applying the MMI formula in the present experiment produced a relatively normal distribution with a mean of 3.15 and standard deviation of 1.25 for 28 participants. This implied that the participants use approximately three media simultaneously in their everyday life.

To identify the high media multitaskers (HMM) and low media multitaskers (LMM) the data was further analyzed. A "mean split approach" was utilized to categorize HMM and LMM. All the participants greater than the group mean were categorized as HMM group and participants less than group mean were categorized as an LMM group (Refer Table 3.1).

3.3.2 Average Response Time for Dot Probe in Facial Stimulus Pair Combinations for HMM and LMM

Average response time for dot probe appearing after two different facial pair combinations was calculated (Tables 3.2, 3.3).

Table 3.1 No. of participants identified as HMM and LMM

Category of media multitaskers	Participants		
	Total	Males	Females
High media multitaskers (HMM)	14	9	5
Low media multitaskers (LMM)	14	8	6

Table 3.2 Average response time for dot probe in facial stimulus pair combinations for HMM

	High media multitaskers (HMM)			
	Neutral-negative trials		Neutral-positive trials	
	Neutral cues	Negative cues	Neutral cues	Positive cues
Average response time (SD) (in ms)	550.55 (77.84)	699.55 (65.86)	698.76 (118.74)	491.49 (86.89)

Table 3.3 Average response time for dot probe in facial stimulus pair combinations for LMM

	Low media multitaskers (LMM)			
	Neutral-negative trials		Neutral-positive trials	
	Neutral cues	Negative cues	Neutral cues	Positive cues
Average response time (SD) (in ms)	484.93 (57.96)	380.60 (83.15)	582.02 (122.22)	598.75 (56.94)

A Mann Whitney *U* test was carried out among HMM and LMM groups with respect to response time in different cues among neutral-negative trials and neutral-positive trials. This was analyzed to understand whether the response time among different cues differ due to difference in media multitasking habits. It was observed that there was a significant difference between HMM and LMM with respect to response time in positive cues during neutral-positive trials; $U = 30.00$, $p < .05$. There was also a significant difference between HMM and LMM with respect to response time in neutral cues during neutral-positive trials; $U = 38.00$, $p < .05$.

Similarly, *U* test had been conducted for negative cues in neutral-negative trials, and the difference found to be significant ($U = 2.00$, $p < .05$). Also for neutral cues in neutral-negative trials, the difference between HMM and LMM was significant; $U = 51.50$, $p < .05$. This suggests that different groups of media multitaskers respond differently to emotional and neutral stimulus.

3.3.3 Attentional Bias Scores for HMM and LMM

To calculate the attention bias for HMM and LMM groups the following criteria was adopted from previous studies (Bullock and Bonanno 2013).

1. Positive Attentional Bias is calculated by subtracting average response time for dot probe appearing after positive facial stimuli from the average response time for dot probe appearing after neutral facial stimuli in neutral-positive stimuli trials. A positive score indicates participant's bias toward positive stimuli. In contrast, negative score reveals participants allocation of attention toward neutral stimuli in neutral-positive stimuli trials.

According to the data, it was found that in case of HMM, the score was 207.27. This reflected that HMM prefer allocation of attention toward positive cues in neutral-positive stimuli trials. However, LMM (−16.73) seemed to allocate attention toward neutral cues in neutral-positive stimuli trials; but the bias seemed to be very small which can be treated as no bias score toward positive or neutral face in neutral-positive trials.

2. Negative Attentional Bias is calculated by subtracting average response time for dot probe appearing after negative facial stimuli from the average response time for dot probe appearing after neutral facial stimuli in neutral-negative stimuli trials. A positive score indicates participant's bias toward negative stimuli. In contrast, negative score reveals participants allocation of attention toward neutral stimuli in neutral-negative stimuli trials.

According to the data, among HMM (score = −149) attentional bias was toward neutral cues in neutral-negative stimuli trials. This reflected the avoidance tendency among HMM toward negative facial stimuli. In case of LMM (score = 104.33), it displayed an attentional bias toward negative facial stimuli in neutral-negative stimuli trials.

3.4 Discussion

The purpose of the study was to understand the selective attention or attentional bias toward emotional facial stimuli among the high and low groups of Media Multitaskers (HMM and LMM) through "Facial dot probe paradigm". The results suggested that in case of "neutral-positive facial pairing", HMM group reflects "positive bias" while there was no significant bias toward neutral or positive stimuli in case of LMM group. This suggests that the HMM orient attention toward positive stimuli in the environment. This is evident from the finding of Song et al. (2013) where participants indulge in media multitasking behavior in order to avoid negative emotions like boredom. In case of "neutral-negative facial pairing" it was found that LMM reflect "negative bias" but HMM reflects bias toward neutral stimuli; with relative to negative stimuli. The negative bias in LMM may be supported by evolutionary theory which suggests that individual pay attention to negative stimuli for survival reasons. But lack of negative bias in HMM may reflect the tendency to avoid negative cues or to look for positive cues in the environment. For example, Burke and Develin (2016) found that on Facebook, posts with positive feelings received more likes than those posts which had negative feelings. Also a research by Greenfield (2010) highlights reduced empathy among college students due to overreliance on technology for communication and relationship building. It can also be argued that in order to reduce anxiety, HMM may adopt an avoidance strategy toward negative stimuli. Besides, the task switching ability among HMM might have facilitated disengagement from negative stimuli due to large time (1000 ms) gap for presentation of facial stimuli pairs.

To sum up, one can say that HMM do not focus upon all the stimuli in a similar way. They indeed have some preferences and attentional bias toward emotional stimuli such that they pay selective attention toward positive emotion when combined with neutral stimuli and display avoidance strategy toward negative stimuli when negative and neutral stimuli are present together.

3.5 Conclusion

It can be said that the HMM reflect an attentional bias for positive stimuli and no bias for negative stimuli with relative to neutral stimuli. The results of the study will be helpful in designing websites or educational content for HMM. However due to the small sample size, the results should be used with caution. Also there are other moderators like emotional status of the individual that should be taken into account in the final results.

Acknowledgments The author thanks Human Factors and Applied Cognition Lab at Indian Institute of Technology Indore for all the technical and experimental support during the execution of this project and acknowledge UGC, Government of India for support.

References

Anderson, J., & Rainie, L. (2013). *Millennials will benefit and suffer due to their hyperconnected lives.* Pew Internet and American Life Project report. Retrieved from http://www.pewinternet.org/2012/02/29/millennials-will-benefit-and-suffer-due-to-their-hyperconnected.

Bar-Haim, Y., Lamy, D., Pergamin, L., Bakermans-Kranenburg, M., & van Ijzendoorn, M. (2007). Threat-related attentional bias in anxious and nonanxious individuals: A meta-analytic study. *Psychology Bulletin, 133*(1), 1–24. doi:10.1037/0033-2909.133.1.1.

Becker, M. W., Alzahabi, R., & Hopwood, C. J. (2013). Media multitasking is associated with symptoms of depression and social anxiety. *Cyberpsychology, Behavior, and Social Networking, 16*(2), 132–135. doi:10.1089/cyber.2012.0291.

Becker, M. W., & Leinenger, M. (2011). Attentional selection is biased toward mood-congruent stimuli. *Emotion*. doi:10.1037/a0023524.

Bullock, A. B., & Bonanno, G. A. (2013). Attentional bias and complicated grief: A primed dot-probe task with emotional faces. *Journal of Expermental Psychopathology, 4*, 194–207. doi:10.5127/jep.020411.

Burke, M., & Develin, M. (2016). Once more with feeling: Supportive responses to social sharing on facebook. In *CSCW '16*. ACM. doi:10.1145/2818048

Carriera, L. M., Cheever, N. A., Rosena, L. D., Beniteza, S., & Changa, J. (2009). Multitasking across generations: Multitasking choices and difficulty ratings in three generations of Americans. *Computers in Human Behavior, 25*(2), 483–489. doi:10.1016/j.chb.2008.10.012.

Economakis, F. (2012). *Media multitasking and depression*. Retrieved from The British Psychological Society. www.bps.org.uk/news/media-multitasking-anxiety-and-depression

Greenfield, P. (2010). Social networking, mental health and human development. *Paper presented at the Lab School of Washington's 15th annual scientific research conference*. Washington, DC. Retrieved from http://test.baltimorelabschool.org/content/scientificconference.

Laine-Hernandez, M., Kinnunen, T., Kusumoto, K., Kätsyri, J., Westman, S., Ravaja, N., & Oittinen, P. (2013). *Multitasking influence on engagement.* WP3, Personal Media Day, Deliverable 2.3.3.7.

Lin, L. (2009). Breadth-biased versus focused cognitive control in media multitasking behaviors. *Proceedings of the National Academy of Sciences of the United States of America, 106*(37), 15521–15522. doi:10.1073/pnas.0908642106.

MacLeod, C., Mathews, A., & Tata, P. (1986). Attentional bias in emotional disorders. *Journal of Abnormal Psychology, 95*(1), 15–20. doi:10.1037/0021-843X.95.1.15.

Mark, G., Wang, Y., & Niiya, M. (2014). Stress and multitasking in everyday college life: An empirical study of online. In *CHI 2014.* Toronto: ACM. doi:10.1145/2556288.2557361

Mathôt, S., Schreij, D., & Theeuwes, J. (2012). OpenSesame: An open-source, graphical experiment builder for the social sciences. *Behavior Research Methods, 44*(2), 314–324. doi:10.3758/s13428-011-0168-7.

Minear, M., Brasher, F., McCurdy, M., Lewis, J., & Younggren, A. (2013). Working memory, fluid intelligence, and impulsiveness in heavy media multitaskers. *Psychonomic Bulletin and Review*. doi:10.3758/s13423-013-0456-6.

Ophir, E., Nass, C., & Wagner, A. D. (2009). Cognitive control in media multitaskers. *Proceedings of the National Academy of Sciences of the United States of America, 106*(37), 15583–15587. doi:10.1073/pnas.0903620106.

Rideout, V., Foehr, U., & Roberts, D. (2010). *Generation M2: Media in the lives of 8–18-year olds.* Menlo Park (CA): The Henry J Kaiser Family Foundation. Retrieved from http://www.kff.org/entmedia/upload/8010.pdf.

Setty, S., Husain, M., Beham, P., Gudavalli, J., Kandasamy, M., Vaddi, R., Hemadri, V., Karure, J. C., Raju, R., Rajan, B., Kumar, V., Jawahar, C. V. (2013). India movie face database: A benchmark for face recognition under wide variations. In *Computer vision, pattern recogniton, image processing and graphics (NCVPRIPG)* (pp. 1–5). Jodhur: IEEE.

Shih, S.-I. (2013). A null relationship between media multitasking and well-being. *PLoS ONE, 8*(5). doi:10.1371/journal.pone.0064508.

Song, K.-S., Nam, S., Lim, H., & Kim, J. (2013). Analysis of youngsters' media multitasking behaviors and effect on learning. *International Journal of Multimedia and Ubiquitous Engineering, 8*(4), 191–198. Retrieved from www.sersc.org/journals/IJMUE/vol8_no4_2013/19.pdf.

Uncapher, M., Thieu, M., & Wagner, A. (2016). Media multitasking and memory: Differences in working memory and long-term memory. *Psychonomic Bulletin Review, 23*(2), 483–490. doi:10.3758/s13423-015-0907-3.

Van der Schalk, J., Hawk, S. T., Fischer, A. H., & Doosje, B. (2011). Moving faces, looking places: Validation of the Amsterdam dynamic facial expression set (ADFES). *Emotion, 4*, 907–920. doi:10.1037/a0023853.

Voorveld, H., Seijn, C., Ketelaar, P., & Smit, E. (2014). Investigating the prevalence and predictors of media multitasking across countries. *International Journal of Communication, 8*, 2755–2777.

Xu, S., Wang, Z., & David, P. (2016). Media multitasking and well-being of university students. *Computers in Human Behavior, 55*, 242–250. doi:10.1016/j.chb.2015.08.040.

Yang, X., Xu, X., & Zhu, L. (2015). Media multitasking and psychological wellbeing in Chinese adolescents: Time management as a moderator. *Computers in Human Behavior, 53*, 216–222. doi:10.1016/j.chb.2015.06.034.

Chapter 4
Cognitive Deficits and Depression Among Diabetic and Nondiabetic Patients with Coronary Heart Disease

Sherin P. Antony, N. Veena, Sanjana Malhotra and Ann Joma Job

Abstract *Aim* The aim of the study was to examine the presence of cognitive deficits and depression among diabetic and nondiabetic patients with coronary heart disease. The differences between the before and the after coronary artery bypass graft surgery of both the diabetic and the nondiabetic patients with coronary heart disease on cognitive abilities were also examined. *Method* The sample consisted of 26 diabetic and 14 nondiabetic patients with coronary heart disease and the tests were administered 3–4 days prior to surgery and 2 weeks after surgery. Both the groups were screened using Edinburgh Handedness Inventory. The participants were administered a battery of neuropsychological tests to assess their cognitive ability, Beck Depression Inventory to assess depression, and the neuropsychological test battery and the depression inventory were administered both before the surgery (pretest) and immediately after the surgery (posttest). Collected data were then analyzed using appropriate statistical analysis. *Results* The results revealed that there was significant difference between the two groups only in the domain of response inhibition. The nondiabetic patient group performed significantly better on response inhibition compared to the diabetic patients. Patients who are diabetic are found to have significantly higher depression score than their nondiabetic counterparts. It was also evidenced that both the diabetic and

S.P. Antony (✉) · N. Veena · S. Malhotra · A.J. Job
Department of Psychology, Jain University, Bengaluru, Karnataka 560027, India
e-mail: sherin.anil@yahoo.com

N. Veena
e-mail: veenakraj@gmail.com

S. Malhotra
e-mail: sanjana326@rediffmail.com

A.J. Job
e-mail: annjjob@gmail.com

S.P. Antony
Department of Psychology, Acharya Institute of Graduate Studies,
Bengaluru, Karnataka 560107, India

M.-T. Leung and L.-M. Tan (eds.), *Applied Psychology Readings*,
DOI 10.1007/978-981-10-2796-3_4

the nondiabetic patients showed a decline in some of the neuropsychological test performances following surgery. The implications of this study were discussed in terms of the need for evaluation of cognitive functions and depression. Further, the usefulness of cognitive retraining, and psychological assistance, as well as the limitations and suggestions for future research were discussed.

Keywords Cognitive deficits · Coronary heart disease · Diabetic · Coronary artery bypass graft surgery

4.1 Introduction

Diabetes is associated with accelerated cognitive decline. It is unclear in which stage of diabetes the cognitive decrement becomes apparent and how they develop over time. Most of the studies have focused on patients with a known history of diabetes of several years. However, type 2 diabetes typically develops insidiously and may often be undiagnosed in the early stages. Therefore, cognitive decrements may start to develop years before the actual diagnosis, even in the prediabetes stages. The detailed neuropsychological data on the early stage of type 2 diabetes are not available and the possible risk factors for early cognitive decrements are not completely known (Ruis et al. 2009).

The prevalence rate of Diabetes mellitus (DM) is continuously rising from 285 million in the year 2010 and the expected rate in 2030 as 438 million (Zheng et al. 2014). The leading cause of patients with DM is cardiovascular disease, which reflects the link between the two. In addition, there have been studies which have portrayed the relationship between cardiovascular disease and depression. Literatures indicate 19–66 % of individuals with myocardial infarction also have the comorbidity with some mental disorder like depressive as well as anxiety states (Khawaja et al. 2009).

Diabetes mellitus and depression are two frequently encountered clinical conditions in primary care. Depression is the highest prevalent clinical disorder with 13.5–21.2 and 5 % of the general population suffering from it. Research has shown depression to be linked with impairment in the executive functioning.

Executive function has been defined as the complex processing of various subprocesses in order to achieve a specific goal. To elaborate these views, executive functions are those that include problem-solving behavior, modification of behavior as an effect of gaining new knowledge and producing strategies. Impairment in the executive functions has been associated with acuteness in major depressive disorder and deficits have been shown on tests measuring inhibition, planning as well as problem solving, mental flexibility (McDermott and Ebmeier 2009) verbal fluency, decision-making, and working memory (Schmid 2015). Individuals with the deficit in executive functioning are unable to segregate external stimuli that need to be facilitated. Few of the studies oppose which exhibit normal executive functioning among Major Depressive Disorder patients (Hammar and Årdal 2009).

Studies have reflected the prevalence of depression among 20 % of both the types of DM patients. There has been a 2.9-fold increase in the incidence of depression among those with DM compared to individuals without. This also increases the incidence of medical morbidity as well as mortality in depressive and DM patients (Zheng et al. 2014) as complications in the retinopathy, nephropathy, neuropathy, macro vascular complications, and sexual dysfunction, have been observed among the patients of DM affected with depression than those who are not affected (de Groot et al. 2000). Depression is linked with inability in glycemic control, that is, hyperglycemia as well as high HbA1c levels. Researchers have found that among diabetic patients, 14.7 % suffer from major depression and 26 % from elevated symptoms of depression. Recent studies have shown that deregulation and hypercortisolism in the HPA axis are related to depression. Therefore across clinical and communities epidemiologists as well as clinicians expect patients with diabetes to be twice more likely to be depressed compared with those of nondiabetic (Anderson et al. 2001). The aggregate estimates based on the literature suggest that major depression and elevated depression symptoms were present, respectively, in 11 and 31 % of individuals with diabetes. Gender is a mediating role in depression among diabetic individuals. The probability of depression is higher among women compared to men which is consistent with epidemiological surveys done in the general population (Gavard et al. 1993).

4.2 Methodology

4.2.1 Objectives

The primary objective of the study was to compare the presence of depression and cognitive deficits in diabetic and nondiabetic patients with coronary heart disease. The second objective was to compare the neuropsychological test performances of both diabetic and nondiabetic patients with coronary heart disease prior and after coronary artery bypass graft surgery (CABG).

4.2.2 Hypotheses

H1 Deficit in mental speed is not related to diabetes among patients with coronary heart disease (Table 4.6).

H2 Deficit in sustained attention is not related to diabetes among patients with coronary heart disease.

H3 Deficit in verbal fluency is not related to diabetes among patients with coronary heart disease.

H4 Deficit in verbal working memory is not related to diabetes among patients with coronary heart disease.

H5 Deficit in response inhibition is not related to diabetes among patients with coronary heart disease.

H6 Deficit in auditory verbal learning and memory is not related to diabetes among patients with coronary heart disease.

H7 Deficit in visual learning and memory is not related to diabetes among patients with coronary heart disease.

H8 Depression is not related to diabetes among patients with coronary heart disease.

H9 There are no significant differences between the before and the after surgery groups of diabetic and nondiabetic patients with coronary heart disease in neuropsychological performances and depression.

4.2.3 Study Sample

As one of the main objectives of the study was to compare diabetic and nondiabetic patients who were diagnosed with coronary heart disease, the study sample necessitated two groups. One group of the study included 26 diabetic patients and another group consisted of 14 nondiabetic patients who were diagnosed with coronary heart disease by cardiologist and scheduled for coronary artery bypass graft surgery (CABG). They were included in the study through purposive sampling on the basis of inclusion and exclusion criteria, from six hospitals in south India, which have cardiothoracic surgery departments.

4.2.4 Procedure

All participants and caregivers were informed about the nature of the study and were included in the sample after obtaining informed consent. The tests were administered 3–4 days before surgery and 2 weeks after coronary artery bypass graft surgery (CABG). The sample selected was within the age range of 30–65 years. Only those who were right handed were included in the sample. Those with other chronic illnesses were not included in the study.

4.2.5 Tools

4.2.5.1 Socio-demographic Data Sheet

Two separate semi-structured socio-demographic data sheets were prepared by the researcher. These were used to document the socio-demographic characteristics of the subjects. The basic details like age, education, and marital status were collected from all the subjects in the two groups.

4.2.5.2 General Health Questionnaire

The General Health Questionnaire developed by Goldberg and Williams (1988) is a self-administered 12-item screening tool, which is used to assess the presence of diagnosable psychiatric disorders in community settings and nonpsychiatric clinical settings. This questionnaire has a total score of 12 and is easy to administer. The tool was used in the present study to screen the subjects for the absence of psychiatric symptoms. The total score ranged from 0 to 36, with higher scores indicating poor psychological well-being. The internal consistency of the GHQ-12 is reported to be .90 by Hankins (2008) and it has high validity, and is not influenced by gender, age, or level of education (Goldberg et al. 1997).

4.2.5.3 Edinburgh Handedness Inventory

Neuropsychological functions are lateralized as left and right hemisphere functions. Handedness is related to the dominance of the cerebral hemispheres. In the present study, handedness inventory is used to avoid the influence of cerebral dominance on neuropsychological performances. Edinburgh Handedness Inventory developed by Oldfield (1971) is a simple and brief method for assessing handedness on a quantitative scale for use in neurological and other clinical and experimental work. This inventory was developed from the results obtained from the reports of 1,100 young adults. Each item of this inventory has been examined from the point of view of gender, culture, and socioeconomic factors related to them. It has 10 simple items which provide a quantitative measure of handedness based on hand preference for everyday activities and takes only about 5–10 min for administration. Handedness is based on a lateral quotient. The tool was used in the present study to screen both the patient groups.

4.2.5.4 Beck Depression Inventory (BDI)

The Beck Depression Inventory developed by Beck 1966 is one of the most widely used instruments for measuring the severity of depression. There are three versions of the BDI—the original BDI, first published in 1961 and later revised in 1978 as BDI-1A, and BDI-II—published in 1966. The scale used in the present study was BDI-II. It consisted of 21 questions with multiple choices and is designed for individuals aged 13 years and above. The inventory is composed of items related to symptoms of depression such as hopelessness and irritability, cognitions such as guilt or feelings of being punished, as well as physical symptoms such as fatigue, weight loss, and lack of interest in sex.

The participants were asked to rate how they have been feeling for the past 2 weeks and each answer is scored on a scale value of 0–3. A higher score indicates higher distress. The scale does not allow one to make a definite diagnosis of depression, but gives a dimensional representation of mood. Carney and associates used BDI score equal to or greater than 10 to diagnose depression in individuals with myocardial infarction, which revealed a moderate sensitivity (78 %) and specificity (90 %). Following this, in the present study a cutoff score of 10 was used to distinguish patients with depression.

The inventory is found to have high 1 week test–retest reliability ($r = .93$), suggesting that it was not overly sensitive to daily variations in mood. It also has high internal consistency ($\alpha = .91$). One measure of an instrument's validity is to see how closely it agrees with another similar instrument that has been validated against clinical interview by a trained clinician. In this respect, the BDI-II is positively correlated with the Hamilton Depression Scale with a Pearson r of .71, showing good agreement.

4.2.5.5 Neuropsychological Tests

Test of Speed: Digit Symbol Substitution Test

Digit symbol substitution test developed by Wechsler (1981) is a test of visuomotor coordination, motor persistence, information processing, and speed. The test consists of a sheet in which numbers one to nine are randomly arranged in four rows of 25 squares each. The subject has to substitute each number with a symbol using a number-symbol key given on top of the page. The first 10 squares are for practice. The test takes about 7 min.

Test of Attention: Digit Vigilance Test

Digit vigilance test developed by Lezak (1995) consists of a sheet containing numbers one to nine randomly ordered and placed in rows on a page. There are 30 digits per row and 50 rows in a test sheet. The subject has to focus on target digits six and nine amongst other distracter digits. Inability to sustain and focus attention leads to increased time to complete the test.

Tests of Executive Function: Controlled Oral Word Association Test

The controlled oral word association test developed by Benton and Hamsher (1989) is a measure of phonemic fluency. In this test, the subject generates words based on phonetic similarity of words. The subject is required to generate words beginning with the letters *F*, *A*, and *S* for 1 min. Proper nouns and names should be excluded. The same word should not be repeated with a different suffix. Subjects who do not know English language were asked to generate words in their own mother tongue commencing with 'ka,' 'pa,' 'ma.' The subject was asked to generate words for 1 min in case of each letter starting with *F*, going unto *A* and ending with *S* or with 'ka,' going on to 'pa' and ending with 'ma' as the case may be.

Animal Names Test

Animal names test is a measure of category fluency developed by Lezak (1995). Category fluency is another form of verbal fluency. In this test, it is the content of the words rather than the phonetic similarity of the words, which is regulated. The subject generates words which belong to a particular semantic category. The animal names test requires the subject to generate names of animals for 1 min.

Verbal N Back Test

The 1 back and 2 back versions of the N back test developed by Smith and Jonides (1999) assess verbal working memory. The 1 back version requires verbal storage and rehearsal while the 2 back version requires in addition to the above, manipulation of information. Therefore, the 1 back version would involve the articulatory loop in the verbal modality and the visuo-spatial sketchpad in the visual modality. The 2 back would involve the central executive in both the modalities.

Stroop Test

Stroop test measures response inhibition was developed by Benson and Struss (1986). It measures the ease with which a perceptual set can be shifted both to conjoin demands and suppressing a habitual response in favor of an unusual one. The prefrontal areas are essential for response inhibition. In this test, the color names 'blue,' 'green,' 'red,' and 'yellow' are printed in capital letters on a paper. The color of the print occasionally corresponds with the color designated by the word. The words are printed in 16 rows and 11 columns.

4.2.5.6 Tests of Learning and Memory

Rey's Auditory Verbal Learning Test (AVLT)

The Rey's Auditory Verbal Learning Test developed by Schmidt (1996) was later adapted for different cultures by WHO. It was also adapted to suit conditions in

Table 4.5 Frequency and percentage of patients with deficit in the domain of verbal fluency in both diabetic and nondiabetic patients

Verbal fluency	Deficit	Diabetic group		Nondiabetic group		Chi-square value
		Frequency	Percentage	Frequency	Percentage	
Phonemic Fluency Test	Yes	7	17.50	3	7.50	0.147 NS
	No	19	47.50	11	27.50	
Animal Names Test	Yes	9	22.50	8	20	1.89 NS
	No	17	42.50	6	15.00	

S significant, *NS* not significant
*Significant at 0.05 level

Table 4.6 Frequency and percentage of patients with deficit in the domain of verbal working memory in both diabetic and nondiabetic patients

Verbal working memory	Deficit	Diabetic group		Nondiabetic group		Chi-square value
		Frequency	Percentage	Frequency	Percentage	
Verbal N back 1 Test	Yes	3	7.50	1	2.50	0.195 NS
	No	23	57.50	13	32.50	
Verbal N back 2 Test	Yes	2	5.00	1	2.50	0.004 NS
	No	24	60	13	32.50	

S significant, *NS* not significant
*Significant at 0.05 level

Table 4.7 Frequency and percentage of patients with deficit in the domain of response inhibition in both diabetic and nondiabetic patients

Response inhibition	Deficit	Diabetic group		Nondiabetic group		Chi-square value
		Frequency	Percentage	Frequency	Percentage	
Stroop effect	Yes	15	37.50	3	7.50	4.83*
	No	11	27.50	11	27.50	

S significant, *NS* not significant
*Significant at 0.05 level

found to have deficit respectively which was not statistically significant. Hence the deficit in the domain of verbal working memory is not related to diabetes among patients with coronary heart disease and the hypothesis 4 is accepted (Table 4.7).

On Stroop test compared to normative scores, 37.5 and 7.5 % of patients in diabetic and nondiabetic groups were found to have deficit respectively which was statistically significant. Hence the deficit in the domain of response inhibition is related to diabetes among patients with coronary heart disease and the hypothesis 5 is rejected (Table 4.8).

On Auditory verbal learning long-term percent retention, compared to normative scores, 20 and 12.5 % of patients in diabetic and nondiabetic groups were found to have deficit respectively which was not statistically significant. On auditory verbal learning immediate recall compared to normative scores 7.5 and 30 %

Tests of Executive Function: Controlled Oral Word Association Test

The controlled oral word association test developed by Benton and Hamsher (1989) is a measure of phonemic fluency. In this test, the subject generates words based on phonetic similarity of words. The subject is required to generate words beginning with the letters *F*, *A*, and *S* for 1 min. Proper nouns and names should be excluded. The same word should not be repeated with a different suffix. Subjects who do not know English language were asked to generate words in their own mother tongue commencing with 'ka,' 'pa,' 'ma.' The subject was asked to generate words for 1 min in case of each letter starting with *F*, going unto *A* and ending with *S* or with 'ka,' going on to 'pa' and ending with 'ma' as the case may be.

Animal Names Test

Animal names test is a measure of category fluency developed by Lezak (1995). Category fluency is another form of verbal fluency. In this test, it is the content of the words rather than the phonetic similarity of the words, which is regulated. The subject generates words which belong to a particular semantic category. The animal names test requires the subject to generate names of animals for 1 min.

Verbal N Back Test

The 1 back and 2 back versions of the N back test developed by Smith and Jonides (1999) assess verbal working memory. The 1 back version requires verbal storage and rehearsal while the 2 back version requires in addition to the above, manipulation of information. Therefore, the 1 back version would involve the articulatory loop in the verbal modality and the visuo-spatial sketchpad in the visual modality. The 2 back would involve the central executive in both the modalities.

Stroop Test

Stroop test measures response inhibition was developed by Benson and Struss (1986). It measures the ease with which a perceptual set can be shifted both to conjoin demands and suppressing a habitual response in favor of an unusual one. The prefrontal areas are essential for response inhibition. In this test, the color names 'blue,' 'green,' 'red,' and 'yellow' are printed in capital letters on a paper. The color of the print occasionally corresponds with the color designated by the word. The words are printed in 16 rows and 11 columns.

4.2.5.6 Tests of Learning and Memory

Rey's Auditory Verbal Learning Test (AVLT)

The Rey's Auditory Verbal Learning Test developed by Schmidt (1996) was later adapted for different cultures by WHO. It was also adapted to suit conditions in

India by Maj et al. (1994). Rey originally developed the test in 1996. It consists of words designating familiar objects like vehicles, tools, animals, and body parts. There are two lists A and B, with 15 different words in each list.

Complex Figure Test (CFT)

The complex figure test developed by Meyers and Meyers (1995) consists of a complex design which is abstract in nature and cannot be named easily. This test measures visuo-constructive ability and visual learning and memory. The figure from the complex figure is copied and subsequently recalled. Immediate and delayed memory scores are obtained.

4.2.6 Analysis of Data

The data obtained were analyzed using the following statistical tests. The statistical analyses were carried out using the statistical software SPSS 16.0. Descriptive statistics such as frequencies and percentages, and mean and standard deviations have been used. Comparison of proportion of subjects falling in the categories of deficits in diabetic and nondiabetic patient groups was carried out using Chi-square test. The comparison between pre- and postsurgery groups of diabetic and nondiabetic patient subgroups were carried out using paired *t* test.

4.3 Results

Characteristics of the present sample are as follows. Table 4.1 summarizes the distribution of the subjects in the sample with respect to the presence of Diabetes.

Of a total of 40 participants that comprised people with coronary heart disease, 26 (65 %) participants had the comorbidity of diabetes and the remaining 14 (35 %) did not suffer from diabetes. Distribution of the sample with respect to sex is given in Table 4.2.

Table 4.1 Distribution of the subjects in the sample with respect to the presence of diabetes

Diabetes	Frequency	Percent
No	26	65.0
Yes	14	35.0
Total	40	100.0

Table 4.2 Gender wise distribution of the study subjects

Sex	Frequency	Percent
Male	28	70.0
Female	12	30.0
Total	40	100.0

Table 4.3 Frequency and percentage of patients with deficit in the domain of mental speed in both diabetic and nondiabetic patients

Mental speed	Deficit	Diabetic group		Nondiabetic group		Chi-square value
		Frequency	Percentage	Frequency	Percentage	
Digit	Yes	11	27.50	6	15.00	0.001 NS
Symbol substitution test	No	15	37.50	8	20.00	

S significant, *NS* not significant
*Significant at 0.05 level

Table 4.4 Frequency and percentage of patients with deficit in the domain of sustained attention in both diabetic and nondiabetic patients

Sustained attention	Deficit	Diabetic group		Nondiabetic group		Chi-square value
		Frequency	Percentage	Frequency	Percentage	
Digit vigilance test	Yes	8	20	1	2.50	2.913 NS
	No	18	45	13	32.50	

S significant, *NS* not significant
*Significant at 0.05 level

Among the total 40 individuals with coronary heart disease in the present sample, 70 % are males and 30 % are females indicating a higher number of male participants in the study (Table 4.3).

On digit symbol substitution test, compared to normative scores, 27 and 15 % of patients in diabetic and nondiabetic groups were found to have deficit respectively which was not statistically significant. Hence the deficit in the domain of mental speed is not related to diabetes among patients with coronary heart disease and the hypothesis 1 is accepted (Table 4.4).

On digit vigilance test, compared to normative scores, 20 and 2.5 % of patients in diabetic and nondiabetic groups were found to have deficit respectively which was not statistically significant. Hence the deficit in the domain of sustained attention is not related to diabetes among patients with coronary heart disease and the hypothesis 2 is accepted (Table 4.5).

On phonemic fluency test, compared to normative scores, 17 and 7 % of patients in diabetic and nondiabetic groups were found to have deficit respectively which was not statistically significant. On animal names test, compared to normative scores, 22 and 20 % of patients in diabetic and nondiabetic groups were found to have deficit respectively which was not statistically significant. Hence the deficit in the domain of verbal fluency is not related to diabetes among patients with coronary heart disease and the hypothesis 3 is accepted (Table 4.6).

On verbal N back 1 test, compared to normative scores, 7.5 and 2.5 % of patients in diabetic and nondiabetic groups were found to have deficit respectively which was not statistically significant. On verbal N back 2 test, compared to normative scores, 5 and 2.5 % of patients in diabetic and nondiabetic groups were

Table 4.5 Frequency and percentage of patients with deficit in the domain of verbal fluency in both diabetic and nondiabetic patients

Verbal fluency	Deficit	Diabetic group		Nondiabetic group		Chi-square value
		Frequency	Percentage	Frequency	Percentage	
Phonemic Fluency Test	Yes	7	17.50	3	7.50	0.147 NS
	No	19	47.50	11	27.50	
Animal Names Test	Yes	9	22.50	8	20	1.89 NS
	No	17	42.50	6	15.00	

S significant, *NS* not significant
*Significant at 0.05 level

Table 4.6 Frequency and percentage of patients with deficit in the domain of verbal working memory in both diabetic and nondiabetic patients

Verbal working memory	Deficit	Diabetic group		Nondiabetic group		Chi-square value
		Frequency	Percentage	Frequency	Percentage	
Verbal N back 1 Test	Yes	3	7.50	1	2.50	0.195 NS
	No	23	57.50	13	32.50	
Verbal N back 2 Test	Yes	2	5.00	1	2.50	0.004 NS
	No	24	60	13	32.50	

S significant, *NS* not significant
*Significant at 0.05 level

Table 4.7 Frequency and percentage of patients with deficit in the domain of response inhibition in both diabetic and nondiabetic patients

Response inhibition	Deficit	Diabetic group		Nondiabetic group		Chi-square value
		Frequency	Percentage	Frequency	Percentage	
Stroop effect	Yes	15	37.50	3	7.50	4.83*
	No	11	27.50	11	27.50	

S significant, *NS* not significant
*Significant at 0.05 level

found to have deficit respectively which was not statistically significant. Hence the deficit in the domain of verbal working memory is not related to diabetes among patients with coronary heart disease and the hypothesis 4 is accepted (Table 4.7).

On Stroop test compared to normative scores, 37.5 and 7.5 % of patients in diabetic and nondiabetic groups were found to have deficit respectively which was statistically significant. Hence the deficit in the domain of response inhibition is related to diabetes among patients with coronary heart disease and the hypothesis 5 is rejected (Table 4.8).

On Auditory verbal learning long-term percent retention, compared to normative scores, 20 and 12.5 % of patients in diabetic and nondiabetic groups were found to have deficit respectively which was not statistically significant. On auditory verbal learning immediate recall compared to normative scores 7.5 and 30 %

Table 4.8 Frequency and percentage of patients with deficit in the domain of auditory verbal learning and memory in both diabetic and nondiabetic patients

Verbal learning and memory	Deficit	Diabetic group		Nondiabetic group		Chi-square value
		Frequency	Percentage	Frequency	Percentage	
Auditory verbal learning long term percent retention	Yes	8	20	5	12.50	0.101 NS
	No	18	45.00	9	22.50	
Auditory verbal learning immediate recall	Yes	3	7.50	12	30.00	0.063 NS
	No	23	57.50	12	30.00	
Auditory verbal learning delayed recall	Yes	5	12.50	2	5.00	0.154 NS
	No	21	52.50	12	30.00	

S Significant, *NS* not significant
*Significant at 0.05 level

Table 4.9 Frequency and percentage of patients with deficit in the domain of visual learning and memory in both diabetic and nondiabetic patients

Recall test	Deficit	Diabetic group		Nondiabetic group		Chi-square value
		Frequency	Percentage	Frequency	Percentage	
Complex Figure Test-Immediate Recall	Yes	7	17.50	0	0.00	4.57*
	No	19	47.50	14	35.00	
Complex Figure Test-Delayed Recall	Yes	8	20.00	0	0.00	5.39*
	No	18	45.00	14	35.00	

S significant, *NS* not significant
*Significant at 0.05 level

of patients in diabetic and nondiabetic groups were found to have deficit respectively which was not statistically significant. On auditory verbal learning delayed recall compared to normative scores 12.5 and 5 % of patients in diabetic and nondiabetic groups were found to have deficit respectively which was not statistically significant. Hence the deficit in the domain of auditory verbal learning and memory is not related to diabetes among patients with coronary heart disease and the hypothesis 6 is accepted (Table 4.9).

On complex figure test-immediate recall compared to normative scores, 17.5 and 0 % of patients in diabetic and nondiabetic groups were found to have deficit respectively which was statistically significant. On complex figure test-delayed recall compared to normative scores, 20 and 0 % of patients in diabetic and nondiabetic groups were found to have deficit respectively which was statistically significant. Hence the deficit in the domain of visual learning and memory is related to diabetes among patients with coronary heart disease and the hypothesis 7 is rejected (Table 4.10).

Table 4.10 Frequency and percentage of patients with depression in both diabetic and nondiabetic patients

Measure depression	Deficit	Diabetic group		Nondiabetic group		Chi-square value
		Frequency	Percentage	Frequency	Percentage	
Depression	Yes	10	25	3	7.50	1.203 NS
	No	16	40	11	27.50	

S significant, *NS* not significant
*Significant at 0.05 level

Beck depression inventory for depression was used as a screening tool in both the groups. Ten patients (25 %) in diabetic group and three patients (7.5 %) in nondiabetic group had depression which was not statistically significant. This indicates there is no significant comorbidity of depression with diabetic patients of coronary heart disease in the present sample. And hence hypothesis 8 is accepted.

4.3.1 Comparison of Neuropsychological Performances and Depression Prior and After Surgery Among Diabetic Patients with Coronary Heart Disease

The differences between the before and the after surgery groups of both the diabetic and the nondiabetic patients on neuropsychological performances and depression were examined. The means and the standard deviations of the scores obtained by the diabetic MI patients before surgery and after surgery in neuropsychological performances and depression were compared using paired '*t*' test, the results of which are given in Table 4.11.

The results revealed that there were significant differences between the two groups of diabetic patients in some of the neuropsychological performances. Compared to their performance before surgery, the diabetic MI patients showed a decline in performance after surgery on mental speed (DST), sustained attention (DVT), phonemic fluency (COWA), verbal working memory (VNB 2), response inhibition (Stroop), and visual memory (CFT-IR and DR). With regard to depression, there was no significant difference between the before and the after surgery groups of diabetic patients.

4.3.2 Comparison of Neuropsychological Performances and Depression Prior and After Surgery Among Nondiabetic Patients with Coronary Heart Disease

The means and the standard deviations of the scores obtained by the nondiabetic patients before surgery and after surgery in neuropsychological performances

Table 4.11 Means and SDs of the scores obtained by the before and the after surgery groups of diabetic patients in neuropsychological performances and depression, and the corresponding '*t*' values

Domains	Tests	Diabetic group				'*t*' value
		Before surgery (N-26)		After surgery (N-26)		
		M	SD	*M*	SD	
Mental speed	DST	290.50	88.42	312.35	105.12	4.23**
Sustained attention	DVT	526.65	134.10	574.81	137.40	3.14**
Category fluency	ANT	11.92	2.60	11.42	2.36	1.34 NS
Phonemic fluency	COWA	12.31	4.79	10.85	4.14	2.94**
Verbal working memory	VNB 1	8.54	.64	8.38	.85	1.69 NS
	VNB 2	7.35	.93	6.77	.99	3.26**
Response inhibition	Stroop test	345.50	135.64	353.35	139.80	4.34**
Auditory verbal learning and memory	AVLT-LTPR	79.80	16.13	81.85	11.18	.25 NS
	AVLT-IR	10.92	1.91	10.73	2.23	.63 NS
	AVLT-DR	10.27	2.27	9.96	2.10	1.18 NS
Visual learning and memory	CFT-IR	19.58	7.20	17.96	7.38	3.43**
	CFT-DR	17.42	7.50	16.23	7.15	2.41*
Depression	BDI	12.03	.43	2.23	7.02	.40 NS

S significant, *NS* not significant
*Significant at 0.05 level

and depression were compared using paired '*t*' test and the results are given in Table 4.12. The results revealed that there were significant differences between the before and the after surgery groups of nondiabetic MI patients in some of the neuropsychological test performances. Compared to their performance before surgery, the nondiabetic patient group showed a decline in performance after surgery on mental speed (DST), sustained attention (DVT), verbal working memory (VNB 1&2), and response inhibition (Stroop), and verbal learning and memory (CFT-IR and DR). With regard to depression, there was no significant difference between the before and the after surgery groups of nondiabetic patients. Therefore hypothesis 9 is rejected.

4.4 Discussion

Comparisons of diabetic and nondiabetic patients with coronary heart disease in neuropsychological test performances and depression showed that both the diabetic and the nondiabetic patients showed a decline in some of the neuropsychological test performances. However in the domain of response inhibition and visual learning and memory, there were significant association between diabetes and deficit. Several studies have linked diabetes to cognitive deficits on measures

Table 4.12 Means and SD scores obtained by the before and the after surgery groups of nondiabetic patients in neuropsychological performances and depression, and the corresponding '*t*' values

Domains	Tests	Nondiabetic group				'*t*' values
		Before surgery ($N = 14$)		After surgery ($N = 14$)		
		M	SD	*M*	SD	
Mental speed	DST	294.21	88.00	316.14	93.75	3.75**
Sustained attention	DVT	533.14	114.92	581.14	125.50	2.70**
Category fluency	A N T	11.93	2.20	11.29	2.23	1.66 NS
Phonemic fluency	COWA	11.86	4.40	10.71	2.92	1.87 NS
Verbal working memory	VNB 1	8.86	.36	8.50	.76	2.11*
	VNB 2	7.79	.97	7.07	.91	2.68**
Response inhibition	Stroop test	249.43	90.69	255.79	90.37	4.11***
Auditory verbal learning and memory	AVLT-LTPR	80.96	19.06	74.71	12.26	1.36 NS
	AVLT-IR	10.36	2.24	9.64	2.09	2.68**
	AVLT-DR	9.86	2.14	9.07	2.55	2.34*
Visual learning and memory	CFT-IR	21.50	5.57	40.00	73.70	.93 NS
	CFT-DR	20.64	5.59	19.29	7.29	1.54 NS
Depression	BDI	12.03	6.43	7.92	3.66	1.00 NS

S significant, *NS* not significant
*Significant at 0.05 level

of complex problem-solving skills (Rennick et al. 1968), mental flexibility and motor speed (Skenazy and Bigler 1984), memory for recent learned information (Franceschi et al. 1984), visuo-spatial deficits and psychomotor slowing (Wredling et al. 1990).

The reasons for this association could be several. It includes diffusely distributed demyelination in the cranial nerves, optic chiasma, and white matter, and extensive gliosis in grey matter, basal ganglia, brain stem, and cerebellum (Reske-Nielsen et al. 1965). Magnetic resonance imaging studies evidenced cortical atrophy (Perros et al. 1997). The increased blood viscosity of diabetics might have contributed to reduced cerebral blood flow (Tatemichi et al. 1992). These reasons might have contributed to the significantly poorer performance in the diabetic group compared to the nondiabetic group. Thus, it may be possible to infer that diabetes significantly affects the executive functions and visual learning and memory of patients with coronary heart disease.

To sum up, the findings in the present study validate previous research findings that diabetes is associated with dysfunction in response inhibition (executive function) and visual learning and memory. Response inhibition is considered to be primarily frontal function. A prefrontal cortex, especially the right prefrontal lobe, is involved to a greater extent in retrieval from episodic memory (Tulving 1999). Lesions in the right temporal lobe disrupt visual learning and memory.

4.5 Conclusion and Implications

Examination of the association between the diabetes and cognitive deficits in patients with coronary heart disease with respect to neuropsychological functions and depression revealed significant association in the deficits of response inhibition and visual learning and memory and diabetes.

The nondiabetic patients performed significantly better than the diabetic patients on response inhibition. With regard to depression there was no such association found. In addition, the differences between the before and after the surgery groups of diabetic and nondiabetic patients in neuropsychological test performances and depression were also examined. Compared to their performances before surgery, both the diabetic and the nondiabetic MI patients showed decline in some of the neuropsychological test performances along with the deterioration in the mood.

Diabetic patients with coronary heart disease may undergo depression which can have a negative impact on recovery and may lead to increased social and occupational dysfunctions. This indicates the need to include psycho-education for both the patient as well as the family members regarding the illness and its prognosis, course of recovery, and the impact of neuropsychological impairment and depression on everyday functioning.

Informing and educating professionals who are involved in the treatment and management of diabetic patients with coronary heart disease along with the mental health professionals about the necessity of having a comprehensive neuropsychological assessment and further plan for a unique cognitive retraining intervention is essential.

References

Anderson, R. J., Freedland, K. E., Clouse, R. E., & Lustman, P. J. (2001). The prevalence of co morbid depression in adults with diabetes a meta-analysis. *Diabetes Care, 24*(6), 1069–1078.

Beck, A. T. (1966). *Manual for the Beck Depression Inventory-II*. San Antonio, TX: Psychological Corporation.

Benson, D. F., & Struss, D. T. (1986). *The frontal lobes*. New York: Raven Press.

Benton, A. L., & Hamsher, K. S. (1989). *Multilingual aphasia examination*. New York: Oxford University Press.

de Groot, M., Anderson, R. J., Freedland, K. E., Clouse, R. E., & Lustman, P. J. (2000). Association of diabetes complications and depression in type 1 and type 2 diabetes: A meta-analysis. *Diabetes, 49*, A63.

Gavard, J. A., Lustman, P. J., & Clouse, R. E. (1993). Prevalence of depression in adults with diabetes: An epidemiological evaluation. *Diabetes Care, 16*, 1167–1178.

Goldberg, D., Gater, R., Sartorious, N., Ustun, T., Piccinelli, M., Gueje, O., et al. (1997). The validity of two versions of the GHQ in the WHO study of mental illness in general health: A stress process model. *Health Psychology, 17*(2), 190–198.

Goldberg, D., & Williams, P. (1988). *A user's guide to the GHQ*. Berkshire: NFER Nelson.

Hammar, Å., & Årdal, G. (2009). Cognitive functioning in major depression—A summary. *Frontiers in Human Neuroscience, 3*, 26.

Hankins, M. (2008). The reliability of the twelve-item general health questionnaire (GHQ-12) under realistic assumptions. *BMC Public Health, 8*, 355.

Kessler, R. C., McGonagle, K. A., Zhao, S., Nelson, C. B., Hughes, M., Eshleman, S., et al. (1994). Lifetime and 12-month prevalence of DSM-III-R psychiatric disorders in the United States: Results from the National Cormorbidity Survey. *Archives of General Psychiatry, 51*, 8–19.

Khawaja, I. S., Westermeyer, J. J., Gajwani, P., & Feinstein, R. E. (2009). Depression and coronary artery disease: The association, mechanisms, and therapeutic implications. *Psychiatry (Edgmont), 6*(1), 38–51.

Lezak, M. D. (1995). *Neuropsychological assessment* (3rd ed.). New York: Oxford University Press.

Lustman, P. J., Anderson, R. J., Freedland, K. E., de Groot, M., & Carney, R. M. (2000). Depression and poor glycemic control: A meta-analytic review of the literature. *Diabetes Care, 23*, 434–442.

McDermott, L. M., & Ebmeier, K. P. (2009). A meta-analysis of depression severity and cognitive function. *Journal of Affective Disorders, 119*(1), 1–8.

Meyers, J., & Meyers, K. (1995). *Rey complex figure and recognition trial: Professional manual.* Florida: Psychological Assessment Resources.

Oldfield, R. C. (1971). The Assessment and analysis of handedness: The Edinburgh Inventory. *Neuropsychologia, 9*, 97–113.

Ruis, C., Biessels, G. J., Gorter, K. J., Van Den Donk, M., Kappelle, L. J., & Rutten, G. E. (2009). Cognition in the early stage of type 2 diabetes. *Diabetes Care, 32*(7), 1261–1265.

Schmid, M. T. (2015). Executive functioning in recurrent—And first episode Major Depressive Disorder: Longitudinal studies.

Schmidt, M. (1996). *Rey auditory verbal learning test: A handbook.* Los Angles: Western Psychological Services.

Smith, E. E., & Jonides, J. (1999). Storage and executive processes in the frontal lobes. *Science, 283*, 1657–1661.

Wechsler, D. (1981). *WAIS-R manual.* New York: The Psychological Corporation.

Zheng, Z., Wu, J., Wang, R., & Zeng, Y. (2014). Diabetes mellitus may induce cardiovascular disease by decreasing neuroplasticity. *Functional Neurology, 29*(1), 7.

Chapter 5
Sex Differences and Emotion in Wayfinding: Using a Map or Verbal Direction (a Pilot Study)

M. Dinah Charlota Lerik, T.D. Hastjarjo and Rini Dharmastiti

Abstract *Objective* The current investigation examined gender differences and emotion in wayfinding behavior. *Background* Looking for a new location or moving from one place to another place is a common everyday task. The ability to find one's way in our complex environments represents one of the most fundamental cognitif function. *Methods* Using survey method in collecting data, this study has 262 students from three universities in Central Java-Indonesia. Age between 17 and 22 years old. Descriptive statistics were used. *Results* Wayfinding behavior dominantly used map and verbal direction almost equally, even on men and women too. There were no positif, neutral, or negatif emotion dominantly effect on wayfinding behavior. Further results are discussed.

Keywords Wayfinding behavior · Map · Verbal direction · Gender · Emotion

5.1 Introduction

Imagine you are driving into the city for the first time you visit. You are looking for a home address and your family for example has spun several times in the same place. You lost. There are two opportunities to be able to find the address,

M. Dinah Charlota Lerik (✉) · T.D. Hastjarjo
Faculty of Psychology, Gadjah Mada University, Yogyakarta 55821, Indonesia
e-mail: charlota@mail.ugm.ac.id
URL: http://www.ugm.ac.id

T.D. Hastjarjo
e-mail: dickyh@ugm.ac.id

R. Dharmastiti
Ergonomic Laboratory, Department Mechanical and Industrial Engineering,
Faculty of Engineering, Gadjah Mada University, Yogyakarta 55821, Indonesia
e-mail: rini@ugm.ac.id

M.-T. Leung and L.-M. Tan (eds.), *Applied Psychology Readings*,
DOI 10.1007/978-981-10-2796-3_5

you can call the homeowner and mention your position at that time and request verbal instructions to the address of the house, or do you stop the vehicle and then ask the people to draw a map to the address you are addressing them. Which is more efficient? The purpose of this research is to answer the question. The term wayfinding was first introduced by Lynch (1960), as the use of sensory signs from the external environment in a consistent and organized.

According to Golledge (1999), wayfinding is the process of determining the location and follow a route that is between the start and destination. Montello (2005) defines wayfinding as the location of a person's body movements trending and aims in an efficient manner, and often it is purpose is not local environment. The author uses the definition of wayfinding as the discovery process finds its way to efficiently move your body to the location in an environment that is recognized or not recognized using the signs in the environment.

Humans perform the task of finding locations each day such as search, exploration, following the planned route or routes both within closed or the environment of the city, in buildings and virtual simulation. Cognitive resources to perform different tasks based on the format and content of spatial knowledge involved, problem-solving strategies, selection perceptual cues from the environment and the final selection of a sequence of movements. Research on spatial representation format, cognitive processes, and strategies for solving problems in different tasks are important issues of spatial cognitive research. Individuals differ in location discovery tasks (Blajenkova et al. 2005; Hegarty et al. 2006; Hugdahl et al. 2006). Gender, experience, age, strategies navigation, and the ability of working memory are some of the factors are consistently found to account for significant variance in the performance of duties discovery location (Cornoldi and Vecchi 2003; Gugerty and Brooks 2004; Lawton 1994; Pazzaglia et al. 2000; Pazzaglia and de Beni 2001; Thorndyke and Hayes-Roth 1982).

Good navigators tend to use strategies that are more flexible and vary from less navigators (Kato and Takeuchi 2003; Lawton 1994; Saucier et al. 2002). Navigator males tend to use cardinal directions, the Euclidean distance, and cognitive maps. This strategy has been called the survey strategy. Instead, the navigator who are less likely to use strategies that rely on ego-centric strategy with reference to the left-right direction and landmarks along the route. Individuals, often women, who rely on the so-called landmark strategy, generally find it difficult to use the navigation strategy-oriented survey (MacFadden et al. 2003). However, a good navigator tends to use a different strategy, in accordance with the demands of siituasi (Saucier et al. 2003). For example, a good navigator can use the navigation directions verbal sequence, such as that provided by many commercial online services (e.g., MapQuest), even when the map and the cardinal directions are not available.

At the same time, the gender differences are often observed in the use of relatively different strategies, different opportunities to gain experience of navigation are also reported (Lawton and Kallai 2002). Using the cardinal directions increases with age (Dabbs et al. 1998), and most people, including women, who grew up in the geo location of the graphic where the streets laid out in a pattern like a grid, reported use cardinal directions greater (Lawton 2001). Therefore, the relative use of two different strategies has emerged based on factors other than gender experience alone. Although most of the literature documenting the existence of individual differences in the strategies used to navigate and learn the route in real-world settings (Hegarty et al. 2006; Kato and Takeuchi 2003; Lawton 1994, 1996, 2001), until now, there has been little research has been striking about the extent to which strategies are observed in real-world settings are the same or different from that used in virtual environments (Chen and Stanney 1999). Hegarty et al. (2006) observed that measures the environmental learning-experience occur after walking through the neighborhood than the experience with a virtual environment. In addition, they observed that the psychometric measures (related to small-scale space) better predict participants' ability to learn in a large-scale environment indirectly through video recordings and not by direct experience.

Gender differences in spatial ability and location of an area that has been of special concern (Coluccia and Louse 2004). Men seem to rely more distal cues such as the line of the hill which provides information about the orientation and direction (Chai and Jacobs 2009; Fortenbaugh et al. 2007). Women are more dependent on cues remain as landmarks to identify sken visual and spatial orientation to form (Chai and Jacobs 2009; Lawton 2010). Men also showed greater accuracy in navigation tasks when given information (Chai and Jacobs 2009; Lawton 2010; Levy et al. 2005), but she has a memory of objects and memory location-object better than men (Levy et al. 2005).

Biological factors are also taken into account the differences in the performance of spatial and spatial ability between the sexes. Levels of testosterone, or testosterone exposure, has been shown to improve performance in the navigation task (Lawton 2010). Brain organization has also been associated with differences in spatial performance. The right hemisphere in men treated the attribute better performance in spatial tasks where this section is a part of the brain involved during the process of spatial (McGlone 1980). However, gender differences in using verbal instructions or map instructions when searching for a new location has not been known well.

Emotion plays a crucial role when people look for a new location. According to Lawton (1994), self-evaluating questionnaires reveal that females are more anxious than males when navigating. The "spatial anxiety" (Lawton 1994, 1996) or "fear to get lost" (Kozloswki and Bryant 1977) can reduce the ability to focus on cues essential to maintain geographical orientation. Many studies find that stress impairs the ability to memorize spatial locations (Evans et al. 1984; Sunanda et al. 2000). In Schmitz (1997), spatial anxiety and fear of the dark negatively correlate with speed in walking through a maze: subjects with high anxiety levels are the slowest. Anxiety about getting lost is likely to inhibit the exploration of unfamiliar places, having a negative impact on self-confidence and on motivation to navigate in new environments (Bryant 1982). So females have few navigational experiences than males, having fewer opportunities to increase their spatial orientation skills.

Moreover, some studies demonstrate a relationship between spatial anxiety, kinds of strategy, and orientation performance. In Schmitz (1997), males show low levels of anxiety and prefer to include more directional elements (configurational strategy) in verbal descriptions of a maze; they also perform better than females when running through a maze. Contrary to this, females show high levels of anxiety and include few directional elements and many landmarks in their descriptions. In agreement with these results, Lawton (1994) finds that the use of survey (configurational) strategies correlates negatively with the level of spatial anxiety. People with high level of spatial anxiety generally do not use this kind of strategy. These individuals are not able to maintain a sense of direction and/or self-position with respect to the surrounding environment (survey strategy). They tend to get lost, confused, and anxious. This research will explore positive, negative, and neutral emotion when people look for a new location.

5.2 Methods

5.2.1 Participants

Participants in this research are the 17–22-year-old students from three universities in Central Java-Indonesia. A total of 264 respondents filled out a questionnaire consisting of, 200 women and 62 men, and 2 samples cannot be analyzed. Sampling was done accidentally.

5.2.2 Measures and Procedures

The data was collected in classical or in group. Participants were first assigned a participant identification number, which was also listed on the questionnaires they were to complete. They were asked to read over they write as a participant. Completing the survey was regarded as informed consent. Every participant was asked to fill out the demographics data. Participant gender and age were collected on this form.

Afterwards, they were given a survey about the last time that they were lost or disoriented by themselves, called the Wayfinding Experience Essay. For this essay they were asked to imagine the last time that they were by themselves and lost or disoriented while finding their way in an environment. As a follow up, they answered questions that were directly relevant to the hypotheses of interest. The questions were: How did you get lost?; What were you feeling?; What did you do to make yourself no longer lost?; Did you look for someone to give you verbal directions or a map? Upon completion of the Wayfinding Experience Essay the participants were thanked, debriefed, and dismissed. Participation took no longer than 15 min.

Information on the situational aspects of the wayfinding experience were extracted from the essays. The essays were coded for situational information along for two dimensions: (a) what kind of cues participant prefer, verbal direction or a map; and (b) whether they made statements about positive, neutral, or negative emotion (e.g., feeling afraid as negative emotion, feeling confused as neutral emotion and feeling better while asking direction as positive emotion). Code made by writers.

5.3 Results

The results of this study showed that when looking for a new location subject utilizing your map as much as 49.2, and 46.2 % verbal cues as well as subjects who seek both verbal and maps are as much as 4.6 %. Thus, only a difference of 3 % among subjects who utilize the map instructions are likely to contain a visual stimulus spatial and verbal cues are likely to contain stimulus words like turn left on the monument, straight, turn right when you arrive at the first red light, when looking for a location new (Fig. 5.1).

Wayfinding by the subject invention utilizing verbal instructions or a map based on sex is as much as 46 % of women chose utilizing verbal cues, while men as much as 48.4 %. The difference between men and women in the use of verbal instructions is only 2.4 %. Meanwhile, the user tapped the map, as many as 49.5 % of women and men as much as 46.8 %, which means that only 2.3 % difference between men and women. As for the women who utilize either verbal instructions or a map as much as 4.5 % and men as much as 4.8 %. This difference can be seen in Fig. 5.2.

The results of descriptive analysis using Chi-square count is worth 2287 with two degrees of freedom and a significant alpha level of 5 %. From the table the obtained Chi-square table is 5.991. Chi-square count < Chi-square

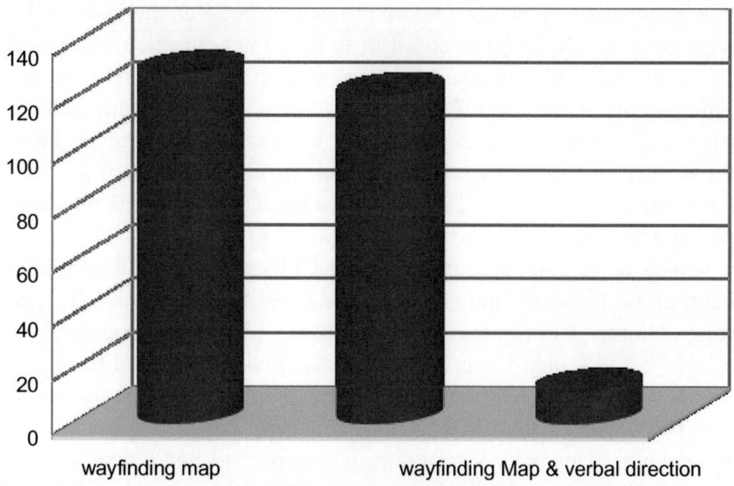

Fig. 5.1 Wayfinding based on user selection of maps or verbal

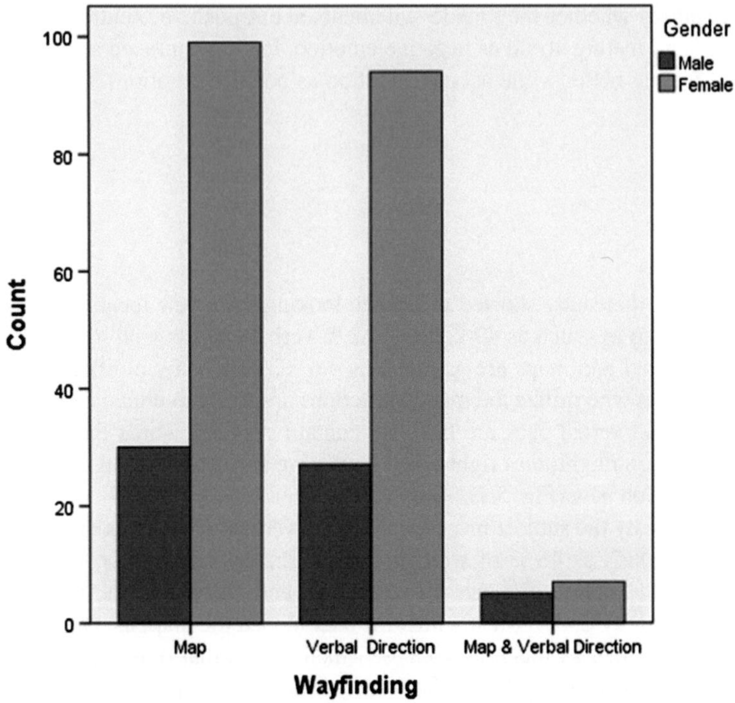

Fig. 5.2 Wayfinding using map or verbal instructions by gender

Table (2.287 < 5.991), then Ho is accepted. Based on the probability or likelihood is found above .319 (.319 > .05). Then Ho received. Based on this analysis, the same can be concluded that there are no differences between the sexes with the use of a maps or verbal direction in an effort to find a new location. This means that both men and women tend to take advantage of both map and verbal instructions.

Wayfinding using map 14.5 % of age 17–18, age 19–20, as many as 33.2 % and as much as 1.5 % ages 21–22. Subjects who use verbal cues aged 17–18 years by 12.6 %, as much as 30.5 % aged 19–20, and 21–22 age as much as 3 %. These results indicate subject in aged 19–20 years old at most tapped the map and verbal instructions when on the move to find a location (Fig. 5.3).

The results of descriptive analysis using Chi-square count worth 2.474 with four degrees of freedom and a significance level of alpha = 5 %. From the table the obtained Chi-Square table is 9.488. Chi-square count < Chi-square Table (2.474 < 4.88), then Ho is accepted. Based on the probability or likelihood is found above .649 .05 (.649 > .05). Then Ho received. Based on this analysis the same can be concluded that there is no relationship between age with the use of manual selection of maps or verbal cues in an effort to find a new location. This means that both subjects aged 17–18 years or 19–20 years old and 21–22 years old, tend to use the two instructions a map and verbal direction (Fig. 5.4).

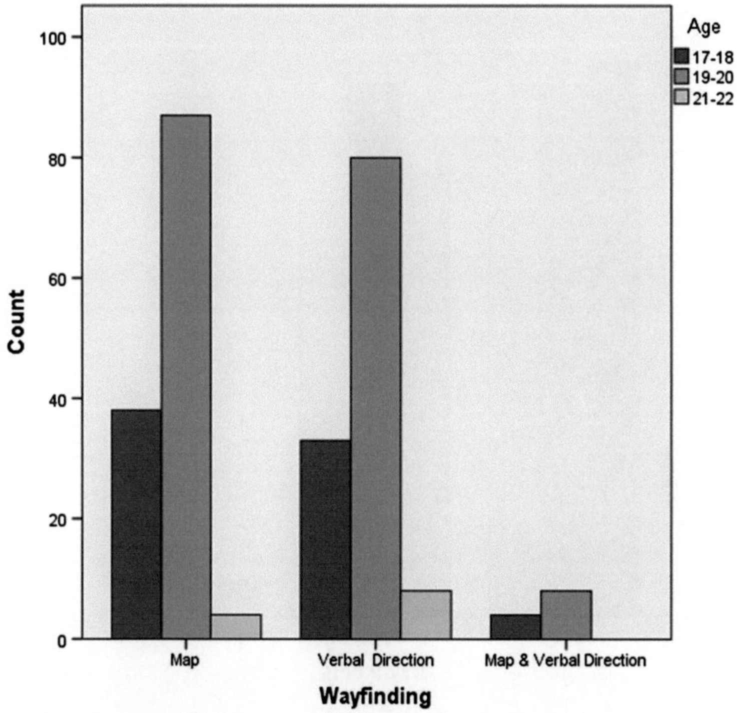

Fig. 5.3 Wayfinding map or verbal direction by age

The results of descriptive analysis using Chi-square count worth 1.595 with four degrees of freedom and a significance level of alpha 5 %. From the table the obtained Chi-square table is 9.488. Chi-square count < Chi-square Table (1.595 < 9. 488), then Ho is accepted. Based on the probability or likelihood is found above .8130 (.810 > .05). Then Ho received. Based on this analysis the same can be concluded that there are no differences between positive, neutral, and negative emotion when using maps or verbal direction in an effort to find a new location. This means that when subjects look for a new location using a map or verbal direction, they can have positive, neutral, or negative emotion (Table 5.3).

5.4 Discussion

The descriptive analysis in Fig. 5.1 have shown that in general subjects seeking new locations tend to use verbal instructions or a map in the presentation are almost the same, namely 49.2 and 46.2 % with only a difference of 3 % only. These results indicate that both the users play almost equivalent and used by subjects in the activities of finding a new location. This is of course contrary to

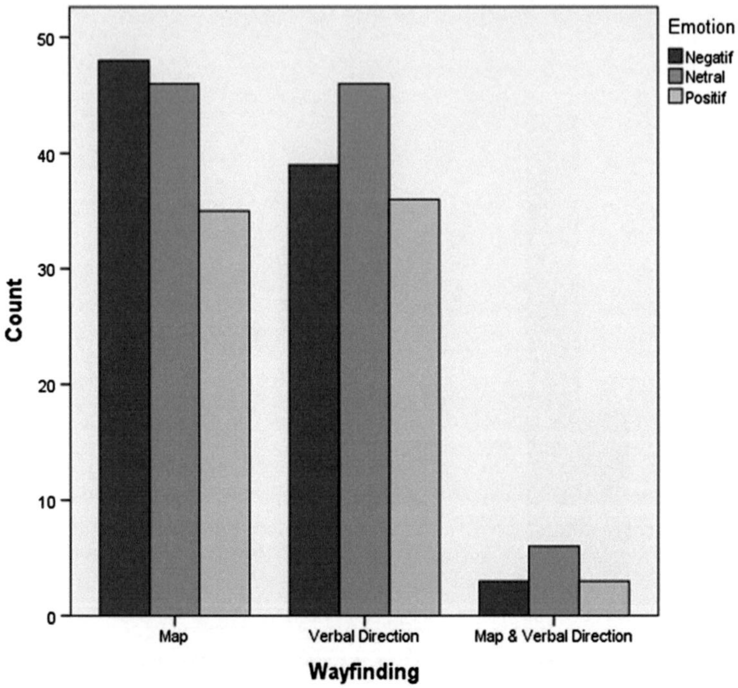

Fig. 5.4 Wayfinding using a map or verbal direction according to subject emotion

Table 5.1 Chi-square tables

	Value	*df*	Asymp. Sig. (two-sided)
Pearson Chi-square	2.287[a]	2	.319
Likelihood ratio	2.028	2	.363
Linear-by-linear association	.449	1	.503
No of valid cases	262		

some theories predict no difference because the imagery or metaphor (Larkin and Simon, 1987; Freksa 1999; Paivio 1971, 1986). A possible explanation of this is happening because of the acquisition of the survey data alone. However, the same result also occurs in research experiments in real environments by Meilinger and Knauff (2008). So we conclude that the results of this survey are very significant, also supported by other studies that found no difference between a map and verbal cues related to the time and errors when searching a new location (Schlender et al. 2000; Pazzaglia and De Beni 2001).

These results as shown in Table 5.1, indicate that there is no relationship between gender differences in subjects with the use of verbal instructions and a map when on the move find a new location. These results are supported by Montello and Sas (2006) mention certain individuals prefer information that describes these in sequence landmark and turn simple acts, whereas there are others who prefer to survey information about the spatial relationships between locations kuantitative in a neighborhood. Other researches like O'Laughlin and Brubaker (1998), Brown et al. (1998), Coluccia and Martello (2004) also showed similar results. Nevertheless, the author argues that the need to do further research on the subject is more numerous so that adequate results are found. This is caused by the results of recent research from Nowak et al. (2015) which mentions gender differences in the utilization of allocentrik strategies (e.g., mental maps) and women utilize strategies route (e.g., turn right, turn left, straight); Collucia et al. (2007) have shown results that men also take advantage of a map from the perspective configuration and women tend to use landmarks when looking for a new location. Annett (1992) also mentions that the dominant pattern in the left hemisphere of the brain that developed first in women so first learn early age, negatively affect the development of spatial skills. It resulted in spontaneous woman picking strategies verbal or verbal cues in an effort to find a new location.

The results in Table 5.2 show that there is no difference in the age of the subject on utilizing maps and verbal instructions were busy finding a new location. This becomes an interesting finding because again exploiting both good map and verbal instructions are relatively similar to the subject. These findings have not gotten corroborating evidence as a result of the lack of research on the use of a map and verbal instructions in the discovery of new locations behavior in subjects aged 17–22-years old. Instead Bosco and Collucia research (2004) shows a decrease in detection function of age on the task of spatial orientation in using maps associated with a decrease in visuospatial working memory function in elderly people. This research compares the participants into three groups, namely group subjects aged 20–30 years old, the group of 60–69 and 70–80 years group. Meneghetti et al. (2011) study about the comparative study of a map in young people aged 20–30-years old with those aged 60–72 years. Head and Isom (2010) also compared the subjects aged 18–22-years old with subjects aged 56–83 years, to see the

Table 5.2 *Chi-square tests*

	Value	*df*	Asymp. Sig. (two-sided)
Pearson Chi-square	2.474[a]	4	.649
Likelihood ratio	2.967	4	.563
Linear-by-linear association	.143	1	.706
No of valid cases	262		

Table 5.3 *Chi-square tests*

	Value	*df*	Asymp. Sig. (two-sided)
Pearson Chi-square	1.595[a]	4	.810
Likelihood ratio	1.576	4	.813
Linear-by-linear association	.618	1	.432
No of valid cases	262		

difference in wayfinding behavior and ability on learning route. Therefore, further research needs to be done to get adequate evidence about age differences.

In this current study, emotion can influence wayfinding behavior as positive, neutral or negative, no difference. Even though, previous research in which higher levels of sense of direction are associated with lower levels of spatial anxiety (McKeen and Roskos-Ewoldsen, 2007). Women also tend to report higher levels of spatial anxiety compared to men (Lawton and Kallai 2002; McKeen and Roskos-Ewoldsen 2007). In the geographical literature, females report anxious, detrimentally emotional reactions to navigational activities, seeing environments as though they were spaces where females are historically victimized (Pain 1997). The lack of emotion differences in wayfinding behavior could be due to differences in the samples of participants across the current and other studies. Lawton and Kallai (2002) tested participants of varying age groups and both genders in a large midwestern city in the US and a similarly sized city in Hungary. The geographical studies came from women of many ages in Europe (Koskela 1999; Pain 1997) and the US (Wesley and Gaarder 2004). In this study, emotion divided into three dimensions, positive, negative, and neutral, this project suggests that emotion lacks adequate construct validity. Perhaps, emotion could be induced when people look for a new location to get adequate evidence about effect of emotion on wayfinding situation. Future research of an experimental or longitudinal nature is needed to answer this question.

References

Annett, M. (1992). Spatial ability in subgroup of left-and right handers. *British Journal of Psychology, 83*(4), 493–515.

Blajenkova, O., Motes, M. A., & Kozhevnikov, M. (2005). Individual differences in the representations of novel environments. *Journal of Environmental Psychology, 25*, 97–109.

Bosco, A., Longoni, A. M., & Vecchi, T. (2004). Gender effects in spatial orientation: Cognitive profiles and mental strategies. *Applied Cognitive Psychology, 18*, 519–532.

Brown, L. N., Lahar, C. J., & Mosley, J. L. (1998). Age and gender related differences in strategy use for route information. A map present direction giving paradigm. *Environment and Behavior, 30*(2), 123–143.

Bryant, K. J. (1982). Personality correlates of sense of direction and geographical orientation. *Journal of Personality and Social Psychology, 43*(6), 1318–1324.

Chai, X., & Jacobs, L. (2009). Sex differences in directional cue use in a virtual landscape. *Behavioral Neuroscience, 123*, 276–283.

Collucia, E., Mammarella, I. C., De Beni, R., Ittyerah, M., & Cornoldi, C. (2007). Remembering object position in the absence of vision: Egocentric, allocentric, and egocentric decentred frames of references. *Perseption, 36*, 850–864.

Coluccia, E., & Louse, G. (2004). Gender differences in spatial orientation: A review. *Journal of Environmental Psychology, 24*, 329–340.

Coluccia, E., & Martello, A. (2004). Il Ruolo Della Memoria Di Lavoro Visuo-Spaziale Nell'Orientamento Geografico: Uno Studio Correlazionale (The Role of VSWM in Geographical Orientation: A correlational study). *Giornale Italiano di Psicologia.*

Cornoldi, C., & Vecchi, T. (2003). *Visuo-spatial working memory and individual differences.* Hove, UK: Psychology Press.

Dabbs, J. M., Chang, L., & Strong, R. A. (1998). Spatial ability, navigation strategy and geographic knowledge among men and women. *Evolution and Human Behavior, 19*, 89–98.

Evans, G. W., Skorpanich, M. A., Garling, T., Bryant, K. J., & Bresolin, B. (1984). The effects of pathway configuration, land-marks and stress on environmental cognition. *Journal of Environmental Psychology, 4*, 323–335.

Fortenbaugh, F., Chaudhury, S., Hicks, J., Hao, L., & Turano, K. (2007). Gender differences in cue preference during path integration in virtual environments. *ACM Transactions on Applied Perception, 4(1), Article 6.*

Freksa, C. (1999). Spatial aspects of task-specific wayfinding maps. In J. S. Gero & B. Tversky (Eds.), *Visual and spatial reasoning in design, key centre of design computing and cognition* (pp. 15–32). Sydney: University of Sydney.

Golledge, R. G. (1999). *Wayfinding behavior: Cognitive mapping and other spatial processes*. Baltimore: The Johns Hopkins University Press.

Gugerty, L., & Brooks, J. (2004). Reference frame misalignment and cardinal direction judgment: Group differences and strategies. *Journal of Experimental Psychology: Applied, 10*(2), 75–88.

Head, D., & Isom, M. (2010). Age effect on wayfinding and route learning skills. *Behavioural Brain Research, 209*(1), 49–58.

Hegarty, M., Montello, D. R., Richardson, A. E., Ishikawa, T., & Lovelace, T. (2006). Spatial abilities at different scales: Individual differences in aptitude-test performance and spatial-layout learning. *Intelligence, 34*, 151–176.

Hugdahl, K., Thamsen, T., & Ersland, L. (2006). Sex differences in visuo-spatial prosesing: An FRMI study of mental rotation. *Neuropsychologia, 44*, 1575–1583.

Kato, Y., & Takeuchi, Y. (2003). Individual differences in wayfinding strategies. *Journal of Environmental Psychology, 23*, 171–188.

Koskela, H. (1999). Gendered Exclusions: Women's fear of violence and changing relations to space. *Geografiska Annaler Series B, Human Geography, 81*, 111–124.

Kozloswki, L. T., & Bryant, K. J. (1977). Sense of direction, spatial orientation, and cognitive maps. *Journal of Experimental Psychology: Human Perception and Performance, 3*(4), 590–598.

Larkin, J. H., & Simon, H. A. (1987). Why a diagram is (sometimes) worth then thousand words. *Cognitive Science, 11*, 64–100.

Lawton, C. (1994). Gender differences in way-finding strategies: Relationship to spatial ability and spatial anxiety. *Sex Roles, 30*, 765–779.

Lawton, C. A. (2001). Gender and regional differences in spatial referents used in direction giving. *Sex Roles, 44*, 321–337.

Lawton, C. A. (2010). Gender, spatial abilities, and wayfinding. In J. C. Chrisler & D. R. McCreary (Eds.), *Handbook of gender research in psychology* (pp. 317–341). New York: Springer.

Lawton, C. A., & Kallai, J. (2002). Gender differences in wayfinding strategies and anxiety about wayfinding: A cross-cultural comparison. *Sex Roles, 47*, 389–400.

Levy, L. J., Astur, R. S., & Frick, K. M. (2005). Men and women differ in object memory but not performance of a virtual radial maze. *Behavioral Neuroscience, 119*, 853–862.

Lynch, K. (1960). *The image of the city*. Cambridge, MA: MIT Press.

MacFadden, A., Elias, L., & Saucier, D. (2003). Males and females scan maps similarly but give directions differently. *Brain and Cognition, 53*, 297–300.

McKeen, J. H., & Roskos-Ewoldsen, B. (2007, May). Spatial and social influences on wayfinding: Predicting gender differences. *Poster presented at the Annual Meeting of the Association for Psychological Science, Washington.*

Meilinger, T., & Kanuff, M. (2008). Ask for direction or use a map: A field experiment on spatial orientation and wayfinding in an urban environment. *Spacial Science, 53*, 2.

Meneghetti, C., Fiore, E., Borelle, F., & De Beni, R. (2011). Learning a map of environment: The rolc of visuo-spatial abilities in young and older adults. *Applied Cognitive Psychology, 25*(6), 952–959.

Montello, D. R. (2005). Navigation. In A. Miyake & P. Shah (Eds.), *The Cambridge handbook of visuospatial thinking* (pp. 257–294). Cambridge: Cambridge University Press.
Montello, D. R., & Sas, C. (2006). Human factors of wayfinding in navigation. In W. Karwowski (Ed.), *International encyclopedia of ergonomics and human factors* (pp. 2003–2008). London: CRC Press/Taylor & Francis, Ltd.
Nowak, N. T., Murali, A., & Driscoll, I. (2015). Factors related to sex differences in navigating a computerized maze. *Journal of Environmental Psychology, 43*, 136–144.
O'Laughlin, E. M., & Brubaker, B. S. (1998). Use of landmarks in cognitive mapping: Gender differences in self report versus performance. *Personality and Individual Differences, 24*(5), 595–601.
Pain, R. H. (1997). Social geographies of women's fear of crime. *Transactions of the Institute of British Geographers, New Series, 22*, 231–244.
Paivio, A. (1971). *Imagery and verbal processes*. New York: Holt, Rinehart and Winston.
Paivio, A. (1986). *Mental representations: A dual coding approach*. New York: Oxford University Press.
Pazzaglia, F., Cornoldi, C., & De Beni, R. (2000). Differenze individuali nella rappresentazione dello spazio e nell'abilità di orientamento: Presentazione di un questionario autovalutativo (In-dividual differences in spatial representation and in orientation ability: Presentation of a self-report questionnaire). *Giornale Italiano di Psicologia, 27*, 627–650.
Pazzaglia, F., & De Beni, R. (2001). Strategies of processing spatial information in survey and landmark-centred individuals. *European Journal of Cognitive Psychology, 13*, 493–508.
Saucier, D., Bowman, M., & Ellias, L. (2003). Sex differences in the effect of articulatory or spatialdual-task interference during navigation. *Brain and Cognition, 53*, 340–350.
Saucier, D. M., Green, S. M., Leason, J., MacFadden, A., Bell, S., & Elias, L. (2002). Are sex differences in navigation caused by sexually dimorphic strategies or by differences in the ability to use strategies? *Behavioral Neuroscience, 116*(3), 403–410.
Schlender, D., Peters, O. H., & Wienhöfer, M. (2000). The effect of maps and textual information on navigation in a desktop virtual environment. *Spatial Cognition and Computation, 2*, 421–433.
Schmitz, S. (1997). Gender related strategies in environmental development: Effect of anxiety on wayfinding in and representation of a three-dimensional maze. *Journal of Environmental Psychology, 17*, 215–228.
Sunanda, B. S., Rao, S., & Raju, T. R. (2000). Chronic restraint stress impairs acquisition and retention of spatial memory task in rats. *Current Science, 79*(11), 1581–1584.
Thorndyke, P. W., & Hayes-Roth, B. (1982). Differences in spatial knowledge acquired from maps and navigation. *Cognitive Psychology, 14*, 560–589.
Wesley, J. K., & Gaarder, E. (2004). The gendered nature of the urban outdoors: Women negotiating fear of violence. *Gender and Society, 18*, 645–663.

Chapter 6
Moral Emotions: An Explorative Study on Elementary School Teachers of Yogyakarta

Ika Widyarini

Abstract Moral emotions are subset of basic emotions and linked to the interests or welfare either of society as a whole or at least of persons other than the judge or agent. These are emotions that respond to moral transgression, or that motivate individuals to choose a certain moral behavior. To encourage children to be considerate and compassion to others, elementary school educators are expected to understand the essential values of adequate moral emotions. Having moral emotions eventually will motivate teachers and students to do good deed. This study is an exploratory qualitative study attempting to build an understanding on the Indonesian school teacher's concepts of moral emotions and their antecedents with an indigenous approach. An open ended survey was conducted to a sample of 121 elementary school teachers from Yogyakarta. The result of this research revealed the perspective of elementary school teachers on moral emotions and the main antecedents of the teachers' moral emotions. This study will be the groundwork of aexperimental research with main objective to study the effect of moral emotions to ethical decision making. Theoretical and applied implementation of this research results also will be discussed.

Keywords Integrity · Values · Moral emotions

6.1 Background

Cultural variance in human emotions is not a novel concept. For decades, scientist studied that events which lead to emotions in people with different cultural background are rather distinctive (Matsumoto et al. 1988). According

I. Widyarini (✉)
Fakultas Psikologi, Universitas Gadjah Mada, Yogyakarta, Indonesia
e-mail: ika.widyarini@ub.ac.id
URL: http://www.ugm.ac.id

M.-T. Leung and L.-M. Tan (eds.), *Applied Psychology Readings*,
DOI 10.1007/978-981-10-2796-3_6

to Mesquita and Frijda (1992) specific event may have elicit different kind of emotions in different cultures because they are coded differently under different schema.

As a subset of basic emotions, moral emotions may also have different cultural-based main antecedents. This study seeks to ensure that the moral emotions be surveyed in the context of culture that surrounded the subjects, especially the antecedents or events that cause the moral emotions. This study is an exploratory study to determine specific events that are antecedent of moral emotions of the people of Java in Indonesia. It will be the groundwork of a experimental research with the main objective to study the effect of moral emotions to ethical decision making. To induce moral emotions and determine the effects on behavior, we should depart from reviewing in detail the events that correspond to potential antecedents of the various moral emotions.

6.1.1 Moral Emotions

Moral emotions arethose emotions that are linked tothe interests or welfare either of society as a whole or at least of persons other than the judge oragent (Haidt 2003). Social intuitionist theory stated that moral emotions play a critical role in individuals' moral intuition, where moral emotions are proposed to precede rational judgment under moral situations. Moral emotions are condition in which individuals react intuitively and emotionally to violation of norms. Moral emotions are triggered when individuals perceive events that violate moral foundations (harm/care, justice/fairness, in-group, authority, and purity) such as suffering, violations of hierarchy, reciprocity, or purity. Each elicits moral emotions such as compassion, guilt, resentment, anger, respect, and disgust.

Two features of moral emotions, which distinguish them from hedonic emotions, are disinterested elicitors and pro-social action tendencies (Haidt 2003). While hedonic emotions such as happiness and fear are elicited when preferable or unfavorable events happen to the agent (or individuals or groups that the agent identifies with), moral emotions can be triggered even when the agent has no self-interest embedded in the event. The second feature refers to the type of action the moral emotions predispose the agents to engage in. While the action tendencies of hedonic emotions are directed toward bringing about a pleasant state for the self, moral emotions put individuals in a motivational state that increases the tendency to engage in pro-social action directed at others' interests.

Haidt (2003) also identifies four moral emotions (anger, elevation, guilt, and compassion) as high on both dimensions of disinterested self and prosocial action tendencies. Others that are within the middle range include gratitude, shame, embarrassment, disgust, and contempt, which vary in their degrees of pro-social action tendency and disinterestedness.

Emotional skill, especially to experience moral emotions as a foundation of moral actions, is an aspect of character that should be taught since early age. It seems that elementary school teacher should also develop adequate competencies of 'feeling the right emotion' in order to foster their student's moral behaviors. In this light, the emphasis of the research will be the events or objects that serve as antecedents of several moral emotions of elementary school teachers.

6.2 Objective of the Study

The objective of the research was to explore the moral emotions and the main antecedents among Indonesia elementary school teachers. The aim of this paper is therefore to establish general conceptual framework that could construct a better understanding about moral emotions in the perspective of Indonesian, and the underlying constructs as a basis for further with the main objective to study the effect of moral emotions to ethical decision making. Practical implication of the findings will be discussed.

6.3 Research Design

6.3.1 Research Approach

This study applies the indigenous psychology approach, by recruiting data analysts culturally in close proximity to the research participants to code the responses in order not to have a perception gap. The data was analyzed using qualitative and quantitative method concurrently. Barrett (2003) stated that reliance solely in the quantitative structuring of a psychological variable may limit the knowledge and theory-generating claims that can be made. Implicitly, a qualitative approach was to understand integrity as a psychological construct in the perspective of Indonesian. A qualitative research approach was therefore considered most efficient in resolving the preceding research objective. Qualitative research provides access to and an understanding at people subjective experiences of psychological phenomenon (Camic et al. 2003).

6.3.2 Research Participant

Due to the availability of the subjects, an incidental sampling method has been applied to draw 121 elementary teachers of Sleman Region in Daerah Istimewa Yogyakarta (29 male; 24 % and 92 female; 76 %).

6.3.3 Data Gathering

Data is obtained through open-ended questionnaire about integrity and moral emotions. Open ended questionnaire has been distributed among participants who should answer 17 questions about moral emotions.

6.3.4 Data Analysis

Data analysis uses a combination of qualitative and quantitative methods. At first stage, the data analysis at broad category stage was done by three elementary teachers who have filled out the questionnaire as research subjects. Data analysis by subjects initially was planned to ensure the proximity of the category to their original responses. However, the categories resulted from the teacher's analysis were unable to adequately answer the original questions. Therefore, data analysis was set up again with three college graduates with psychology degree who were Javanese, familiar with Sleman region or Yogyakarta culture and also accustomed to psychological terms used by Javanese.

At second stage of the data analysis, a descriptive quantitative method was applied to identify broad categories and selective categories to be further summarized into main themes. One of the most common ways to describe variables is with a frequency distribution. Based on the open ended questions asked to the research participants, frequency distributions will be developed to display the percentages particular notion in the participant's responses. The keywords and broad categories, which are produced by this second group of analysts and have answered the questions suitably, are the basis for descriptive statistics presented. Subsequently, based on the selective categories main themes will be developed to identify the antecedents of moral emotions in the perspective of Indonesian elementary school teachers.

6.4 Results

6.4.1 Antecedents of Inspiration (Ordinary Events)

In everyday life we can encounter inspirational event, without going to movie theatre or buying books. What kind of everyday occurrence most inspirational for subjects are probed with question: "Give an example of one everyday life event that inspire you to do good deeds or applying virtues!" (Table 6.1).

Noticeably most subjects agreed that observing people doing good deed (31.15 %) are more inspirational than witnessing other's misery (24.59 %) or disaster (12.30 %). Further, positive outcome such as success despite of facing obstacles (10.66 %) is also decided on by respondent being inspirational (Table 6.2).

Table 6.1 Inspiring event (broad category)

Category	Frequency (%)
People doing good deed	31.15
Observing other's misery	24.59
Disaster	12.30
Success despite obstacle	10.66
Children doing good deed	7.38
People doing evil	4.10
Being helped by others	2,46
Environment condition	2.46
Inspirational talk show	1.64
Other	3.28

Table 6.2 Inspiring event (selective category)

Category	Frequency (%)
Positive behavior	55.74
Unfortunate event	40.16
Negative behavior	4.10

Inconclusion, most subjects perceived that factual positive behavior lead to inspiration in others (55.74 %) which is significantly higher than unfortunate events (40.16 %) and negative behavior (4.10 %). This means observing positive behavior of others has more motivational effect than sad about adverse events or anger caused by bad behavior.

6.4.2 Moral Emotions

To clearly detach moral emotion form hedonic emotion, participant was asked: "How do you feel when experiencing such inspiring events?" (Table 6.3).

When being probed further on the issue of inspiring events, the subjects mostly describe positive emotions (38.98 %), along with feeling touched (29.66 %) and being motivated to do something good (19.44 %) (Table 6.4).

Selective coding specified the description above into positive moral emotions (61.86 %), which significantly higher number than general positive emotion (27.12 %) induced by inspiring events.

Table 6.3 Feelings resulted from inspiring events (broad category)

Category	Frequency (%)
Positive emotion	38.98
Touched	29.66
Motivated	19.49
Negative emotion	7.63
Other	4.24

Table 6.4 Feelings resulted from inspiring events (selective category)

Category	Frequency (%)
Positive moral emotion	61.86
Positive emotion	27.12
Negative emotion	5.93
Developed	3.39
Negative moral emotion	1.69

6.4.3 Type of Moral Emotions

To clarify whether emotion can motivate the participant to do good deed or strongly defend values, this question was asked to participants: "What kind of feelings will inspire a person to consistently do virtue?" (Table 6.5).

Positive emotions definitely lead to virtues (30.56 %) which significantly higher than negative emotions (14.29 %) or empathy (10.71 %). This finding is interesting since empathy seems a strong stimulus of affection to motivate individual to act positively (Table 6.6).

Selective category further emphasizes the positive emotions (59.26 %) as major stimulations to attempts doing positive deeds. Sense of obligation (25.93 %) is also a key factor which inspires a person to make favorable act, while negative emotions (14.81 %) may also contribute to such positive act.

Table 6.5 Feelings lead to virtues (broad category)

Category	Frequency (%)
Positive emotions	30.56
Negative emotions	14.29
Empathy	10.71
Togetherness	8.33
Religious	7.94
Positive values	7.94
Feeling useful	7.14
Feedback	5.56
Responsible	2.38
Being exemplary	1.59
Other	3.57

Table 6.6 Feelings lead to virtues (selective category)

Category	Frequency (%)
Positive emotions	59.26
Obligation	25.93
Negative emotions	14.81

6.4.4 Antecedents of Embarrassment (Shame)

Antecedents of embarrassment (shame) for the elementary school teachers were identified by unfinished sentence: "I feel embarrassed when …" (Table 6.7).

The antecedents of embarrassment (shame) for Indonesian mostly are negative behavior (44.92 %), significantly more than when their expectation was not met (26.27 %) or when caught in awkward situation caused by tardiness (17.8 %) (Table 6.8).

In selective category the results of broad category are being punctuated; negative behavior especially done by the individual himself is the main source of embarrassment (95.73 %). Physical appearance (2.56 %) and facing new situation (1.71 %) noticeably is not main factors of embarrassment.

6.4.5 Antecedents of Guilt

Antecedents of guilt for the elementary school teachers were identified by unfinished sentence: "I feel guilty when …" (Table 6.9).

Bad behavior to others (34.45 %) exceeds other factors as main antecedents of guilt for Indonesian. When personal behavior was not as expected (24.37 %) by him or others, an individual may also develop a guilt feeling. Guilt as well incited when a person's statement doesn't match his behavior (16.81 %) or a responsibility has not been performed (11.76 %) (Table 6.10).

Evidently, inconsistency (41.53 %) exceeds other factors as main antecedents of guilt for Indonesian. Indonesian apparently feels guilty when there is

Table 6.7 Antecedents of embarrassment/shame (broad category)

Category	Frequency (%)
Negative behavior	44.92
Expectation not met	26.27
Tardiness	17.80
Irresponsibility	4.24
Poor physical appearance	2.54
Burdening other	1.69
Facing new situation	1.69
Other	0.85

Table 6.8 Antecedents of embarrassment/shame (selective category)

Category	Frequency (%)
Negative behavior	95.73
Appearance	2.56
New situation	1.71

Table 6.9 Antecedents of guilt (broad category)

Category	Frequency (%)
Bad behavior to others	34.45
Behavior not met expectation	24.37
Inconsistency between statement and behavior	16.81
Unfulfilled responsibility	11.76
Breaking rules	6.72
Bad words	5.04
Other	0.84

Table 6.10 Antecedents of guilt (selective category)

Category	Frequency (%)
Inconsistency	41.53
Negative behavior to others	39.83
Inconformity	18.64

discrepancy between reality and expectation, between obligation and fulfillment or between statement and behavior. Negative behavior to others also a significant factor (39.83 %) to incite guilt, while inconformity (18.64 %) to rules or standard may as well be a guilt factor.

6.4.6 Antecedents of Anger

Antecedents of anger for the elementary school teachers were identified by unfinished sentence: "I feel angry when …" (Table 6.11).

Being hurt or disrespected by others (43.59 %) equally strong to provoke anger as observing other people not behaving correspond to (personal or social) expectation (43.59 %). Personal behavior does not meet individual's expectation also a rather significant source of anger. This result illustrates that anger mostly provoked by others than self irritated.

6.4.7 Antecedents of Pity

Antecedents of pity for the elementary school teachers were identified by unfinished sentence: "I feel pity when …" (Tables 6.12, 6.13).

Table 6.11 Antecedents of anger (broad category)

Category	Frequency (%)
Hurt by others	43.59
Others do not do as expected	43.59
Behavior not met expectation	10.26

Table 6.12 Antecedents of pity (broad category)

Category	Frequency (%)
The suffering of others	80.83
Bad manners of others	5.83
Inability to help other	5.00
Other having problem	4.17
Potential is not maximized	4.17

Table 6.13 Antecedents of pity (selective category)

Category	Frequency (%)
The suffering of others	89.17
Bad manners of others	5.83
Inability to help other	5.00

Other person's affliction seems to be primarily causing pity of Indonesian (89.17 %) whether the distress caused by unfortunate events or failure.

6.4.8 Antecedents of Sympathy

Antecedents of sympathy for the elementary school teachers were identified by unfinished sentence: "I feel sympathy when …" (Table 6.14).

Antecedents of sympathy to others have diverse origins. Even though mostly Indonesian feel sympathy when observing other person' bad condition (30.7 %), observing good natured people's characteristics (21.93 %) also bring about sympathy. Positive action (18.42 %) and hard work (14.91 %) of other also stimulate the sympathetic quality of an individual (Table 6.15).

Table 6.14 Antecedents of sympathy (broad category)

Category	Frequency (%)
Other's bad condition	30.70
Good nature of people	21.93
Action of others	18.42
Other's hard work	14.91
Success of others	9.65
Touched by something	2.63
Good condition	1.75

Table 6.15 Antecedents of sympathy (selective category)

Category	Frequency (%)
Applied positive values	44.74
Other's bad condition	30.70
Achievement	24.56

As a deduction from broad category, positive values applied in other person's behavior (44.74 %) is a major stimulation to be sympathetic, compared to other's bad condition (30.7 %). Achievement by other also incites sympathy especially those of resulted from hard work (24.56 %). Positive behavior of other predominantly initiates sympathy not necessarily has to be tagged along with other's misfortunes.

6.4.9 *Antecedents of Compassion*

Antecedents of compassion for the elementary school teachers were identified by unfinished sentence: "I feel touched when …" (Table 6.16).

According to the broad category, witnessing other person suffering directly or through media (24.79 %) may cause major compassion along with success (20.51 %) and accepting an act of kindness (11.11 %) (Table 6.17).

Compassion after all is taking place when an Indonesian sees achievement after hard work and eradication of obstacles (37.5 %). Perceiving positive values being applied in actions (33.04 %) is also a main cause of compassion in others. Ambiguous responses categorized as 'other' in broad category mostly are negative situation faced by other (29.46 %) is serving as the third main cause for compassion.

Table 6.16 Antecedents of compassion (broad category)

Category	Frequency (%)
Suffering of other	24.79
Other's success	20.51
Accept other people favor	11.11
Hard work	9.40
Good deed of other	9.40
Good character of other	6.84
Success despite of shortcoming	5.98
See good things	2.56
Other	9.40

Table 6.17 Antecedents of compassion (selective category)

Category	Frequency (%)
Achievement after hard work	37.50
Applied positive values	33.04
Negative situation	29.46

6.4.10 Antecedents of Sadness

Antecedents of sadness for the elementary school teachers were identified by unfinished sentence: "I'm sad when…" (Table 6.18).

The sadness mostly developed when there is difference between other person's behavior and personal expectation (32.5 %), significantly higher than when observing other's suffering (21.67 %). Perceiving inability to fulfill an obligation (19.17 %) or to help other in need (10.83 %) as a failure to accomplish personal responsibility may also serve as a cause of sadness (Table 6.19).

In conclusion, an Indonesian's reason for sadness is mostly personal suffering (47.46 %), but the perceived incapability to do something useful (30.51 %) and other people' suffering (22.03 %) also notably trigger sadness.

6.4.11 Antecedents of Pride

Antecedents of pride for the elementary school teachers were identified by unfinished sentence: "I am proud when …" (Table 6.20).

Table 6.18 Antecedents of sadness (broad category)

Category	Frequency (%)
Other's behavior not met expectation	32.50
Other's suffering	21.67
Unfulfilled responsibility	19.17
Not being able to do good	10.83
Suffered	8.33
Unmet expectation	5.83
Other	1.67

Table 6.19 Antecedents of sadness (selective category)

Category	Frequency (%)
Personal suffering	47.46
Not doing good	30.51
Other's suffering	22.03

Table 6.20 Antecedents of pride (broad category)

Category	Frequency (%)
Student's achievement	35.00
Achievement	20.83
Able to do good	18.33
Succeed in teaching	15.00
Other's do good	6.67
Other	4.17

Table 6.21 Antecedents of pride (selective category)

Category	Frequency (%)
Personal achievement	71.43
Righteousness	26.89
Being respected	1.68

All subjects of this research are elementary school teachers, so unavoidably their student's achievement (35 %) is the main source of their pride besides their personal achievement (20.83 %), perceived ability to do positive feat (18.33 %) as well as succeed in teaching (15 %) which is basically all round up in personal achievement (Table 6.21).

The main source of pride of the subjects is their personal achievement (71.43 %) through success in teaching and educating their student to accomplishment. Being respected (1.68 %) apparently not an issue of pride, because righteousness or doing something good (26.89 %) is higher in the possibility to be the basis of pride.

6.4.12 Antecedents of Elevation

Antecedents of inspiration (elevation) for the elementary school teachers were identified by unfinished sentence: "I am inspired by …" (Table 6.22).

Inspiring moments might lead to a development of virtues and the main source of inspiration is observing other's act of kindness or doing something good (28.21 %), feeling touched by something positive (19.66 %) as well as learning about someone's success (16.24 %) (Table 6.23).

Table 6.22 Antecedents of elevation (broad category)

Category	Frequency (%)
Other's doing good deed	28.21
Being moved/touched	19.66
Other's success	16.24
Expectation to act	9.40
Media	8.55
Succeed despite shortcoming	6.84
Situation	5.13
Other's struggle	4.27
Experience good thing	1.71

Table 6.23 Antecedents of elevation (selective category)

Category	Frequency (%)
Kindness	37.72
Enthusiasm	32.46
Achievement	29.82

Evidently people are inspired mostly by kindness (37.72 %), enthusiasm to accomplish something (32.46 %) and the achievement (29.8 %) after struggling through obstacles.

6.4.13 Antecedents of Admiration

Antecedents of amazement for the elementary school teachers were identified by unfinished sentence: "I am amazed at …" (Table 6.24).

Aligned with inspiration, admiration was drawn from observing other's act of kindness or virtues (28.7 %). This percentage is significantly higher than being amazed by success (18.26 %) or by the behavior of an idolized person (15.65 %) (Table 6.25).

Specifying further the responses of the subject, it become apparent that Indonesian are mostly amazed by virtues being applied in manners (63.25 %) and accomplishment of a goal through hard work and perseverance (28.21 %).

6.4.14 Antecedents of Hate

Antecedents of hate for the elementary school teachers were identified by unfinished sentence: "I hate …" (Table 6.26).

Table 6.24 Antecedents of admiration (broad category)

Category	Frequency (%)
Good people	28.70
Successful people	18.26
Idolized person	15.65
Competence	7.83
Social spirit	6.96
People struggle despite shortage	6.09
Leader	4.35
God	4.35
Courage	2.61
Hardworking people	2.61
Something good	2.61

Table 6.25 Antecedents of admiration (selective category)

Category	Frequency (%)
Applied virtues	63.25
Achievement through hard work	28.21
Competence	4.27
Religiosity	4.27

Table 6.26 Antecedents of hate (broad category)

Category	Frequency (%)
Other's negative character	22.81
Dishonesty	16.67
Evil done by others	14.91
Vanity	11.40
Bad situation	9.65
Evil	7.89
Bad words	6.14
Hurt by others	4.39
Other	6.14

Table 6.27 Antecedents of hate (selective category)

Category	Frequency (%)
Bad character	99.12
Bad condition	9.65

As expected considering the inclination of admiration feeling, the main antecedents of hate are observing the negative character of others (22.81 %), dishonesty (16.67 %), malevolence act (14.91 %) and vanity (11.4 %) (Table 6.27).

So, mostly Indonesian hate bad character (99.12 %), significantly more than loathing bad situation or condition (9.65 %).

6.4.15 Antecedents of Regret

Antecedents of regret for the elementary school teachers were identified by unfinished sentence: "I feel regret when …" (Table 6.28).

Making mistake or doing negative things is the absolute reason Indonesian having regret (51.67 %). While not doing task or duty as expected (25 %) and not accomplishing task at best possible way (10 %) are the next main factors to create regret feelings (Table 6.29).

Classifying the original responses further, it become apparent that two major antecedents that may generate regret are making mistakes (55 %) and not to making the best attempts to meet personal expectation (40.83 %).

Table 6.28 Antecedents of regret (broad category)

Category	Frequency (%)
Making mistake/doing negative things	51.67
Not doing as expected	25.00
Not optimal task completion	10.00
Other	6.67
Unmet expectation	4.17
Not heeded advice	2.50

Table 6.29 Antecedents of regret (selective category)

Category	Frequency (%)
Making mistake/doing negative things	55.00
Not doing as expected	40.83
Not respected	3.33
Other	0.83

Table 6.30 Antecedents of disgust (broad category)

Category	Frequency (%)
Unclean condition	43.64
Immorality	36.36
No respect	10.91
Animal	5.45
Laziness	1.82
Mistakes	1.82

Table 6.31 Antecedents of disgust (selective category)

Category	Frequency (%)
Negative behavior	50.91
Unclean conditions	43.64
Animal	5.45

6.4.16 Antecedents of Disgust

Antecedents of disgust for the elementary school teachers were identified by unfinished sentence: "I am disgusted when …" (Table 6.30).

In this broad category low hygiene seems to be the main cause of disgust (43.64 %), while immorality or profanity also serves as a major cause (36.36 %). Observing a failure to respect other people is the third main reason (10.91 %) to feel disgusted (Table 6.31).

It can be concluded that negative behavior draws more disgust (50.91 %) than unclean condition (43.64 %).

6.5 Discussion

In this research, the participant demonstrates the tendency of moral emotions to be mostly affected by other people's behavior rather than non social conditions i.e. bad conditions of environment or situation.

Participants of this research seem agree that moral emotions positively motivate people to do good deeds. Positive moral emotions have a higher chance to motivate people than negative moral emotions. Moral emotions' possibility leading to positive behavior is on the basis of a well recognized notion that emotion tends to close the gap between having an impression of the situation and acting on the impression. Frijda (1988) who stated a term of 'action tendencies' to describe the connection of emotion and behavior argued that tendencies to act in particular (biologically significant) ways were integral to emotion and were central to distinguishing among emotions with a direct biological significance—tendency to approach is the root of desire, tendency to avoid is the root of fear, tendency to reject is the root of disgust, and so on. Moral emotions may serve as tendencies submitting to human conscience or moral intuition as it is a root to lead a person to act with integrity. The premise is similar to the nature of moral emotions that move subject as disinterested elicitors to engage in pro-social action (Haidt 2003).

Research results showed that most of moral emotions of the Indonesian school teacher are caused by similar objects or events as general population in the world. Admiration for example, admiration strikes by observing a deserved success. The participants seem admire achievement after hard work or well-deserved success; however they seem admiring others who can carry out good deeds more than worldly success. Elevation and admiration seems interchangeable in the conception of Indonesian.

In Indonesian language the term of embarrassment and shame are expressed in one word "malu". Therefore the concept of embarrassment and shame is interchangeable for Indonesian. According to Tangney et al. (2007) when describing shame-inducing situations, respondents expressed more concern with others' evaluations of the self. The source of shame of Indonesian is rather distinct; appearance seems not an essential factor of embarrassment. Behaving badly toward others or bad character is the main factor of Indonesian school teachers' shame. In a collective society like Javanese, behaving badly toward others raises a concern with how other will evaluate their character.

In opposition to shame (Tangney et al. 2007), a person experiencing guilt is already relatively "decentered"—focusing on a negative behavior somewhat separate from the self. In focusing on a bad behavior, rather than a bad self, a person in the middle of a guilt experience is more likely to recognize (and have concerns about) the effects of that behavior on others rather than on others' evaluations. Correspond to the general knowledge, the main antecedents of guilt of the research participants' controllable actions are in inconsistencies, negative behavior to other and inconformity to prevailing norms. The concern is more toward the effects of behavior to themselves not to others.

Regret, in a manner similar to guilt, also evokes desires to "kick oneself and to correct one's mistake, and wanting to undo the event and get a second chance" (van Dijk and Zeelenberg 2002). According to Berndsen, van der Pligt, Doosje, and Manstead (2004) unlike guilt, regret resulted from intrapersonal harm, whereas guilt is more associated with interpersonal harm. Accordingly, the results of the research the regret of Indonesia school teachers are mostly intrapersonal concerns due to making mistakes and not doing as expected.

Pity and compassion are known for altruistic emotions (Carr 1999), therefore they can be regarded as the main moral emotions. They are directed at the needs of others and a foundation for social virtues. In this research, pity and compassion for Indonesian are relatively one construct. The main antecedents for both moral emotions are suffering of others.

On the other hand, feeling of sadness resulted from personal suffering which is a complete opposite to pity and compassion. The self-directed nature of sadness as emotion is not too strong in affecting behavior of individual to do good deed. As reported by Schnall et al. (2008) that sadness may not influence individual moral judgment as severe as disgust.

Anger has often been studied in animals and inhumans as a nonmoral emotion, a reaction to frustration or goalblockage, linked to an action tendency that gather togetherthe resourcesrequired to accumulatean aggressive response to the blockage (Rozin et al. 1999). Indonesian feel anger when they are hurt by others, not so similar to Rozin et al. (1999) argument. The cultural background may play a perceptive and regulation role in this dissimilarity.

Pride is member of a family of "self-conscious emotions" that are evoked by self-reflection and self-evaluation (Tangney et al. 2007). When we "do the right thing," positive feelings of pride and self-approval are likely to result. Accordingly, the research participant' pride is mostly affected by their personal achievement and good deed. Pride is a moral emotion when the projection of positive consequence leads the individual to engage in positive action.

As for hate and disgust, participants of this research mostly are affected by the bad behavior of other person to another, apparently both emotions can be classified as indignation for unfairness. The experience of the emotion need not be personally involved in the social transgression. For example, we may feel indignant at the bad treatment of B by A. Indignation (sometimes used synonymously with resentment) is in part based on the controllability of harm and requires perceived responsibility on the part of the harm-doer. This indignation appears to be generated only by moral concerns, with "virtue as its own reward" (Turillo et al. 2002).

This research has come into conclusion that the antecedents of positive moral emotions (sympathy, pity, compassion, pride, admiration, elevation) are achievement through hardship, enthusiasm and perseverance, applied positive values by others, unfortunate events. The antecedents of negative moral emotions (embarrassment, regret, guilt, anger, sadness, disgust, hate) are negative values, negative behavior, mistakes.

Further research should be done to verify the effect of moral emotions to ethical behavior or integrity. The specific cultural background of the research participants is proved to provide a slightly different interpretation of events as elicitor of moral emotions. The antecedents observed in this research will be the basis of several methods of moral emotions stimulation (i.e. vignettes, short clips or films). The stimulations will serve as treatments for an experimental study tolearn the causal effect of moral emotions to ethical decision making.

Acknowledgments This research is funded by Center of Indigenous and Cultural Psychology, Psychology Department of Gadjah Mada University Yogyakarta, Indonesia.

References

Barnard, A., Schurink, W., & De Beer, M. (2008). A conceptual framework of integrity. *SA Journal of Industrial Psychology, 34*(2), 40–49.

Barrett, P. (2003). Beyond psychometrics: Measurement, non-quantitative structure, and applied numerics. *Journal of Managerial Psychology, 18*(5), 421–439.

Berndsen, M., van der Pligt, J., Doosje, B., & Manstead, A. (2004). Guilt and regret: The determining role of interpersonal and intrapersonal harm. *Cognition and Emotion, 18*(1), 55–70.

Camic, P. M., Rhodes, J. E., & Yardley, L. E. (2003). *Qualitative research in psychology: Expanding perspectives in methodology and design*. American Psychological Association.

Carr, B. (1999). Pity and compassion as social virtues. *Philosophy, 74*(3), 411–429.

Frijda, N. H. (1988). The laws of emotion. *American Psychologist, 43*(5), 349.

Haidt, J. (2003). The moral emotions. *Handbook of Affective Sciences, 11*, 852–870.

Matsumoto, D., Kudoh, T., Scherer, K., & Wallbott, H. (1988). Antecedents of and reactions to emotions in the United States and Japan. *Journal of Cross-Cultural Psychology, 19*(3), 267–286.

Mesquita, B., & Frijda, N. H. (1992). Cultural variations in emotions: A review. *Psychological Bulletin, 112*(2), 179.

Rozin, P., Lowery, L., Imada, S., & Haidt, J. (1999). The CAD triad hypothesis: A mapping between three moral emotions (contempt, anger, disgust) and three moral codes (community, autonomy, divinity). *Journal of Personality and Social Psychology, 76*(4), 574.

Schnall, S., Haidt, J., Clore, G. L., & Jordan, A. H. (2008). Disgust as embodied moral judgment. *Personality and Social Psychology Bulletin*.

Tangney, J. P., Stuewig, J., & Mashek, D. J. (2007). Moral emotions and moral behavior. *Annual Review of Psychology, 58*, 345.

Turillo, C. J., Folger, R., Lavelle, J. J., Umphress, E. E., & Gee, J. O. (2002). Is virtue its own reward? Self-sacrificial decisions for the sake of fairness. *Organizational Behavior and Human Decision Processes, 89*(1), 839–865.

Turner, J. H., & Stets, J. E. (2006). Moral emotions. In *Handbook of the sociology of emotions* (pp. 544–566). Springer, New York.

Van Dijk, W. W., & Zeelenberg, M. (2002). Investigating the appraisal patterns of regret and disappointment. *Motivation and Emotion, 26*(4), 321–331.

Chapter 7
A Structural Equation Model of WhatsApp's Addiction, Emotion Regulation, Personality, Academic Performance Decrement, and Social Connection of WhatsApp's Attitude

So-Fong Chan and Man-Tak Leung

Abstract WhatsApp is the most popular smartphone messenger application all over the world in 2015, which have more than 700 million users in the world. Nowadays, it is common to find people addicted to the WhatsApp because they text any time at any place. Confirmatory factor analysis was conducted to evaluate the construct validity of the questionnaires, whereas reliability was indicated by Cronbach's alpha. The researchers establish the relationship among several variables and constructs by using structural equation model. This study has included 203 participants in Hong Kong. The researchers examined the relationship among WhatsApp's addiction, emotion regulation, personality, academic performance decrement, and social connection of WhatsApp's attitude. It is found that personality (neuroticism) is significantly associated with emotion regulation, while emotion regulation is significantly associated with WhatsApp addiction and finally WhatsApp's addiction is significantly associated with academic performance decrement and social connection of WhatsApp's attitude. The result of the model indicates that emotion regulations were the risk factors of WhatsApp's addiction and WhatsApp's addiction would affect the academic and social connection.

Keywords Whatsapp's addiction · Emotion regulation · Social connection of WhatsApp's attitude

---

S.-F. Chan (✉) · M.-T. Leung
Counselling and Psychology Department, Hong Kong Shue Yan University, Hong Kong, China
e-mail: sfchan1992@yahoo.com.hk

M.-T. Leung
e-mail: mtleung@hksyu.edu

M.-T. Leung and L.-M. Tan (eds.), *Applied Psychology Readings*,
DOI 10.1007/978-981-10-2796-3_7

7.1 Introduction

WhatsApp addiction is a social problem, which increasingly affects people in Hong Kong. More people tend to use WhatsApp instead of face-to-face communication, which indicates that face-to-face communication skills of people deteriorate. Nowadays, most of the university and secondary school students and half of the primary school students have smartphone and use WhatsApp, so they all have better opportunity to develop WhatsApp addiction.

This study can provide the scientific evidence for the teachers, social workers, and psychologists about how to eliminate the WhatsApp addiction or other similar instant social messaging applications. For example, psychologists can provide more emotion regulation training for people with WhatsApp addiction in order to resolve WhatsApp addiction.

The aim for this research is to investigate the structural equation model between WhatsApp addiction, emotional regulation, personality, academic performance decrement, social capital, and social connection of WhatsApp's attitude. Most previous researches investigated the relationship related to internet addiction, smartphone addiction, instant messaging addiction, and Facebook addiction, but none of these investigated the relationship related to WhatsApp addiction. Those variables, namely: Emotional regulation, self-esteem, personality, self-control, academic performance decrement, social capital, were found that had a significant relationship with another kind of addiction. This model has added the new concept of WhatsApp addiction. Thus, this research is going to find out whether WhatsApp addiction is similar to another kind of addiction.

7.2 Research Question

Are there significant structural relationship between WhatsApp addiction (obsession, neglect and control disorder), emotional regulation (nonaccept, goals, impulse, aware, strategies and clarity), personality (extraversion, neuroticism and psychoticism), academic performance decrement, and social connection of WhatsApp's attitude?

7.3 Literature Review

7.3.1 WhatsApp Addiction

WhatsApp messenger is a cross-platform smartphone online messenger application for exchanging text, pictures, and video without payment, which is the most popular CMC application (WhatsApp.com 2015). With the increasing smartphone users, more people adapt to using WhatsApp as a daily real-time messenger application (Church and de Oliveira 2013). WhatsApp addiction means the extreme excessive use and having poor control in using WhatsApp that lead to impairment and negative repercussions, according to the internet addiction (Block 2008).

7.3.2 Emotion Regulation

Koole et al. (2009) define emotion regulation as self-regulation of emotion because self-regulation and emotion regulation are interfaced. Self-regulation was correlated to different kinds of addictions such as gambling, drug addiction, and smartphone addiction (Abolghasemi and Rajabi 2013; Yan Deursen et al. 2015; Moore et al. 2012).

Healthy emotion development has been recognized vital to a person's psychological and physical well-being (Oktan 2011). Emotion regulation was one of the emotion management skills which includes emotion encoding, emotion decoding, and emotional understanding (Oktan 2011). Koole et al. (2009) define emotional regulation as the ability to regulate specific emotions along with pressure and situation.

Kober (2014) argued that deficient emotional regulation in young age was the risk factor of individual to develop and constantly suffer from substance use disorder in the later so that emotion regulation and inability in emotional regulation were the causal factors. The research found that there was significant correction between addiction potential and emotion regulation, which indicated that people with poorer emotional regulation had higher addiction potential (Nikmanesh et al. 2014).

Emotion regulation was negatively significantly correlated to the internet addiction and smartphone addiction (Yu et al. 2013; Choi et al. 2014; Hormes et al. 2014). Emotion management skills are the predictor and negatively correlated to internet addiction, which meant that people with internet addiction had poor emotional management skills such as anger management, coping, and showing emotion (Oktan 2011).

Emotion regulation were significantly negatively associated with academic motivation and academic success (Singh and Singh 2013; Gumora and Arsenio 2002). Students with lower competence in emotion regulation would allow their arousal affect their academic achievement (Singh and Singh 2013).

7.3.3 Personality

Personality is the generally stable pattern of behavior, thinking, and feeling of an individual (Kendler 1963). Some researchers described personality of an individual in term of traits or dimensions (Krueger and Reckless 1931). For example,

Eysenck defined personality in four traits, namely psychoticism, lie, extraversion, and neuroticism (Eysenck and Eysenck 1964). In big five personality, there are five dimensions, namely, extraversion, emotional stability, agreeableness, conscientiousness, and openness (Barrick and Mount 1991). According to Davis (2001), cognitive behavioral model of problematic internet use was related to personality trait.

In internet addiction, researchers found that internet addiction was positively correlated to neuroticism and psychoticism and negatively correlated to extraversion (Yan et al. 2014; Yao et al. 2014; Xiuqin et al. 2010; Anolli et al. 2005). In instant messaging addiction, there was contradiction since Ehrenberg et al. (2008) reported that neuroticism positively predicted the instant messaging addiction and Wang et al. (2012) found that neuroticism had no relationship to instant messaging use. In smartphone addiction, there was significantly positive relationship between social extroversion (Hong et al. 2012). In Facebook addiction, researchers found that neuroticism was positively correlated to Facebook use; however, some researches did not find the correlation (Pettijohn et al. 2012). The nature of WhatsApp was more similar to instant messaging, so the personality traits of an individual with WhatsApp's addiction were uncertain.

7.3.4 Academic Performance Decrement

Academic performance decrement refers to the destructive impact of addiction to the academic work and academic performance such as not doing homework, falling asleep in classes, and shrinking grades (Kubery et al. 2001; Jiang 2014).

Jiang (2014) found that there was significant positive correlation between academic performance decrement and both internet addiction and online gaming addiction, which meant that the internet addiction and playing online games interfered the academic performance (Jiang 2014). Instant messaging addiction was the strongest predictor of academic performance decrement (Huang and Leung 2009). According to Huang (2011), instant messaging addiction was negatively correlated to academic performance. Students with addiction would certainly bring negative influence to their academic result.

There was negative correlation between grade point average (GPA) and time spent on internet, which indicated internet addiction would lower the GPA among college students (Mishra et al. 2014). There was negative significant correlation between GPA and internet addiction (Akhter 2013).

7.3.5 Social Connection of WhatsApp's Attitude

WhatsApp attitude refers to the cognitive and emotional orientation that foster and inhibit an individual's preference to use WhatsApp (Ledbetter 2009). Excessive use of text messaging is due to social support function of WhatsApp (Sultan 2014). Social connection of the WhatsApp affects the WhatsApp attitude the most (Sultan 2014). Social connection of WhatsApp's attitude refers to the effect of losing WhatsApp on people's social connection and social network.

Social connection is positively correlated to online communication technology, especially instant messaging and Facebook (Ledbetter 2009). The mediated effect of WhatsApp addiction is significant between extraversion and WhatsApp's attitude (Sultan 2014). People with internet addiction developed more favorable social connection of WhatsApp's attitude (Sultan 2014).

7.3.6 Participants

This study has included 203 undergraduate students who use WhatsApp on their smartphone in their daily life from different Hong Kong universities.

7.3.7 Instruments

The research designs are survey questionnaire, using convenient sampling. There are total five scales including WhatsApp addiction scale, difficulties in emotion regulation scale (DERS), Eysenck Personality Questionnaire-Revised, Short Scale for Chinese (EPQ-RSC), social connection of WhatsApp's attitude scale, and academic decrement scale. The items and sample items are shown in Table 7.1.

7.3.7.1 WhatsApp Addiction Scale

This scale is from the BBM and WhatsApp addiction scale modified by Sultan (2014). The original scale is the three factor model of problematic internet use questionnaire developed by Demetrovics et al. (2008). This scale is to measure the intension of WhatsApp addiction. Participants are asked to rate on a five-point scale, ranging from 1= "Never" to 5= "Always." The higher score means heavier addiction on WhatsApp. The Reported reliability of WhatsApp addiction scale was .91 (Sultan 2014). The reliability of problematic internet use scale were from .76 to .80 and the test–retest correlation was .90 (Koronczai et al. 2011). The items and sample items are shown in Table 7.1.

7.3.7.2 Difficulties in Emotion Regulation Scale (DERS)

This scale is developed by Gratz and Roemer (2004), which was translated to Chinese by 文永沁 (2006). This scale is to measure emotion dysregulation of an

Table 7.1 Number of items and sample items of the eight scales

Scales and subscales	No. of items	Sample item
WhatsApp addiction scale	17	
Obsession	5	How often do you daydream about WhatsApp?
Neglect	6	How often do you neglect household chores to spend more time on WhatsApp?
Control disorder	6	How often do you try to conceal the amount of time spent on WhatsApp?
Difficulties in emotion regulation scale	36	
Nonaccept	6	When I'm upset, I feel like I am weak?
Goals	5	When I'm upset, I have difficulty concentrating?
Impulse	6	When I'm upset, I feel out of control?
Aware	6	When I'm upset, I acknowledge my emotions?
Strategies	8	When I'm upset, it takes me a long time to feel better?
Clarity	5	I know exactly how I am feeling.
EPQ-RSC	34	
Extraversion	12	你是個健談的人嗎?
Neuroticism	12	你是個容易被激怒的人嗎?
Psychoticism	10	你是否努力是自己對人不粗魯?
Social connection of WhatsApp's attitude scale	5	Without WhatsApp, my social life would be drastically different.
Academic decrement scale	3	How often did you sleep late because of using WhatsApp?

individual (Simón et al. 2014). Participants are asked to rate on five-point scale from 1 = "Almost never" to 5 = "Almost always." The higher the score is in this scale, the greater the difficulties are in emotion regulation. The reliability of difficulties in emotion regulation scale were reported from .80 to .89 (Gratz and Roemer 2004). Gratz and Roemer (2004) reported that DERS has adequate construct and predictive validity. The items and sample items are shown in Table 7.1.

7.3.7.3 The Eysenck Personality Questionnaire-Revised, Short Scale for Chinese (EPQ-RSC)

The original scale is developed by Eysenck et al. (1996.) This scale was modified by Mingyi et al. (2000), which was translated into Chinese version. This study uses three dimensions (36 items), namely extraversion, neuroticism, and psychoticism, because these three dimensions are mainly related to addiction. The higher score of extraversion means sociable, optimistic, and extrovert. The higher score of neuroticism means emotional, depressive, and excitable. The higher score of psychoticism means aggressive, self-centered, and masculine. Participants are asked to response yes or no question only. A previous study reported that the reliability of EPQ-RC is .78 (neuroticism), .66 (extraversion) and .75 (psychoticism) (Yan et al. 2014). The items and sample items are shown in Table 7.1.

7.3.7.4 Social Connection of WhatsApp's Attitude Scale

This scale is reconstructed by Sultan (2014). The original is the measuring online communication attitude (MOCA) developed by Ledbetter (2009). Social connection is one of the subscales of MOCA, having five dimensions such as self-disclosure, miscommunication, and ease (Ledbetter 2009). Participants are asked to rate Likert-type scale from 1 = "strongly disagree" to 5 = "strongly agree." The higher score meant better attitude toward WhatsApp. The reliability of this scale is .82 in a recent study (Sultan 2014). The items and sample items are shown in Table 7.1.

7.3.7.5 Academic Decrement Scale

This scale is developed by Kubery et al. (2001). Participants are asked to rate five-point scale from 1 = "Never" to 5 = "Always." The higher score meant higher academic decrement due to the use of WhatsApp. This study used the three questions from Huang and Leung (2009), which modified the scale from Kubery et al. (2001). Those questions had been used in measuring the relationship between academic performance decrement and instant messaging. The items and sample items are shown in Table 7.1.

7.3.8 Descriptive Statistics

The mean, standard deviation, sample size, and with the correlations between all variables for this study are shown in Table 7.2.

7.3.9 Reliability

In this study, for the WhatsApp addiction scale, the coefficient alphas of three subscales are higher than .70. For the Difficulties in emotion regulation scale, the coefficient alphas of six subscales are higher than .60. For the EPQ-RSC, the coefficient alphas of three subscales are higher than .60. The coefficient alphas of social connection of WhatsApp's attitude scale are .81. The coefficient alphas of academic decrement scale are .84. The detail of coefficient alphas of the main study is shown in Table 7.3.

Table 7.2 Descriptive statistics

Variables	1	2	3	4	5	6	7	8	9	10	11	12	13	14
1. Obsession	–													
2. Neglect	.668**	–												
3. Control disorder	.636**	.773**	–											
4. Nonaccept	.274**	.307**	.303**	–										
5. Goals	.309**	.370**	.348**	.538**	–									
6. Aware	.057	.110	.063	−.175*	−.165*	–								
7. Impulse	.369**	.396**	.370**	.596**	.671**	.005	–							
8. Strategies	.328**	.369**	.316**	.686**	.758**	−.214**	.691**	–						
9. Clarity	.162*	.242**	.236**	.455**	.436**	.309**	.476**	.430**	–					
10. Psychoticism	−.141*	−.106	−.165*	−.086	−.018	.108	.032	−.058	.110	–				
11. Neuroticism	.180*	.205**	.221**	.502**	.492**	.002	.576**	.609**	.394**	−.025	–			
12. Extraversion	.145*	.055	−.027	−.207**	−.262**	−.011	−.218**	−.271**	−.164*	−.022	−.327**	–		
13. Social connection of WhatsApp's attitude	.335**	.385**	.329**	.152*	.291**	−.060	.092	.162*	.010	−220**	.062	−.014	–	
14. Academic Performance decrement	.543**	.767**	.680**	.257**	.325**	.057	.333**	.330**	.264**	−.111	.216**	.091	.377**	–
Mean	2.011	2.13	2.28	2.70	3.05	2.41	2.45	2.72	2.39	.18	.54	.60	3.21	2.31
SD	.601	.643	.752	.756	.771	.51	.78	.70	.58	.17	.28	.28	.83	.89

* $p < 0.05$; ** $p < 0.01$

Table 7.3 Coefficient alphas of the main study

Scales	α
WhatsApp addiction scale	
1. Obsession	.730
2. Neglect	.773
3. Control disorder	.822
Difficulties in emotion regulation scale	
1. Nonaccept	.837
2. Goals	.837
3. Impulse	.871
4. Aware	.663
5. Strategies	.861
6. Clarity	.739
EPQ-RSC	
1. Extraversion	.841
2. Neuroticism	.824
3. Psychoticism	.607
Social connection of WhatsApp's attitude scale	.810
Academic decrement scale	.846

7.3.10 Validity

In this study, CFA has been used to examine the validity of WhatsApp addiction, EPQ-RSC, self-control, and social capital. These indicate a good fit of items representing the instruments which are confirmed to be valid. The goodness of fit indices is as follows for WhatsApp addiction: the ration between $\chi^2/df = 3.45$; GFI = .91; CFI = .96; RMSEA = .11. The goodness of fit indices is as follows for EPQ-RSC: the ration between $\chi^2/df = 2.22$; GFI = .92; CFI = .92; RMSEA = .06. The goodness of fit indices is as follows for self-control scale: the ration between $\chi^2/df = 2.21$; GFI = .94; CFI = .87; RMSEA = .07. The goodness of fit indices is as follows for social capital scale: the ration between $\chi^2/df = 3.20$; GFI = .93; CFI = .94; RMSEA = .10.

7.3.11 Structural Equation Modeling (SEM)

SEM includes personality, emotion regulation, WhatsApp addiction, Social connection of WhatsApp's attitude, and Academic performance decrement. The structural model for this study was shown in Fig. 7.1. This model is used to show the relationship between five latent variables, including personality, emotion regulation, WhatsApp addiction, Social connection of WhatsApp's attitude, and Academic performance decrement, to their observable variables/indicators. The

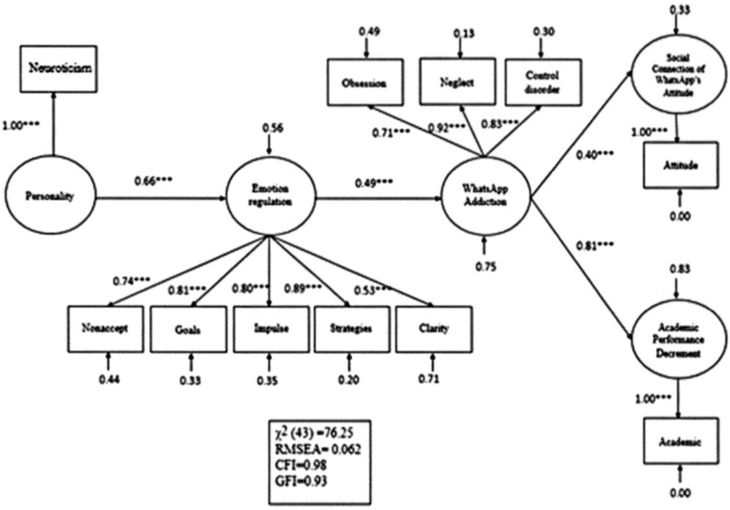

Fig. 7.1 The structural modeling of the relationship between personality, emotion regulation, WhatsApp addiction, social connection of WhatsApp's attitude, and academic performance decrement. *Note* χ^2 = maximum fit function Chi-square; *df* degree of freedom; *RMSEA* root mean square error of approximation; *GFI* goodness of fit index; *CFI* comparative fit index. $^{*}p < .05$; $^{**}p < .01$; $^{***}p < .001$

goodness of fit indices for this model is satisfactory, with the $\chi^2(43) = 76.25$; the chi-square ratio $\chi^2/df = 1.77$; GFI = .93; CFI = .98; RMSEA = .062.

Personality only includes neuroticism because all three subscales are not correlated that effect the fitness of the model. It is found that neuroticism is the most significant factor among three factors. Personality is significantly related to neuroticism ($\beta = 1.00, p < .001$).

Emotion regulation includes five observed variables, including nonaccept, goals, impulse, strategies, and clarity. However, emotion regulation does not include aware because aware is negatively correlated to other factors, which affect the fitness of the model. Emotion regulation is significantly correlated to nonaccept ($\beta = 0.74, p < .001$), goals ($\beta = 0.81, p < .001$), impulse ($\beta = 0.80, p < .001$), strategies ($\beta = 0.89, p < .001$), and clarity ($\beta = 0.53, p < .001$).

WhatsApp addiction includes three observed variables, including obsession, neglect, and control disorder. WhatsApp addiction is significant correlated to obsession ($\beta = 0.71$, $p < .001$), neglect ($\beta = 0.92$, $p < .001$), and control disorder ($\beta = 0.83, p < .001$).

Social connection of WhatsApp's attitude only includes attitude. Social connection of WhatsApp's attitude is significantly related to attitude ($\beta = 1.00, p < .001$).

Academic performance decrement has one observable variable only, which is academic. Academic performance decrement is significant related to academic ($\beta = 1.00, p < .001$).

As for the latent variables, five of the latent variables are significantly correlated with $p < .001$. Personality was positive related to emotion regulation

($\beta = .66$, $p < .001$), whereas emotion regulation would positive and significantly related to WhatsApp addiction ($\beta = .49$, $p < .001$). Finally, WhatsApp addiction positively and significantly gives rise to social connection of WhatsApp's attitude ($\beta = .40, p < .001$) and academic performance decrement ($\beta = .81, p < .001$).

7.4 Discussion

The primary purpose of this study is to investigate structural relationship among WhatsApp's addiction, emotion regulation, personality, academic performance decrement, and social connection of WhatsApp's attitude. The result showed significant relationship between variables.

In the structural equation model, emotion regulation is the mediator between personality (neuroticism) and WhatsApp addiction (obsession, neglect and control disorder). Individuals with difficulties in emotion regulation are prone to engage in addictive behaviors to suppress difficult emotion and seek out instant emotion gratification (Yu et al. 2013). Importantly, emotion regulation is the significant predictor of WhatsApp addiction. The fundamental characteristic of addiction is the deficiency of self-regulation (Demetrovics et al. 2008; Yu et al. 2013 and Kober 2014). If people have a deficit in self-regulation, they cannot regulate their behavior and emotion in a stressful situation, which lead to addiction for finding instant gratification.

People with high neuroticism suffer from a lack of emotion stability and are more capricious, anxious and prone to be agitated, so they would be more engages to internet addiction (Ge et al. 2014; Yan et al. 2014). Neuroticism is associated with a greater tendency to experience negative affect and a diminished capacity to downregulate negative emotions. Neuroticism is positively significant predictor of emotion regulation (Harenski et al. 2009). Neuroticism indirectly predicts WhatsApp addiction through emotion regulation by the result of structural equation modeling. Their emotional instability and sensitivity to WhatsApp would prompt that they neglect other issues and have difficulties in controlling using WhatsApp.

In personality, not only neuroticism is significant indirect predictor of WhatsApp addiction, but also extravision is significant direct predictor of WhatsApp addiction. However, comparing with the emotion regulation, the influence of extravision toward WhatsApp addiction is mild. Extravision is the significant predictor of WhatsApp addiction when extravision is the only predictor in the structural equation model.

There was significant positive relationship between WhatsApp addiction and academic performance decrement, thus supporting the study's hypothesis by the result in structural equation modeling. Instant messaging addiction was the strongest predictor of academic performance decrement (Huang and Leung 2009; Huang 2011). People spent a larger amount of time on social media and they often use social media before doing their homework, so social media addiction has a negative impact on academic performance (Huang 2011). People, who neglect another important issue due to increasing use of WhatsApp, would neglect the academic performance and homework. If people have difficulties in controlling the use of WhatsApp, they cannot control themselves to do homework and review.

WhatsApp addiction was the positive significant predictor of social connection of WhatsApp's attitude, thus supporting the study's hypothesis by the result in structural equation modeling. The more addictive to WhatsApp people are, the more important they perceive WhatsApp to their social connection. According to the social influence model, the opinion of surrounding peers and superiors dictate appropriate media choice, so there is strong connection between the social media and social connection (Ledbetter 2009). Attitude of social connection was positively associated with the online communication, particularly instant messenger (Ledbetter 2009).

7.5 Suggestion for the Future Study

This study gives the basic understanding of the relationship between WhatsApp addiction, emotion regulation, personality, social connection of WhatsApp's attitude, Academic performance, self-control, and self-esteem. For the further direction of studies, researcher can still try to explore about WhatsApp addiction by adding some variables such as locus of control, attachment style, and parenting style.

This study is specific to the Hong Kong. However, WhatsApp is an international smartphone application that people all over the world use it. It is worth testing whether these findings are generalizable to other cultures. WhatsApp are similar to other smartphone applications such as Line, Wechat, BBM. Sultan (2014) uses the test WhatsApp addiction and BBM addiction together, which reported the relationship between WhatsApp and BBM addiction and extraversion. It is worth testing whether these findings are generalizable to other smartphone application.

References

Abolghasemi, A., & Rajabi, S. (2013). The role of self-regulation and affective control in predicting interpersonal reactivity of drug addicts. *International Journal of High Risk Behaviors & Addiction, 2*(1), 28.

Akhter, N. (2013). Relationship between internet addiction and academic performance among university undergraduates. *Educational Research and Reviews, 8*(19), 1793–1796.

Anolli, L., Villani, D., & Riva, G. (2005). Personality of people using chat: An on-line research. *Cyberpsychology & Behavior, 8*(1), 89–95.

Barrick, M. R., & Mount, M. K. (1991). The big five personality dimensions and job performance: A meta-analysis. *Personnel Psychology, 44*(1), 1–26.

Block, J. J. (2008). Issues for DSM-V: Internet addiction. *American Journey of Psychiatry, 165*(3), 306–307.

Choi, J. E., Seo, E. J., Lee, E. H., & Yoo, M. S. (2014). Smartphone addiction, emotional intelligence and self control on college students. *Journal of Korean Academic Society of Home Care Nursing, 21*(1), 44–51.

Church, K., & de Oliveira, R. (2013, August). What's up with WhatsApp? Comparing mobile instant messaging behaviors with traditional SMS. In *Proceedings of the 15th international conference on human–computer interaction with mobile devices and services* (pp. 352–361). Toronto: ACM.

Davis, R. A. (2001). A cognitive-behavioral model of pathological internet use. *Computers in Human Behavior, 17*, 187–195.

Demetrovics, Z., Szeredi, B., & Rózsa, S. (2008). The three-factor model of Internet addiction: The development of the problematic internet use questionnaire. *Behavior Research Methods, 40*(2), 563–574.

Ehrenberg, A., Juckes, S., White, K. M., & Walsh, S. P. (2008). Personality and self-esteem as predictors of young people's technology use. *Cyber Psychology & Behavior, 11*(6), 739–741.

Eysenck, H. J., et al. (1996). *Manual of the Eysenck Personality Scales (EPS adult)*. London: Hodder & Stoughton Publishers.

Eysenck, H. Y., & Eysenck, S. B. G. (1964). *Manual of the Eysenck Personality Inventory*. San Diego: Educational and Industrial Testing Services.

Ge, Y., Se, J., & Zhang, J. (2014). Research on relationship among internet-addiction, personality traits and mental health of urban left-behind children. *Global Journal of Health Science, 7*(4), 60.

Gratz, K. L., & Roemer, L. (2004). Multidimensional assessment of emotion regulation and dysregulation: Development, factor structure, and initial validation of the difficulties in emotion regulation scale. *Journal of Psychopathology & Behavioral Assessment, 26*(1), 41–54.

Gumora, G., & Arsenio, W. F. (2002). Emotionality, emotion regulation, and school performance in middle school children. *Journal of School Psychology, 40*(5), 395–413.

Harenski, C. L., Kim, S. H., & Hamann, S. (2009). Neuroticism and psychopathy predict brain activation during moral and nonmoral emotion regulation. *Cognitive, Affective, & Behavioral Neuroscience, 9*(1), 1–15.

Hong, F. Y., Chiu, S. I., & Huang, D. H. (2012). A model of the relationship between psychological characteristics, mobile phone addiction and use of mobile phones by Taiwanese University female students. *Computers in Human Behavior, 28*(6), 2152–2159.

Hormes, J. M., Kearns, B., & Timko, C. A. (2014). Craving Facebook? Behavioral addiction to online social networking and its association with emotion regulation deficits. *Addiction, 109*(12), 2079–2088.

Huang, H. (2011). *Social media addiction among adolescents in urban China: An examination of socio-psychological traits, uses and gratifications, academic performance, and social capital*. Doctoral dissertation. Hong Kong: Chinese University of Hong Kong.

Huang, H., & Leung, L. (2009). Instant messaging addiction among teenagers in China: Shyness, alienation, and academic performance decrement. *Cyber Psychology & Behavior, 12*(6), 675–679.

Jiang, Q. (2014). Internet addiction among young people in China Internet connectedness, online gaming, and academic performance decrement. *Internet Research, 24*(1), 2–20.

Kendler, H. H. (1963). Personality. *Basic psychology*, (pp. 439–493). Appleton-Century-Crofts. doi:10.1037/13107-013.

Kober, H. (2014). Emotion regulation in substance use disorders. In *Handbook of emotion regulation* (2nd ed.). (pp. 428–446). New York, NY: Guilford Press. Retrieved from http://search.proquest.com/docview/1617245225?accountid=14548

Koole, S., Dillen, L. F., & Sheppes, G. (2009). Self-regulation of emotion. In K. D. Vohs & F. R. Baumeister (Eds.), *Handbook of self-regulation* (Vol. 2). New York: Guilford Press.

Koronczai, B., Urbán, R., Kökönyei, G., Paksi, B., Papp, K., Kun, B., et al. (2011). Confirmation of the three-factor model of problematic internet use on off-line adolescent and adult samples. *Cyber Psychology, Behavior, and Social Networking, 14*(11), 657–664.

Krueger, E. T., & Reckless, W. C. (1931). *Traits of personality*. New York: Longmans Green and Co. doi:10.1037/11036-012.

Kubery, R., Lavin, M., & Barrows, J. (2001). Internet use and collegiate academic performance decrements: Early findings. *Journal of Communication, 51*(2), 366.

Ledbetter, A. M. (2009). Measuring online communication attitude: Instrument development and validation. *Communication Monographs, 76*(4), 463–486.

Mingyi, Q., Guocheng, W., Rongchun, Z., & Shen, Z. (2000). Development of the revised Eysenck Personality Questionnaire short scale of Chinese (EPQ-RSC). *Journal of Chinese Psychology Acta Psychological Sinica, 32*(3), 317–323.

Mishra, S., Draus, P., Goreva, N., Leone, G., & Caputo, D. (2014). The impact of internet addiction on university students and its effect on subsequent academic success: A survey based study. *Issues in Information Systems, 15*(1). 344–352.

Moore, S. M., Thomas, A. C., Kyrios, M., & Bates, G. (2012). The self-regulation of gambling. *Journal of Gambling Studies, 28*(3), 405–420.

Nikmanesh, Z., Kazemi, Y., & Khosravy, M. (2014). Study role of different dimensions of emotional self-regulation on addiction potential. *Journal of Family & Reproductive Health, 8*(2), 69.

Oktan, V. (2011). The predictive relationship between emotion management skills and Internet addiction. *Social Behavior and Personality: An International Journal, 39*(10), 1425–1430.

Pettijohn, T. F., LaPiene, K. E., & Horting, A. L. (2012). Relationships between Facebook intensity, friendship contingent self-esteem, and personality in US college students. *Cyberpsychology, 6*(1), 1–7.

Simón, I. G., Penelo, E., & de la Osa Chaparro, N. (2014). Factor structure and measurement invariance of the Difficulties Emotion Regulation Scale (DERS) in Spanish adolescents. *Psicothema, 26*(3), 401–408.

Singh, P., & Singh, N. (2013). Difficulties in emotion regulation: A barrier to academic motivation and performance. *Journal of the Indian Academy of Applied Psychology, 39*(2), 289–297.

Sultan, A. J. (2014). Addiction to mobile text messaging applications is nothing to "lol" about. *Social Science Journal, 51*(1), 57–69. doi:10.1016/j.soscij.2013.09.003.

Wang, W., Ngai, E. W., & Wei, H. (2012). Explaining instant messaging continuance intention: The role of personality. *International Journal of Human–Computer Interaction, 28*(8), 500–510.

WhatsApp.com. (2015). WhatsApp—How it works. Retrieved from: http://www.whatsapp.com

Xiuqin, H., Huimin, Z., Mengchen, L., Jinan, W., Ying, Z., & Ran, T. (2010). Mental health, personality, and parental rearing styles of adolescents with Internet addiction disorder. *Cyberpsychology, Behaviour, and Social Networking, 13*(4), 401–406.

Yan Deursen, A. J., Bolle, C. L., Hegner, S. M., & Kommers, P. A. (2015). Modeling habitual and addictive smartphone behavior: The role of smartphone usage types, emotional intelligence, social stress, self-regulation, age, and gender. *Computers in Human Behavior, 45*, 411–420.

Yan, W., Li, Y., & Sui, N. (2014). The relationship between recent stressful life events, personality traits, perceived family functioning and Internet addiction among college students. *Stress and Health, 30*(1), 3–11.

Yao, M. Z., He, J., Ko, D. M., & Pang, K. (2014). The influence of personality, parental behaviors, and self-esteem on Internet addiction: A study of Chinese college students. *Cyberpsychology, Behavior, and Social Networking, 17*(2), 104–110.

Yu, J. J., Kim, H., & Hay, I. (2013). Understanding adolescents' problematic Internet use from a social/cognitive and addiction research framework. *Computers in Human Behavior, 29*(6), 2682–2689.

文永沁。(2006)。低成就學生的情緒調節對學業情緒與偏差行為的影響。(碩士論文,國立政治大學)

Chapter 8
The Relationship Between Personality Traits, School Climate, Parental Relationship, Anxiety, Depression, Self-esteem, and Cyber-Victimization

Wilmon Kwan and Man-Tak Leung

Abstract With the rapid bloom in the use of Information and Communication Technologies (ICTs), the human lives have actually becoming more and more convenient. However, the unpleasant incident cyber-victimization (CV) has also appeared which means people would possibly become the victim of bully cases via the ICTs platforms. The objective of the present study is to examine the association between CV, personality traits, parental relationship and school climate, and some psychological consequences, which includes anxiety, depression, and self-esteem. In the study, questionnaires were disturbed with the year 1–4 undergraduate students studying in one Hong Kong University. There are 196 participants, which aged from 17 to 24 years old ($M = 20.16$, SD = 1.78) and the participants consisted of 58 male (29.6 %) and 138 female (70.4 %). The findings indicate that extraversion and psychoticism have positive association with CV, while agreeableness and student commitment have negative association with CV. The variables also significantly predict CV. Also, CV has positive relationship with and significantly predicts anxiety and depression. Intervention and preventive strategies would be discussed based in the research findings.

Keywords Cyber-victimization (CV) · Personality traits · School climate · Parental relationship · Psychological impacts

W. Kwan (✉) · M.-T. Leung
Department of Counselling and Psychology, Hong Kong Shue Yan University, North Point, Hong Kong
e-mail: wilmonkwan@gmail.com

M.-T. Leung
e-mail: mtleung@hksyu.edu

M.-T. Leung and L.-M. Tan (eds.), *Applied Psychology Readings*,
DOI 10.1007/978-981-10-2796-3_8

8.1 Introduction

8.1.1 Research Background

Up to November, 2015, there are over 3.3 billion of Internet users in the world (Internet World Stats 2015). Compare the number with 2005, which are around 1 billion, this rapid bloom in the figure suggests that the role of the Information and Communication Technologies (ICTs) in people's daily lives is becoming more and more important. In the present time, the ICTs has offered people with easier ways of living as they could simply learn, communicate, and shop via the Internet without even leaving their home. Though ICTs would provide people with a lot of convenience and benefits, it could still bring a lot of troubles. The most notorious one is the cyber-bullying, which is the new form of bullying behaviors that appear on the platforms of the ICTs (Li 2007). According to Ngai and Chan (2010), there are around one-third of the 2978 secondary school students being surveyed who reveal that they had the experience of being cyber-bullied in 2009. This survey indicates that the problem of cyber-bullying has become very serious among the secondary school students in Hong Kong and it is worthwhile to further investigate the issue.

8.1.2 Literature Review

8.1.2.1 Personality Traits and Cyber-Victimization

Personality traits is the persisting features and patterns of the ways an individual perceives, reasons, and links oneself and the surrounding people and environment (APA 2000). Cyber-victimization (CV) is defined as the experience of cyber-bullying, which means intentionally and repeating to perform hurtful behaviors on others through the ICTs (Akbulut et al. 2010). According to Corcoran et al. (2012), the students that are the victims of traditional bullying and cyber-bullying had significantly higher level of neuroticism than the students that are not related to cyber-bullying behaviors. Another study found that the experience of cyber-victimization has a positive correlation with emotional instability, which also compatible with the term neuroticism, and has a negative relationship with conscientiousness (Kokkinos et al. 2013). Celik et al. (2012) also found that the status of cyber-victimization has positive correlations with emotional instability and agreeableness.

Research suggests that psychoticism has a positive association with cyber-victimization (Ozden and Icellioglu 2014). Furthermore, the research also found that there is a strong positive association between psychoticism and a specific category of cyber-victimization, which is people spreading hurtful rumor of the cyber-bullied victims. Similarly, Fanti et al. (2012) found that cyber-victimization is positively associated with narcissistic, callous–unemotional and impulsive traits.

Ayas and Deniz (2014) also found that psychoticism is positively associated with the experience of cyber-victimization among the elementary school students in Turkey. According to Kokkinos et al. (2014), impulsive/irresponsible traits have a positive association with the status of cyber-victimization among university students in Europe. In Eysenck's three factor model of personality (i.e., PEN), impulsivity is classified as the component of psychoticism (as cited in Whiteside and Lynam 2001). Therefore, the findings in the studies support the positive association between cyber-victimization experience and psychoticism. Contradicting with the above findings, Arıcak (2009) found that there is a negative association between psychoticism and the exposure of cyber-bullying behaviors among colleague students. It indicates that with higher psychoticism, experience of cyber-victimization could be reduced. To conclude, the personality traits, psychoticism, neuroticism, and conscientiousness are expected to have significant relationship with cyber-victimization and further investigation would be carried on in the present research.

8.1.2.2 School Climate and Cyber-Victimization

Apart from personality traits, the social aspects of individuals should be also considered to understand cyber-victimization because of its crucial roles in ones' development (Festl and Quandt 2013). School climate is defined as the combination of the learning environment at school, school rules, school commitment, and the relationships with schoolmates and teachers (Brand et al. 2003). The great amount of time spent with peers in school makes them one of the most influential parties towards ones' development and growth. The individuals would try to imitate and learn from each other in order to gain affirmation and develop a sense of belonging and identity. According to Davis and Koepke (2014), there is a negative association between cyber-victimization and school climate. In the research, the students' attitudes and thoughts on their schools and the environment is counted as the school climate. Surprisingly, the researchers found that the likelihood of the students to be cyber-victimized would be increased with the increase of restrictions among the use of cell phone in school. This finding suggests that cyber-victimization is related to the policies and attitudes of school among the uses of ICTs. Another research suggests that the students that are not a cyber-bully and have not been cyber-bullied would have more optimistic opinions on their schools and teachers than the students that are only involved in cyber-bullying and students involved in both cyber-bullying and victimization. The finding suggests that the view of students towards their schools and teachers may help to screen out individuals that are more vulnerable to be the cyber-victims and bullies. According to Sourander et al. (2010), the experience of cyber-victimization would have a positive association with the problems with peers and the perceived unsafety at the school among adolescents. Similarly, Casas et al. (2013) also found that there is a positive association between perceived security problem in school and cyber-victimization and a negative association between cyber-victimization and the perceived positive peer interaction. To conclude, the results support that school factors would influence students' experience of being cyber-victimized.

8.1.2.3 Parental Relationship and Cyber-Victimization

Parental relationship relates to the quality of connection of the children with their parents and their attachment, which developed since the infancy stage as the infants would try to absorb the caregivers' patterns of behaviors and thinking towards the surroundings as well as themselves (Ma and Huebner 2008, p. 178). According to Özdemir (2014), cyber-victimization experience is positively associated with the individuals' communication with mother, which was measured the times of communication. Another research in the U.S. suggests that the support from parents has a negative association with the cyber-victimization experience among students in middle school (Wang et al. 2009). With higher support of parents, the students could have more opportunities to combat the unpleasant experience. According to Accordino and Accordino (2011), there is a negative association between cyber-victimization and the relationship with parents. A close relationship with parents could reduce the chance of the students to be cyber-bullied.

According to Davis and Koepke (2014), there is a negative correlation between cyber-victimization, which included Nasty type (people saying hurtful things related to the cyber-victims) and the Aggressive type (cyber-victims receiving hostile e-mails), and the quality of the parental relationship. However, in the study, only the mother–child relationship correlates with the cyber-victimization experience significantly. The correlation of the experience and father–child relationship is only near significance. The finding suggests that relationship with mother and father may have different extent on influence the cyber-victimization experience.

8.1.2.4 Psychological Impacts and Cyber-Victimization

Self-esteem is defined as the attitude of an individual on perceiving the worth and values towards oneself, which could be negative or positive (Patchin and Hinduja 2010). Several research conducted in the U.S. suggests that there is a negative correlation between cyber-victimization and self-esteem and a positive correlation between depressive symptoms and anxiety (Aoyama et al. 2011; Kowalski and Limber 2013; Wigderson and Lynch 2013). Similarly, many studies also find that self-esteem is negatively correlated with the cyber-victimization experience (Özdemir 2014; Patchin and Hinduja 2010).

According to Schenk and Fremouw (2012), the victims of cyber-bullying score higher in the level of phobic anxiety, general anxiety, and depressive symptoms compare with individuals who have no experience of being a cyber-bully or victim among the university students. Sahin et al. (2012) also reported that the increase in the engagement of cyber-victimization would result in scoring higher in depression and anxiety. Research suggests that having cyber-victimization experience would increase the opportunity of having depressive symptoms for almost two times. Suicidal ideation and depression is also found to have a positive association with the cyber-victimization experience (Bonanno and Hymel 2013). In the findings of the literatures, the effect of cyber-victimization on the symptoms of anxiety, depression, and self-esteem are constant.

Yet, a research discovered that cyber-victimization experience is positively correlated with social anxiety but it has no significant association with depressive symptoms (Dempsey et al. 2009). Brown et al. (2014) also reported that cyber-victimization experience correlate with depressive symptoms among female participants.

8.1.3 Research Hypotheses

With respect to the studies reviewed, a theoretical model is estimated, it is hypothesized that the variables would have the following relationships:

(i) H_1: Individuals that have higher in psychoticism and neuroticism and lower in conscientiousness would have higher level of cyber-victimization experience.
(ii) H_2: Individuals that perceive their school climate more positively would have lower level of cyber-victimization experience.
(iii) H_3: Individuals that have poor parent–child relationship would have higher level of cyber-victimization experience.
(iv) H_4: Individuals that have higher level of cyber-victimization experience would have higher level of anxiety.
(v) H_5: Individuals that have higher level of cyber-victimization experience would have more depressive symptoms.
(vi) H_6: Individuals that have higher level of cyber-victimization experience would have lower level in self-esteem.

8.2 Methods

8.2.1 Participants

The current study recruited 196 participants, who were all year 1 to year 4 undergraduate students studying in one Hong Kong (HK) university. The age of the participants ranged from 17 to 24 years old ($M = 20.16$, SD = 1.78) and the participants consisted of 58 male (29.6 %) and 138 female (70.4 %).

8.2.2 Research Design

The current research was a quantitative research. Hard copies of the questionnaire were distributed in the campus of the HK university with the method of convenient sampling. In questionnaire, there were 179 items in total and consent forms were attached.

8.2.3 Research Procedure

A pilot study was carried out before main study ($n = 30$). In the main study, the participants were selected in one HK university campus. The participants were first informed with the purpose and the potential harm of the study. After signing two informed consent forms, the participants were given a set of the questionnaire. The participants mainly required around 20 min to complete the whole set of questionnaire. After finishing the study, one of the consent forms was given to them for any inquiry in the future. All of the data collection and analysis was done by the same person.

8.2.4 Instruments

The scales utilized in the study were translated from English to Chinese.

8.2.4.1 Personality Traits

The revised version of the Eysenck Personality Questionnaire (EPQ-R; Eysenck et al. 1985) and the Chinese version of the Big Five Inventory (BFI; John et al. 2008) were used in the study. For the BFI, it includes five subscales, which are the neuroticism (N), conscientiousness (C), extraversion (E), openness (O), and agreeableness (A). There are 44 items in the BFI, which are eight items for N, nine items for C, 10 items for O, eight items for E and eight items for N. Based on a Likert-scale with five points (1 = strongly disagree, 5 = strongly agree), the participants responded according to the level of fitness that the statements could define them, for instance, "I can be moody" and "I am sociable and outgoing." The internal consistencies were .82, .73, .85, .82, and .70 for N, C, E, O, and A respectively.

For the EPQ-R, only the Psychoticism subscale (P) was utilized as the other dimensions of personality traits in the EPQ-R could be measured by the BFI. Based on the scoring scale on yes or no, which scored with 1 and 0 respectively, the participants responded to the questions, for example "Do you try not to be rude to people?". The internal consistency was .68 for the P scale.

8.2.4.2 School Climate

The Inventory of School Climate-Student (ISC-S; Brand et al. 2003) was used to examine the perceived school climate. In the present research, only four subscales, which consisted of 21 items, were included in the questionnaire, which were the six items of Teacher Support (TS; "Teachers help students to organize their work"), five items of Consistency and Clarity of Expectation and Rules (CR; "When teachers make a rule, they mean it"), five items of Student Commitment/Achievement Orientation (SC; "Grades are very important to students") and five items of Positive Peer Interaction (PPI; "Students in this school are very interested in getting to know other students"). The scale was rated based on a Likert-scale with four points (5 = All of the time, 1 = none of the time). The internal consistencies were .79, .72, .80, and .82 for TS, CR, SC, and PPI, respectively.

8.2.4.3 Parental Relationship

The Chinese version of the Inventory of Parent and Peer Attachment (IPPA; Armsden and Greenberg 1987) was included. In present study, the two subscales of parent trust (PT) and parent communication (PC) were utilized. There are nine items in the PC subscale ("If my parent knows something is bothering me, she asks me about it") and 10 items in the PT sub-scale ("When I am angry about something, my parent tries to be understanding"). The participant responded a Likert-scale with five points (5 = always true or all of the time, 1 = never true or nearly never). The internal consistency was .88 for PC and .90 for PT.

8.2.4.4 Cyber-Victimization

The cyber-victimization scale established by Akbulut et al. (2010) was used to examine the participant's experience of cyber-victimization. The scale was a single factor model and it consisted of 28 items. In the current research, 26 items were adopted, which included "Facing with people using my personal information without my consent" and "Receiving insulting e-mails or instant messages." The participants responded based on a Likert-scale with five points (5 = most of the time, 1 = never). The internal consistency was .96.

8.2.4.5 Anxiety

The Generalized Anxiety Disorder 7 (GAD-7; Spitzer et al. 2006) was utilized to examine the severity of symptoms related to anxiety. The Chinese version of the scale was adopted. The scale is a single factor and it consisted of seven items, which included "Worrying too much about different things." The items were rated base on a Likert-scale with four points (3 = almost every day, 0 = none of the days). The internal consistency for the scale was .94.

8.2.4.6 Depression

The Center for Epidemiologic Studies Depression Scale (CES-D; Radloff, 1977) was used to measure the severity of symptoms related to depression. There are 20 items in the CES-D, which includes "My sleep was restless," "People were unfriendly." Items were rated based on a Likert-scale with four points (3 = all of the time, 0 = never or none of the time). The internal consistency was .91.

8.2.4.7 Self-esteem

The Rosenberg's Self-esteem Scale (Rosenberg, 1965) would be used for measuring the participants' self-esteem. The instrument contains of 10 items, which included "I certainly feel useless at times" and "I feel that I'm a person of worth, at least on an equal plane with others." The participant responded based on a Likert-scale with four points, (4 = agree strongly, 1 = disagree strongly). The internal consistency was .85.

8.2.5 Data Analysis

All data was analyzed with the Version 19 of the IBM SPSS statistics. After the data collection of the main study, the descriptive statistics were calculated. The distribution of the data could be examined through the results. The Cronbach's alpha (α) is calculated to examine the reliability of subscales. The correlational analysis was computed by the Pearson's coefficients (r) in order to examine the associations among the 16 variables. The hypotheses of the present research could be investigated through the analysis. Also, multiple regression analysis was carried out to examine the predictive relationships of the variables.

8.3 Results

8.3.1 Descriptive Statistics and Correlational Analysis

For the sake of clarity, the means, standard deviations, and correlations of the cyber-victimization (CV) and the other variables were presented in the Table 8.1.

8.3.2 Regression Analysis

In order to examine the predicting relationships of CV with the other variables, regression analysis was computed. Furthermore, three path models had been constructed based on the findings.

Table 8.1 Mean, standard deviation and correlations among variable

	1	2	3	4	5	6	7	8	9	10	11	12	13	14	15	16
1. E	–															
2. A	.01	–														
3. C	−.03	.10	–													
4. N	−.30**	−.36**	−.28**	–												
5. O	.30**	.01	.14*	−.17*	–											
6. P	.33**	−.39**	−.13	.03	.09	–										
7. TS	.13	.21**	.06	−.12	.10	−.02	–									
8. CR	−.01	.13	−.03	−.04	.23**	−.07	.37**	–								
9. SC	−.12	.14*	.04	.09	.04	−.26**	.43**	.42**	–							
10. PPI	.19**	.09	−.03	−.08	.18*	.00	.44**	.34**	.33**	–						
11. PT	.20**	.23**	.06	−.18*	.13	−.25**	.37**	.22**	.25**	.28**	–					
12. PC	.09	.06	.03	−.06	.13	−.26**	.28**	.15*	.19**	.29**	.71**	–				
13. CV	.22**	−.14*	.03	−.11	.07	.23**	−.04	−.10	−.19**	.01	−.05	.05	–			
14. AXN	−.07	−.24**	−.11	.45**	−.10	.16*	−.10	−.09	.02	.02	−.09	.02	.15*	–		
15. DEP	−.11	−.26**	−.17	.48**	−.15*	.22*	−.14*	−.18*	.07	.10	−.23**	−.07	.25**	.76**	–	
16. SES	.31**	.24**	.24**	−.50**	.26**	−.09	.24**	.14	.02	.17*	.31**	.15*	−.04	−.37**	−.63**	
M	3.05	3.51	3.00	3.20	3.20	.22	3.37	3.70	3.60	3.47	3.67	3.13	1.63	1.05	.95	2.84
SD	.68	.47	.49	.66	.61	.11	.52	.48	.57	.67	.67	.76	.59	.72	.49	.45

E, extraversion; A, agreeableness; C, conscientiousness; N, neuroticism; O, openness; P, psychoticism; TS, teacher support; CR, consistency and clarity of rules and expectations; SC, student commitment/achievement orientation; PPI, positive peer interactions; PT, parent trust; PC, parent communication; CV, cyber-victimization; AXN, anxiety; DEP, depression; SES, self-esteem

** $p < .001$; *$p < .05$

Regression was conducted with CV predicting Anxiety. The regression is significant ($F(1,193) = 4.46$, $p < .05$), which CV also significantly predicts anxiety ($\beta = .15, p < .05$). Regression was conducted with CV predicting Depression. The regression is significant ($F(1,191) = 12.62$, $p < .001$), CV significantly predicts depression ($\beta = .25, p < .05$). However, self-esteem could not be predicted by CV ($\beta = -.18, p > .05$).

As shown in Fig. 8.1, Regression was conducted with personality traits predicting CV. The regression is significant ($F(5,189) = 3.34$, $p < .05$). It was found that CV could be significantly predicted by extraversion ($\beta = .19, p < .05$) and agreeableness ($\beta = -.19, p < .05$).

Regression was conducted with psychoticism predicting CV. The regression is significant ($F(1,193) = 10.88$, $p < .001$). As shown in Fig. 8.2, psychoticism also was found to be a significant predictor of the CV experience ($\beta = .23, p < .001$).

Regression was conducted with school climate predicting CV. The regression is found to be insignificant ($F(5,189) = 3.340$, $p > .05$). As shown in Fig. 8.3, although the model is found to be statistically insignificant, student commitment/achievement orientation was a significant predictor of CV ($\beta = -.23, p < .001$).

Regression was conducted with parental relationship predicting CV. The regression is found to be insignificant ($F(2,191) = 1.76$, $p > .05$, $R^2 = .02$). Also, CV could not significantly be predicted by parent trust ($\beta = -.18, p = .084 > .05$) and parent communication ($\beta = -.18, p = .085 > .05$).

8.4 Discussion

The major purpose for the present study is to investigate the association between personality traits, school climate, parental relationship with cyber-victimization (CV) and also the relationship between CV and certain negative psychological consequences, which includes anxiety, depression, and self-esteem. From the research findings, personality traits and student commitment/achievement orientation are the factors that could predict CV. Also, anxiety and depression could be predicted as the negative psychological consequences by the unpleasant experience.

From the research findings, the experience of CV had a positive relationship with the students' level of extraversion (E) and psychoticism (P), while having a negative relationship with agreeableness (A). H_1 was only partially supported as there were no significant findings on the relationship between level of neuroticism, conscientiousness, and cyber-victimization. The research findings were mainly consistent with the prior studies (Arıcak, 2009; Ozden and Icellioglu, 2014; Kokkinos et al. 2013), except for A, which was found to be positively related to CV in the study of Celik et al. (2012). The inconsistency could be contributed by the cultural difference among the subjects and prior study was conducted among Turkish and with half of the participants using the distance education as the means to receive education. The habits and attitudes of participants on using of ICTs

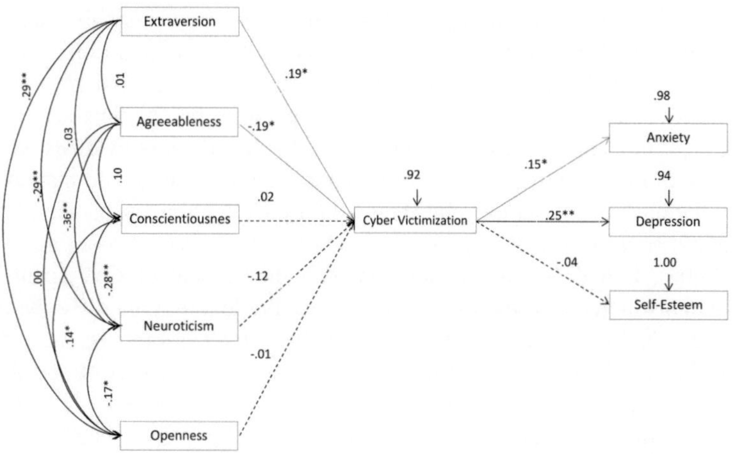

Fig. 8.1 Final model for personality traits, cyber-victimization and psychological impacts

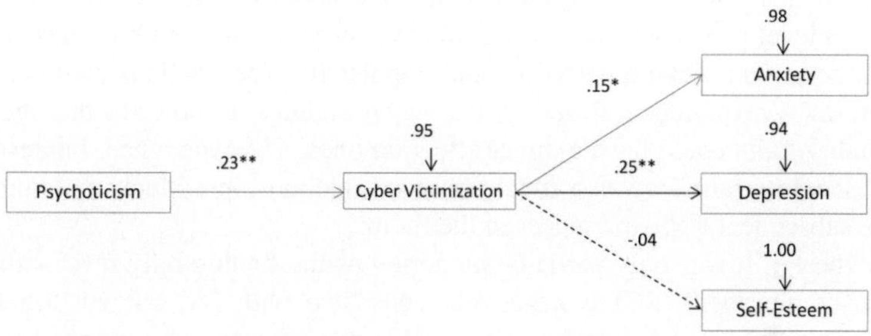

Fig. 8.2 Final model for psychoticism, cyber-victimization and psychological impacts

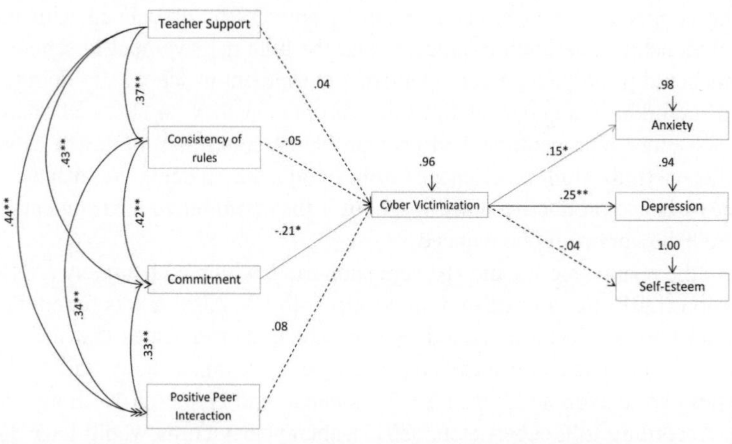

Fig. 8.3 Final model for school climate, cyber-victimization and psychological impacts

could contribute to the inconsistency. According to Jensen-Campbell et al. (2002), the trait of A and E had a strong positive impact on the peer friendship and acceptance and individuals with higher A would reported lesser peer victimization. Also, ones' positive and unaggressive response actions towards conflicts also increase with A (Jensen-Campbell and Graziano 2001). In such case, individuals with high level in A would encounter lesser cyber-victimization as they could maintain harmony relationship with others and they would have higher acceptance and positive justification towards the aggressive acts of cyber-bullies. According to Kraut et al. (2002), E had positive association with the amount of time spent in the Internet. This increase of the use of Internet would definitely increase the chance of an individual to become the target of a cyber-victim. Moreover, the individuals with higher level in E would tend to be a more frequent user of social media (Correa et al. 2010). In such case, the chance of facing the cyber-bullies would be higher among the more extraverted people. Therefore, CV could be predicted by E positively. For P, Campbell and Morrison (2007) found that people with more symptoms of psychoticism would report their interpersonal environment more negatively, which related to frequent rejection and hostility from peer. The reason for this could relate to the troublesome actions performed by the people with high level in P. Those people would have more conflicts with friends because of their sensation seeking behaviors and impulsivity. Their actions could result in the future CV experience. Based on the above findings, it indicates that the three personality traits could have a direct effect on ones' CV experience. Interestingly, the personality traits may also affect the social relationships, which could possibly induce subsequent CV experiences in the future.

For the H_2, it was only partially supported as the finding only reveals that the student commitment (SC) is negatively correlated with CV, but not the school climate. According to Schneider et al. (2012), the students who reported a lower school performances would be more likely to be cyber-victimized. On the other hand, Roseth et al. (2008) found that the students with high achievement would experience cooperative goal structure in school rather than competitive structure, also the cooperative goal structure would positively be associated with positive peer relationship. The finding indicates that the high achievement in school of the students could promote a less competitive environment in school. By doing so, the students could have a better relationship with peer as they do not need to compete with each other. The conflicts and peer problems could then be lower as well as the cyber-victimization experience. Furthermore, the students could have higher tendency to have productive aims in school if they committed as a students. Other problem behaviors could be reduced.

From the results, the H_4 and H_5 were supported, which both anxiety (ANX) and depression (DEP) has a positive relationship with CV. Also, it was found that both ANX and DEP could be predicted by CV, which also indicates that they are the negative psychological consequences. The results are consistent with the majority of studies (Wigderson and Lynch 2013; Bonanno and Hymel 2013; Bannink et al. 2014). According to Goebert et al. (2011), the cyber-victims would have suicidal ideation after the facing the CV in a long period of time. Apart from the AXN,

DEP and suicidal ideation, the CV is also related to delinquencies and problems in school, emotional distress, and substance abuse (Goebert et al. 2011; Brown et al. 2014). The studies indicate that the psychological consequences of CV could affect the individuals' psychological well-being at an extremely large extent.

H_3 and H_6 were not supported by the findings as the parental relationship and self-esteem was found to have no association with CV. The outcome of study was inconsistent with some of the prior research as they do find a significant predicting role of the above factors on CV (Wang et al. 2009; Özdemir 2014; Patchin and Hinduja 2010). The inconsistency could be contributed by the contextual different among samples. Since the above studies were conducted in the western countries, which are mainly individualism, and among the primary and secondary school students, the effects of the above factors could be minimized.

8.5 Limitation

The small sample size of study was one of the major limitations. In the 196 participants, more than 19 % of the participants only had a mean score of 1.12 with the score ranged from 1 to 5 in the CV scale, which 1 and 2 represent never and seldom, respectively. The prevalence of the CV among the participants was relatively low and the CV experience could only take place accidentally. Apart from the sample size, the selection of CV scale as well as the inadequacy of studies and measurements in CV also contributes to the insignificant findings. Since topics of CV only arose with the bloom in ICTs' use during the past 10 years (Griezel et al. 2012), measurements and the mechanism of related to CV still needs time to be developed and validated. The insufficiency of validation in the CV scale used could lead to the insignificance relationship among variables.

The self-report measurement on the experience of cyber-victimization could affect the research findings. According to Li (2010), the victim of cyber-bullying would tend to use avoidance and neglecting the coping strategies to deal with the unpleasant incident rather than seeking help from others. Issues like underreporting and volunteer bias could occur and it may interfere with the results.

8.6 Future Direction and Applications

Majority of the researchers had found that the experience of being cyber-bullied would increase the likelihood of an individual to become another cyber-bully and induce the acts on others (Beran and Li 2007; Celik et al. (2012); Dilmac 2009; Norret and Rivers 2006). After years of exposure, the victims may have learnt the act and become insensitive to the negative feelings of being cyber-bullied. In such case, a vicious cycle would be occurred as the cyber-victims would become one of the bullies themselves and create more sufferers. As mentioned above, the victims of cyber-bullying may not want to seek help (Li 2010). Therefore, interventions and prevention must be taken by the educational providers and social workers actively. Since the personality of individual is hard to alter after ones' early development, some practical skills like interpersonal skills and coping strategies could be taught. As for the schools, they could organize activities and programs that could increase the motivation of student in committing to school. Most importantly, the educational providers should also be educated and have better understanding about CV before offering help to the victims. Also, longitudinal studies could also been carried on in order to understand the long-term effect of the factors that affect CV and understand the topic in-depth. The experience of being a cyber-bully could also be examined along with CV in order to understand a more thorough picture behind the cyber-bullying.

8.7 Conclusion

To conclude, the personality factors and school factors are the most crucial factors in stopping cyber-bullying behaviors. Individuals that are more extraverted and psychotic in personality would more prone to be cyber-bullied, while being more agreeable could help to reduce the chance of being cyber-bullied. Students that are committed to their school and wanted to strive for achievement would less likely to become a cyber-victim. Having the CV experience could affect the well-being of people as it increases the severity of the symptoms of anxiety and depression. Therefore, the topic should be addressed properly in order to promote the welfare and caring atmosphere in society.

References

Accordino, D. B., & Accordino, M. P. (2011). An exploratory study of face-to-face and cyberbullying in sixth grade students. *American Secondary Education, 40*(1), 14–30.

Akbulut, Y., Sahin, Y. L., & Eristi, B. (2010). Development of a scale to investigate cybervictimization among online social utility members. *Online Submission, 1*(1), 46–59.

Amercan Psychiatric Association. (2000). *Diagnostic and statistical manual of mental disorders, text revision* (4th ed.). Washington DC: American Psychiatric Association.

Aoyama, I., Saxon, T. F., & Fearon, D. D. (2011). Internalizing problems among cyberbullying victims and moderator effects of friendship quality. *Multicultural Education and Technology Journal, 5*(2), 92–105.

Arıcak, O. T. (2009). Psychiatric symptomatology as a predictor of cyberbullying among university students. *Eurasian Journal of Educational Research, 34*(1), 169.

Armsden, G. C., & Greenberg, M. T. (1987). The inventory of parent and peer attachment: Individual differences and their relationship to psychological well-being in adolescence. *Journal of Youth and Adolescence, 16*(5), 427–454.

Ayas, T., & Deniz, M. (2014). Predicting the exposure levels of cyber bullying of elementary students with regard to psychological symptoms. *Procedia-Social and Behavioral Sciences, 116*, 4910–4913.

Bannink, R., Broeren, S., van de Looij-Jansen, P. M., de Waart, F. G., & Raat, H. (2014). Cyber and traditional bullying victimization as a risk factor for mental health problems and suicidal ideation in adolescents. *PLoS ONE, 9*(4), e94026.

Beran, T., & Li, Q. (2007). The relationship between cyber-bullying and school bullying. *Journal of Student Wellbeing, 1*(2), 15–33.

Bonanno, R. A., & Hymel, S. (2013). Cyber bullying and internalizing difficulties: Above and beyond the impact of traditional forms of bullying. *Journal of Youth and Adolescence, 42*(5), 685–697.

Brand, S., Felner, R., Shim, M., Seitsinger, A., & Dumas, T. (2003). Middle school improvement and reform: Development and validation of a school-level assessment of climate, cultural pluralism, and school safety. *Journal of Educational Psychology, 95*(3), 570.

Brown, C. F., Demaray, M. K., & Secord, S. M. (2014). Cyber victimization in middle school and relations to social emotional outcomes. *Computers in Human Behavior, 35*, 12–21.

Campbell, M. L., & Morrison, A. P. (2007). The relationship between bullying, psychotic-like experiences and appraisals in 14–16-year olds. *Behaviour Research and Therapy, 45*(7), 1579–1591.

Casas, J. A., Del Rey, R., & Ortega-Ruiz, R. (2013). Bullying and cyberbullying: Convergent and divergent predictor variables. *Computers in Human Behavior, 29*(3), 580–587.

Celik, S., Atak, H., & Erguzen, A. (2012). The effect of personality on cyberbullying among university students in Turkey. *Egitim Arastirmalari—Eurasian. Journal of Educational Research, 49*, 129–150.

Corcoran, L., Connolly, I., & O'Moore, M. (2012). Cyberbullying in Irish schools: An investigation of personality and self-concept. *The Irish Journal of Psychology, 33*(4), 153–165.

Correa, T., Hinsley, A. W., & De Zuniga, H. G. (2010). Who interacts on the Web?: The intersection of users' personality and social media use. *Computers in Human Behavior, 26*(2), 247–253.

Davis, K., & Koepke, L. (2014). Risk and protective factors associated with cyberbullying: Are relationships or rules more protective? *Learning, Media and Technology*, 1–25. doi: 10.1080/17439884.2014.994219.

Dempsey, A. G., Sulkowski, M. L., Nichols, R., & Storch, E. A. (2009). Differences between peer victimization in cyber and physical settings and associated psychosocial adjustment in early adolescence. *Psychology in the Schools, 46*(10), 962–972.

Dilmac, B. (2009). Psychological needs as a predictor of cyber bullying: A preliminary report on college students. *Educational Sciences: Theory and Practice, 9*(3), 1307–1325.

Eysenck, S. B., Eysenck, H. J., & Barrett, P. (1985). A revised version of the psychoticism scale. *Personality and Individual Differences, 6*(1), 21–29.

Fanti, K. A., Demetriou, A. G., & Hawa, V. V. (2012). A longitudinal study of cyber bullying: Examining risk and protective factors. *European Journal of Developmental Psychology, 9*(2), 168–181.

Festl, R., & Quandt, T. (2013). Social relations and cyberbullying: The influence of individual and structural attributes on victimization and perpetration via the Internet. *Human Communication Research, 39*(1), 101–126.

Goebert, D., Else, I., Matsu, C., Chung-Do, J., & Chang, J. Y. (2011). The impact of cyber bullying on substance use and mental health in a multiethnic sample. *Maternal and Child Health Journal, 15*(8), 1282–1286.

Griezel, L., Finger, L. R., Bodkin-Andrews, G. H., Craven, R. G., & Yeung, A. S. (2012). Uncovering the structure of and gender and developmental differences in cyber bullying. *The Journal of Educational Research, 105*(6), 442–455.

Internet World Stats. (2015). World internet users and 2015 population stats. Retrieved December 18, 2015, http://www.internetworldstats.com/stats.htm

Jensen-Campbell, L. A., & Graziano, W. G. (2001). Agreeableness as a moderator of interpersonal conflict. *Journal of Personality, 69*(2), 323–362.

Jensen-Campbell, L. A., Adams, R., Perry, D. G., Workman, K. A., Furdella, J. Q., & Egan, S. K. (2002). Agreeableness, extraversion, and peer relations in early adolescence: Winning friends and deflecting aggression. *Journal of Research in Personality, 36*(3), 224–251.

John, O. P., Naumann, L. P., & Soto, C. J. (2008). Paradigm shift to the integrative big-five trait taxonomy: History, measurement, and conceptual issues. In O. P. John, R. W. Robins, & L. A. Pervin (Eds.), *Handbook of personality: Theory and research* (pp. 114–158). New York, NY: Guilford Press.

Kokkinos, C. M., Antoniadou, N., & Markos, A. (2014). Cyber-bullying: An investigation of the psychological profile of university student participants. *Journal of Applied Developmental Psychology, 35*(3), 204–214.

Kokkinos, C. M., Antoniadou, N., Dalara, E., Koufogazou, A., & Papatziki, A. (2013). Cyber-bullying, personality and coping among pre-adolescents. *International Journal of Cyber Behavior, Psychology and Learning (IJCBPL), 3*(4), 55–69.

Kowalski, R. M., & Limber, S. P. (2013). Psychological, physical, and academic correlates of cyberbullying and traditional bullying. *Journal of Adolescent Health, 53*(1), S13–S20.

Kraut, S., Kiesler, B., Boneva, J., Cummings, J., Helgeson, V., & Crawford, A. (2002). Internet paradox revisited. *Journal of Social Issues, 58*, 49–74.

Li, Q. (2007). Bullying in the new playground: Research into cyberbullying and cyber-victimisation. *Australasian Journal of Educational Technology, 23*(4), 435–454.

Li, Q. (2010). Cyberbullying in high schools: A study of students' behaviors and beliefs about this new phenomenon. *Journal of Aggression, Maltreatment and Trauma, 19*(4), 372–392.

Ma, C. Q., & Huebner, E. S. (2008). Attachment relationships and adolescents life satisfaction: Some relationships matter more to girls than boys. *Psychology in the Schools, 45*(2), 177.

Ngai, A. & Chan, S. C. (2010). A Study on Cyber-bullying among Hong Kong Secondary Students. *Youth Study Series, 44*. Retrieved from http://yrc.hkfyg.org.hk/files/yrc/yrc_ys44.pdf

Norret, N., & Rivers, I. (2006). The prevalence of bullying by text message or email: Result of a four year study. Poster presented at *British Psychological Society Annual Conference*, Cardiff.

Özdemir, Y. (2014). Cyber victimization and adolescent self-esteem: The role of communication with parents. *Asian Journal of Social Psychology, 17*(4), 255–263.

Ozden, M. S., & Icellioglu, S. (2014). The perception of cyberbullying and cyber-victimization by university students in terms of their personality factors. *Procedia-Social and Behavioral Sciences, 116*, 4379–4383.

Patchin, J. W., & Hinduja, S. (2010). Cyberbullying and self-esteem. *Journal of School Health, 80*(12), 614–621.

Radloff, L. S. (1977). The CES-D scale a self-report depression scale for research in the general population. *Applied Psychological Measurement, 1*(3), 385–401.

Rosenberg, M. (1965). *Society and the adolescent self-image* (p. 326). Princeton, NJ: Princeton University Press.

Roseth, C. J., Johnson, D. W., & Johnson, R. T. (2008). Promoting early adolescents' achievement and peer relationships: The effects of cooperative, competitive, and individualistic goal structures. *Psychological Bulletin, 134*(2), 223.

Şahin, M., Aydin, B., & Sari, S. V. (2012). Cyber bullying, cyber victimization and psychological symptoms: A study in adolescents. *Cukurova University Faculty of Education Journal, 41*(1), 53–59.

Schenk, A. M., & Fremouw, W. J. (2012). Prevalence, psychological impact, and coping of cyberbully victims among college students. *Journal of School Violence, 11*(1), 21–37.

Schneider, S. K., O'Donnell, L., Stueve, A., & Coulter, R. W. (2012). Cyberbullying, school bullying, and psychological distress: A regional census of high school students. *American Journal of Public Health, 102*(1), 171–177.

Sourander, A., Klomek, A. B., Ikonen, M., Lindroos, J., Luntamo, T., Koskelainen, M., et al. (2010). Psychosocial risk factors associated with cyberbullying among adolescents: A population-based study. *Archives of General Psychiatry, 67*(7), 720–728.

Spitzer, R. L., Kroenke, K., Williams, J. B., & Löwe, B. (2006). A brief measure for assessing generalized anxiety disorder: The GAD-7. *Archives of Internal Medicine, 166*(10), 1092–1097.

Wang, J., Iannotti, R. J., & Nansel, T. R. (2009). School bullying among adolescents in the United States: Physical, verbal, relational, and cyber. *Journal of Adolescent Health, 45*(4), 368–375.

Whiteside, S. P., & Lynam, D. R. (2001). The five factor model and impulsivity: Using a structural model of personality to understand impulsivity. *Personality and Individual Differences, 30*(4), 669–689.

Wigderson, S., & Lynch, M. (2013). Cyber-and traditional peer victimization: Unique relationships with adolescent well-being. *Psychology of Violence, 3*(4), 297.

Chapter 9
Differences in Participant Motivation Based on Category of Body Mass Index and Gender

I.T. Heazlewood, J. Walsh, M. Climstein, K. Adams, T. Sevene and Mark DeBeliso

Abstract Motivation is defined as "the directions and intensity of one's effort" and is a significant factor in the selection of exercise and sport. Participant motivation evaluates those factors that enhance or inhibit motivation to participate and is represented by factors as health orientation, weight concern/weight loss and personal goal achievement. The research aim was to evaluate the differences in nine participant motivation factors based on health risk categories of body mass index (BMI) using four BMI categories of underweight, normal, overweight and obese and related to athlete gender. The nine participant motivation factors utilized in the study were health orientation, weight concern, personal goal achievement, competition, recognition, affiliation, psychological coping, life meaning and self-esteem. Male and female athletes competing at the 2009 World Masters Games, Sydney, Australia volunteered for the research (male; $n = 3687$; mean age = 53.72; SD = 10.05 and female; $n = 3488$; mean age = 49.39; SD = 9.15). Athletes

I.T. Heazlewood (✉) · J. Walsh
School of Psychological and Clinical Science, Charles Darwin University, Darwin, NT 0909, Australia
e-mail: ian.heazlewood@cdu.edu.au
URL: http://www.cdu.edu.au/

M. Climstein
Exercise, Health and Performance Faculty Research Group, University of Sydney, Sydney, NSW 2006, Australia
e-mail: mike.climstein@sydney.edu.au

K. Adams · T. Sevene
Kinesiology Department, California State University, 100 Campus Center, Valley Hall, Seaside, CA 93955-800, USA
e-mail: kadams@csumb.edu

M. DeBeliso
College of Education and Human Development, Southern Utah University, 351 W. University Blvd., Cedar City, UT 84720, USA
e-mail: markdebeliso@suu.edu

M.-T. Leung and L.-M. Tan (eds.), *Applied Psychology Readings*,
DOI 10.1007/978-981-10-2796-3_9

completed an online survey using the Limesurveytm interactive survey system where they responded to a 56 item sport psychological instrument, the Motivations of Marathoners Scale. Results for male athletes significant differences ($p < .001$) were identified for BMI category with health orientation, weight concern, personal goal achievement, competition, affiliation, life meaning and self-esteem, although eta^2 values were small (η^2 values .002–.020). For female athletes significant differences ($p < .001$) were identified for BMI category with health orientation, weight concern, personal goal achievement, competition, affiliation and self-esteem, although eta^2 values were small (η^2 values .001–.017). No significant differences occurred for recognition, life meaning or psychological coping.

Keywords Masters sport · BMI · Participant motivation · Gender

9.1 Introduction

Motivation is defined as "the directions and intensity of one's effort" and is a significant factor in the selection of exercise and sport. Participant motivation evaluates those factors that enhance or inhibit motivation to participate and is represented by factors as health orientation, weight concern/weight loss and personal goal achievement (Masters et al. 1993; Marcus and Forsyth 2009). These motivating factors are identified to influence the quantity of physical activity in people. Some research has been conducted on participant motivation factors displayed by 2009 World Masters Games (WMG) athletes based on issues of gender and comparisons between different international competition cohorts (Heazlewood et al. 2011, 2012, 2015).

9.1.1 Body Mass Index

Body mass index (BMI units in kg m^{-2}) or Quetelet index (American College of Sports Medicine 2010) and research indicates that obesity related health problems and health risks increase above a BMI value of 25. According to American College of Sports Medicine (2010) criteria scores athletes would be underweight (BMI < 18.5), normal (BMI = 18.5–24.9), overweight (BMI = 25.0–29.9) and obese (BMI > 30.0) scores. BMI scores of 25.0–29.9 increases disease risk for females and high risk for males and greater than 30 results in high risk for females and very high risk for males.

Research has indicated the following trends that link BMI with nutrition and physical activity behaviours across different populations. BMI was used to predict dietary risk and race in a study of university women (Anderson 2006) which indicated that at risk eating behaviours were somewhat linked to BMI. A study of the effects of effects of self-efficacy, body mass, and cardio respiratory fitness on exercise motives in Chinese college students (Shen and Xu 2007) and discovered physical and psychological variables have both independent and specialized functions on exercise motives. Future motivational studies in exercise should focus attention to ecological approaches that account for physical, psychological, and social factors. Ecological approaches reflect the context of the behaviours such as sports competition. Sicilia et al. (2014) evaluated the relationship of exercise motivation and social physique anxiety in secondary education male and female adolescents and included BMI and gender as potential predictors of motivation and social physique anxiety.

Caperchione et al. (2008) evaluated mediating relationship between body mass index and the direct measures of the theory of planned behaviour on physical activity intention, and the findings indicated that the direct measure of attitude and perceived behavioural control mediated the relationship between BMI and physical activity intention. The current research problem is what influence BMI categories in predicting participant motivation factors as health orientation, weight concern, personal goal achievement, competition, recognition, affiliation, psychological coping, life meaning and self-esteem in terms of these factors being important to masters athletes at international level competitions.

9.1.2 Research Aim

The research aim was to evaluate the differences in nine participant motivation factors based on health risk categories of body mass index (BMI), using four BMI categories of underweight, normal, overweight and obese (American College of Sports Medicine 2010) and related to athlete gender. To assess if BMI differentiated the level of importance and difference in nine participant motivation factors of health orientation, weight concern, personal goal achievement, competition, recognition, affiliation, psychological coping, life meaning and self-esteem and enable the development of specific intervention programs based on the different dimensions of participant motivation interacting with gender to enhance participation in sport and physical activity by masters athletes.

9.2 Methods

9.2.1 Sample and Instruments

The study was approved by a university human research ethics committee. Male and female athletes competing at the 2009 World Masters Games, Sydney, Australia volunteered to participate in the research project (male; $n = 3687$; mean age = 53.72; SD = 10.05 and female; $n = 3488$; mean age = 49.39; SD = 9.15). Athletes completed an online survey using the Limesurveytm interactive survey system where they responded to a 56 item sport psychological instrument, the Motivations of Marathoners Scale (MOMS) with a 7-point Likert scale response to each item. The range was 1 = least important to 7 = most important reason. The MOMS instrument focused on nine participant motivation factors related to health orientation, weight concern, personal goal achievement, competition, recognition, affiliation, psychological coping, life meaning and self-esteem.

The MOMS instrument displays high internal consistency good test–retest reliability, factor validity, construct validity, convergent validity and discriminant validity (Masters et al. 1993; Ogles and Masters 2000). The nine factors represented the dependent variable set in the analysis. The four categories for body mass index (BMI units in kg m^{-2}), where weight is divided by height squared were based on American College of Sports Medicine (2010) criteria where underweight (<18.5), normal (18.5–24.9), overweight (25.0–29.9) and obese (>30.0) scores. The additional obesity class categories of I (30–34.9), II (35.0–39.9) and III (>40.0) were not applied. The BMI categories were the independent nominal level variables used in the ANOVA using SPSS Statistics version 22 software.

9.2.2 Statistical Analysis

The research design was a cross-sectional non experimental design using a cohort of athletes who competed at the 2009 World Masters Games, Sydney Australia. Cross tabulations were applied to assess the frequency distribution for the four BMI categories with gender. Mean and standard deviation for participant motivation factor scores by gender were calculated to assess trends. One-way ANOVAs were conducted on each of the nine factors by BMI factor using gender separately in the analyses. A two-way ANOVA with gender and BMI category had insufficient cell counts for an adequate solution and was not applied. The effect sizes eta^2 or η^2 were calculated for the ANOVA solutions where .01 is considered small, .06 medium and .14 large (Cohen 1988). Post hoc tests included least significant difference (LSD), Scheffe and Tamhane's T^2 (unequal variance).

9.3 Results

Table 9.1 displaying the cross tabulations were applied to assess the frequency distribution for the four BMI categories with gender to understand the frequency distribution of the sample. There were significant different (Chi-square = 177.5, $df = 3$, $p < .001$).

Table 9.2 indicates the general differences in participant motivation factors of health orientation, weight concern, personal goal achievement, competition, recognition, affiliation, psychological coping, life meaning and self-esteem for male and female athletes.

Table 9.1 Frequency distribution for gender with BMI category

WMG data	Classification			
	Underweight	Normal	Overweight	Obese
Male	11	1317	1399	430
Female	44	1656	879	347
Total	55	2973	2278	777

American College of Sports Medicine (2010) criteria for BMI Scores
Underweight (<18.5)
Normal (18.5–24.9)
Overweight (25.0–29.9)
Obese (>30.0)

Table 9.2 Mean and standard deviation for participant motivation factors and gender

Participant motivation factor	Gender	Mean	SD
Weight concern	Male	3.86	1.39
	Female	3.93	1.48
Competition	Male	4.06	1.45
	Female	3.57	1.45
Health orientation	Male	4.79	1.50
	Female	4.79	1.51
Goal achievement	Male	4.89	1.45
	Female	4.71	1.52
Recognition	Male	2.84	1.49
	Female	2.61	1.45
Affiliation	Male	4.37	1.42
	Female	4.84	1.40
Psychological coping	Male	2.74	1.45
	Female	2.79	1.50
Life meaning	Male	3.02	1.50
	Female	3.06	1.53
Self-esteem	Male	3.86	1.44
	Female	3.97	1.50

The results indicated some paradoxical effects. For male athletes significant differences ($p < .001$) were identified for BMI category with health orientation, weight concern, personal goal achievement, competition, affiliation, life meaning and self-esteem, although eta^2 values were small (η^2 values .002–.020). No significant differences occurred for recognition or psychological coping. The post hoc analyses (LSD, Scheffe and Tamhane's T^2) indicated weight concern was identified as a moderate motivation factor for overweight and obese athletes, competition as a high motivator for underweight athletes, health orientation as moderate for normal BMI values, goal achievement as very high for underweight athletes, affiliation as moderate for obese athletes, life meaning low for most BMI categories and self-esteem marginally important for overweight athletes. The ANOVA output for participant motivation factors, F ratio and significance for males are displayed in Table 9.3 using BMI category as independent variable.

For female athletes significant differences ($p < .001$) were identified for BMI category with health orientation, weight concern, personal goal achievement, competition, affiliation and self-esteem, although eta^2 values were small (η^2 values .001–.017). No significant differences occurred for recognition, life meaning or psychological coping. Weight concern was identified as a moderate motivation factor for overweight and obese athletes, competition as a moderate motivator for normal BMI athletes, health orientation as moderate for normal BMI values, goal achievement as high for underweight athletes, affiliation as high for obese athletes and self-esteem marginally important for underweight and normal BMI athletes. The ANOVA output for participant motivation factors, *F* ratio and significance for males are displayed in Table 9.4 using BMI category as independent variable.

Tables 9.5 and 9.6 indicate the means and standard deviations for male and female athletes based on the four BMI categories: the independent variable and the nine participant motivation factors as the dependent variables in the nine one-way ANOVA analyses. To reiterate the total scale for each factor is a seven point Likert scale where 1 represents not an important reason to 7 a most important reason.

Table 9.3 ANOVA output for participant motivation factors, *F* ratio and significance for males using BMI as independent variable

Factor	*F* ratio	Significance
Weight concern	16.209	<.000
Competition	5.778	.001
Health orientation	16.047	<.000
Goal achievement	13.478	<.000
Recognition	1.480	.218
Affiliation	3.865	.009
Psychological coping	1.415	.236
Life meaning	5.853	.001
Self-esteem	6.107	<.000

Table 9.4 ANOVA output for participant motivation factors, *F* ratio and significance for females using BMI as independent variable

Factor	*F* ratio	Significance
Weight concern	6.894	<.000
Competition	4.142	.006
Health orientation	6.439	<.000
Goal achievement	13.293	<.000
Recognition	.194	.900
Affiliation	2.691	.045
Psychological coping	.464	.707
Life meaning	1.215	.303
Self-esteem	3.619	.013

Table 9.5 Means and standard deviations for the BMI category with each participant motivation factor for male athletes

BMI category		Weight concern	Competition	Health orientation	Goal achievement	Recognition	Affiliation	Psychological coping	Life meaning	Self-esteem
Underweight	Mean	2.96	5.09	4.00	6.18	2.31	4.07	2.68	2.89	3.54
	SD	1.36	1.12	2.27	.96	1.83	2.10	2.05	2.30	2.25
Normal	Mean	3.66	4.17	4.93	5.07	2.92	4.26	2.82	3.15	3.99
	SD	1.30	1.44	1.43	1.41	1.50	1.42	1.49	1.53	1.44
Overweight	Mean	4.06	4.00	4.83	4.81	2.81	4.42	2.71	2.99	3.82
	SD	1.401	1.47	1.49	1.46	1.40	1.41	1.42	1.46	1.42
Obese	Mean	3.89	3.88	4.30	4.58	2.79	4.52	2.67	2.76	3.62
	SD	1.48	1.38	1.62	1.47	1.47	1.42	1.43	1.46	1.46

Table 9.6 Means and standard deviations for the BMI category with each participant motivation factor for female athletes

BMI category		Weight concern	Competition	Health orientation	Goal achievement	Recognition	Affiliation	Psychological coping	Life meaning	Self-esteem
Underweight	Mean	3.19	3.71	4.61	5.17	2.77	4.59	2.74	3.05	4.12
	SD	1.20	1.56	1.50	1.38	1.63	1.54	1.55	1.79	1.54
Normal	Mean	3.87	3.64	4.91	4.86	2.61	4.80	2.80	3.09	4.05
	SD	1.41	1.44	1.44	1.41	1.43	1.42	1.47	1.51	1.47
Overweight	Mean	4.09	3.48	4.71	4.54	2.60	4.86	2.73	2.98	3.85
	SD	1.53	1.46	1.54	1.51	1.45	1.37	1.47	1.49	1.47
Obese	Mean	3.94	3.36	4.51	4.35	2.59	5.04	2.83	2.94	3.83
	SD	1.58	1.40	1.63	1.57	1.48	1.29	1.59	1.55	1.56

Table 9.7 Male and female comparison for BMI category with participant motivation factor

Factor	Male	Female
Weight concern	Moderate motivator for overweight and obese athletes	Moderate motivator for overweight and obese athletes
Competition	High motivator for underweight athletes	Moderate for normal BMI athletes
Health orientation	Moderate for normal BMI values	Moderate for normal BMI values
Goal achievement	Very high for underweight athletes	High for underweight athletes
Recognition	ns	ns
Affiliation	Moderate for obese athletes	High for obese athletes
Psychological coping	ns	ns
Life meaning	Low for most BMI categories	ns
Self-esteem	Marginally important for overweight athletes	Marginally important for underweight and normal BMI values

Table 9.7 indicates the male and female comparisons for BMI category with participant motivation factor based on post hoc tests. It can be observed that weight concern, health orientation, goal achievement, affiliation show similar trends across both genders in terms of BMI category and level of motivation.

The same situation is relevant to recognition and psychological coping which were not related to BMI category for both genders. In terms of completion is serves at a high motivator for underweight males and a moderate motivator for normal BMI females, whereas self-esteem is marginally important for overweight males and underweight and normal BMI females.

These results indicate some complexity in terms of specific responses for the nine participant factors of health orientation, weight concern, personal goal achievement, competition, recognition, affiliation, psychological coping, life meaning and self-esteem.

9.4 Discussion

Although effect sizes were categorized as small, however, statistically significant differences were observed for both genders for BMI categories with the nine participant motivation. Both genders displayed health orientation, weight concern, personal goal achievement, competition, affiliation and self-esteem as sources of difference interacting with four BMI categories from marginal, moderate to large importance. In males, competition was a high motivator and goal achievement was a very high motivator for underweight athletes. In females goal achievement was high for underweight athletes and affiliation as high for obese athletes. It is important to highlight that participant motivation in terms of rccognition or psychological coping in males and recognition, life meaning or psychological coping in females were not differentiated by BMI category. The findings indicate that complex interactions occur between gender and the four BMI categories and the nine participant motivation factors evaluated in this study.

As a consequence of these findings marketing and encouraging athlete participation at international level masters competitions to different genders and interacting with the different BMI categories and linked to participant motivation profiles based on BMI will require more complex sport psychological marketing strategies as follows:

1. Strategies relevant to both genders should focus on weight concern issues for overweight and obese athletes, health orientation for normal BMI athletes, goal achievement for underweight athletes and affiliation for obese athletes.
2. In the context of gender specific strategies focus on competition for underweight males and for normal BMI females, life meaning for most BMI categories in males with no distinction for females and self-esteem for overweight males and underweight and normal BMI females.
3. Life meaning and psychological coping were not differentiated by BMI categories and were not identified as important factors for motivating both genders at this level of competition.

9.5 Conclusion

These findings based on a large cohort of male and female athletes competing at the 2009 World Masters Games suggest that BMI categories interaction with gender and influence participation motivation responses that subsequently influence participation in international masters sport competitions.

References

American College of Sports Medicine. (2010). *ACSM' guidelines for exercise testing and prescription* (8th ed.). Alphen aan den Rijn: Wolters Kluwer Health.

Anderson, V. E. (2006). *Utility of health belief model constructs in predicting dietary behaviors among female university students: A pilot investigation*. Electronic Theses & Dissertations. Paper 629.

Caperchione, C. M., Duncan, M. J., Mummery, K., Steele, R., & Schofield, G. (2008). Mediating relationship between body mass index and the direct measures of the Theory of Planned Behaviour on physical activity intention. *Psychology, Health and Medicine, 13*(2), 168–179.

Cohen, J. (1988). *Statistical power analysis for the behavioral sciences* (2nd ed.). Hillsdale, NJ: Erlbaum.

Heazlewood, I. T., Walsh, J., Climstein, M., Burke, S., Kettunen, J., Adams, K. J., et al. (2011). Sport psychological constructs related to participation in the 2009 World Masters Games. *World Academy of Science, Engineering and Technology, 7*, 2027–2032.

Heazlewood, I. T., Walsh, J., Climstein, M., Burke, S., Kettunen, J., Adams, K. J., et al. (2012). Athlete motivations to participate in the 2010 Pan Pacific Masters Games. In: *ICSEMIS 2012 Pre-olympic conference: sport inspiring a learning legacy*. 19–24 July, 2012 Glasgow, UK.

Heazlewood, I. T., Walsh, J., Climstein, M., Burke, S., Kettunen, J., Adams, K. J., et al. (2015). Participant motivation: A comparison of male and female athletes competing at the 2009 World Masters Games. In: *Conference proceedings of the 2015 Asian congress of applied psychology (ACAP 2015): Applied Psychology* 19 and 20 May 2015, Holiday Inn-Concorde Hotel, Singapore. Applied Psychology: 291–297. doi:10.1142/9789814723398_0016.

Marcus, B. H., & Forsyth, L. A. (2009). *Motivating people to be physically active* (2nd ed.). Champaign, IL: Human Kinetics.

Masters, K. S., Ogles, B. M., & Jolton, J. A. (1993). The development of an instrument to measure motivation for marathon running: The motivations of marathoners scales (MOMS). *Research Quarterly for Exercise and Sport, 64*(2), 134–143.

Ogles, B. M., & Masters, K. S. (2000). Older versus younger adult male marathon runners: Participative motives and training habits. *Journal of Sport Behavior, 23*(3), 1–14.

Shen, B. & Xu, C. (2007). Effects of self-efficacy, body mass, and Cardio respiratory fitness on exercise motives in Chinese college students. *Journal of Physical Activity and Health, 5*(5), 706–718.

Sicilia, A., Sáenz-Alvarez, P., González-Cutre, D., & Ferriz, R. (2014). Exercise motivation and social physique anxiety in adolescents. *Psychologica Belgica, 54*(1), 111–129. doi:10.5334/pb.ai.

Chapter 10
Participant Motivation Predicting Training Sessions and Training Type in Male and Female Athletes Competing at 2010 Pan Pacific Masters Games

I.T. Heazlewood, J. Walsh, M. Climstein, K. Adams, T. Sevene and Mark DeBeliso

Abstract Participant motivation evaluates those factors that enhance or inhibit motivation to participate and is represented by factors as health orientation, weight concern/weight loss, and personal goal achievement. The research aim was to evaluate the relationship between participant motivation predicting the quantity of training and training types completed by male and female athletes. The total weekly session in males were predicted by goal achievement and affiliation, whereas in females the predictor set was goal achievement, affiliation, health orientation, and psychological coping.

Keywords Participant · Motivation · Masters athletes · Gender

---

I.T. Heazlewood (✉) · J. Walsh
School of Psychological and Clinical Science, Charles Darwin University, Darwin, NT 0909, Australia
e-mail: ian.heazlewood@cdu.edu.au

M. Climstein
Exercise, Health and Performance Faculty Research Group, University of Sydney, Sydney, NSW 2006, Australia
e-mail: mike.climstein@sydney.edu.au

K. Adams · T. Sevene
Kinesiology Department, California State University, 100 Campus Center, Valley Hall, Seaside, CA 93955-800, USA
e-mail: kadams@csumb.edu

M. DeBeliso
College of Education and Human Development, Southern Utah University, 351 W. University Blvd., Cedar City, UT 84720, USA
e-mail: markdebeliso@suu.edu

M.-T. Leung and A.L.M. Tan (eds.), *Applied Psychology Readings*,
DOI 10.1007/978-981-10-2796-3_10

10.1 Introduction

10.1.1 Participant Motivation

Motivation is defined as "the directions and intensity of one's effort" and is a significant factor in the selection of exercise and sport. Participant motivation evaluates those factors that enhance or inhibit motivation to participate and is represented by factors as health orientation, weight concern/weight loss, and personal goal achievement (Masters et al. 1993; Marcus and Forsyth 2009). These motivating factors are identified to influence the quantity of physical activity in people. Some research has been conducted on participant motivation factors displayed by 2009 World Masters Games (WMG) athletes based on issues of gender and comparisons between different international competition cohorts (Heazlewood et al. 2011a, b, 2012, 2015).

Factors such as human exercise physiology, motor skill learning, sports biomechanics, and kinathropometry sets to limits on overt human motor performance; however, exercise and sport psychology in the context of motivation will assist in reaching these limits, especially via the construct of participant motivation. It is easy for athletes to underperform and very difficult for athletes to over perform in all sports situations, and commitment in training and competition are very dependent on an athlete's level of motivation. The construct of participant motivation evaluates those factors that enhance or impede motivation to participate in sport and are represented by such factors as health orientation, weight concern/weight loss, and personal goal achievement (Masters et al. 1993; Marcus and Forsyth 2009; Weinberg and Gould 2011).

Previous research based on international level competition at the World Masters Games and Pan Pacific Masters Games levels identified multiple factors in master's athletes to be significant in motivating their participation and adherence to sport. These factors included type of sport, gender, age, and intrinsic versus extrinsic motivation (Heazlewood et al. 2011a, b, 2012, 2015; Ogles and Masters 2000). The most significant factors promoting participation with WMG masters athletes were the socializing environment of sport, getting physically fit and improving competitive personal best performances. Both male and female athletes at the 2009 World Masters Games displayed similar participant motivations factors, such as goal achievement, health orientation, and affiliation as the most important factors. The discriminant function analysis indicated in terms of differences between male and females athletes affiliation, and competition were the most significant discriminators with females having higher affiliation scores than males, whereas males displayed higher competition scores and suggests some slight underpinning differences motivating them to compete at this level (Heazlewood et al. 2015). Strategies to increase participation in masters sport should focus on these factors as other factors such as weight loss, improving mental health, and living longer were not identified as important determinates of sports participation at the World

Masters level. However, the relationship between training frequency and training type linked to participant motivation at this point in time has not been explored fully. What strategies should be applied to motivate athletes to train in terms of frequency and training type should be evaluated to asses if any trend exist between the different dimensions of participant motivation and the different constructs of training frequency and type to develop effective psychological strategies to enhance training motivation.

10.1.2 Research Aim

The research aim was to evaluate the relationship between participant motivation factors of health orientation, weight concern, personal goal achievement, competition, recognition, affiliation, psychological coping, life meaning, and self-esteem and predict the quantity of training and training types completed by athletes prior to competing in the 2010 Pan Pacific Masters Games.

10.2 Methods

10.2.1 Research Design

The research design was action research integrated with correlation and regression analysis. Action research is conducted in the context or setting where the research outcomes will be applied. In this context, to masters athletes with an interest in competing in an international level competitions, the correlation analysis will serve as the initial starting point to evaluate the relationship between the participant motivation factors of health orientation, weight concern, personal goal achievement, competition, recognition, affiliation, psychological coping, life meaning, and self-esteem with training factors of total training sessions, aerobic sessions, resistance sessions, and anaerobic sessions per week. The regression analysis will follow correlation analysis if the relationships between participant motivation factors and training factors are substantive. If substantive, it is hypothesized that the regression models and relevant regression equations will predict training session frequency and training type, the dependent variables, by the participant motivation factors, the independent variables.

10.2.2 Sample and Instruments

The study was approved by a university human research ethics committee. Male and female athletes competing at the 2010 Pan Pacific Masters Games, Gold

Coast, Australia volunteered to participate in the research project (male; $n = 739$; mean age = 50.82; SD = 9.4 and female; $n = 851$; mean age = 47.63; SD = 8.4). Athletes completed an online survey using the Limesurveytm interactive survey system where they responded to a 56 item sport psychological instrument, the Motivations of Marathoners Scale (MOMS) with a 7-point Likert scale response to each item. The range was 1 = least important to 7 = most important reason. The MOMS instrument focused on nine participant motivation factors related to health orientation, weight concern, personal goal achievement, competition, recognition, affiliation, psychological coping, life meaning, and self-esteem. The MOMS instrument has been subjected to reliability and validity analysis displays high internal consistency (Cronbach alpha range .80–.93), good test–retest reliability (intraclass correlations, R range .71–.90), factor validity, construct validity, convergent validity, and discriminant validity (Masters et al. 1993; Ogles and Masters 2000). The training was quantified based on the self-reports of the athletes within the survey total using number of training sessions, aerobic sessions, resistance sessions, and anaerobic sessions per week.

10.2.3 Statistical Analysis

Statistical analysis compared training session differences between gender using independent t tests, Pearson bivariate correlation to explore any relationships between training sessions and type with the nine participant motivation factors and finally stepwise multiple linear regression with the participant motivation factors as the predictor variables and training frequency and type as the dependent variables and using SPSS Statistics version 22 software.

10.3 Results

10.3.1 Descriptive Statistics

The descriptive statistics for male and female athletes are displayed in Table 10.1 for age, training sessions and type and for the nine participant motivation factors. The independent t test analyses are displayed in Table 10.2. Based on training frequency and type there was no difference in total sessions per week (male = 3.97/week; females = 4.04/week), aerobic training (male = 3.51/week; females = 3.26/week), anaerobic training (male = 2.63/week; females = 2.63/week). The only significant difference occurred in resistance training (male = 3.24/week; females = 2.49/week; $p < .001$) (Table 10.3). The correlation analysis for both male and females athletes are displayed in Tables 10.4 and 10.5.

Table 10.1 The descriptive statistics for male and female athletes for age, training session, frequency, and type and the nine participant motivation factors

Variable	Female mean	SD	Male mean	SD
Age (years)	47.63	8.41	50.82	9.38
Days/week training for Pan Pacific Masters	4.04	1.70	3.97	1.68
Sessions/week resistance training	2.49	1.67	3.24	2.84
Sessions/week aerobic training	3.26	1.99	3.51	2.33
Sessions/week anaerobic training	2.63	1.34	2.93	2.20
Psychological coping	2.62	1.42	2.62	1.42
Self-esteem	3.76	1.47	3.76	1.47
Life meaning	2.75	1.48	2.72	1.53
Health orientation	4.57	1.60	4.36	1.66
Weight concern	3.53	1.71	3.35	1.67
Affiliation	4.87	1.36	4.55	1.38
Recognition	2.40	1.42	2.68	1.45
Competition	3.27	1.39	3.75	1.44
Goal achievement	4.31	1.56	4.34	1.62

Table 10.2 Independent *t* test for mean, standard deviation, and standard error of the mean

Training sessions and type	Sex of athlete	*N*	Mean	Std. deviation	Std. error mean
Days/week training	Female	830	4.04	1.70	.059
	Male	712	3.97	1.68	.063
Sessions/week resistance training	Female	266	2.49	1.67	.103
	Male	229	3.24	2.84	.188
Sessions/week aerobic training	Female	590	3.26	1.99	.082
	Male	472	3.51	2.33	.108
Sessions/week anaerobic training	Female	196	2.63	1.34	.096
	Male	173	2.93	2.20	.168

Table 10.3 Independent *t* tests for training sessions and type of training

Training sessions and type of training	*t*	*df*	Sign.
Days/week training			
Equal variances assumed	.751	1540	.453
Equal variances not assumed	.752	1510.148	.452
Sessions/week resistance training			
Equal variances assumed	−3.610	493	.000
Equal variances not assumed	−3.482	357.121	.001
Sessions/week aerobic training			
Equal variances assumed	−1.870	1060	.062
Equal variances not assumed	−1.838	927.683	.066
Sessions/week anaerobic training			
Equal variances assumed	−1.589	367	.113
Equal variances not assumed	−1.544	276.970	.124

Table 10.4 Correlations for male athletes for training sessions and type and the nine participant motivation factors

Training type	Psychological coping	Self-esteem	Life meaning	Health orientation	Weight concern	Affiliation	Recognition	Competition	Goal achievement
Days/week training	.061	.156**	.106**	.267**	.144**	−.147**	.050	.133**	.295**
	.144	.000	.010	.000	000	.000	.230	.001	.000
Session/week resistance training	.046	.094	.074	.194**	.093	−.009	−.004	.076	.138
	.532	.213	.308	.006	.192	.907	.955	.294	.058
Session/week aerobic	.012	−.034	.018	.110*	.029	−.089	.055	.078	.118*
	.812	.493	.706	.021	.542	.063	.255	.098	.013
Session/week anaerobic	.005	−.066	.029	.165*	.051	−.099	.019	.083	−.003
	.949	.440	.729	.048	.542	.234	.817	.320	.971

Table 10.5 Correlations for female athletes for training sessions and type and the nine participant motivation factors

Training type	Psychological coping	Self-esteem	Life meaning	Health orientation	Weight concern	Affiliation	Recognition	Competition	Goal achievement
Days/week training	.091*	.170**	.148**	.227**	.177**	−.044**	.066	.195**	.320**
	.046	.000	.001	.000	.000	.324	.145	.000	.000
Session/week resistance training	No significant correlations								
Session/week aerobic training	No significant correlations								
Session/week anaerobic training	No significant correlations								

10.3.2 Correlations

Days per week training in males were correlated from highest to lowest correlations with gaol achievement, health orientation, competition, weight concern, self-esteem, life meaning, and psychological coping ($r = .320–.091$, $p < .001–.046$). It is interesting to note that none of the participant motivations factors were correlated training sessions per week for resistance, aerobic, or anaerobic training. It is important to note the coefficient of determination or common variance between variables is small for most of these correlations.

Days per week training in females had significant correlations from highest to lowest correlations with goal achievement, health orientation, self-esteem, affiliation, weight concern, competition, and life meaning ($r = .295–.106$, $p < .001–.01$). Sessions per week for resistance training correlated only with health orientation ($r = .194$, $p = .006$). Session per week or aerobic training correlated with goal achievement ($r = .118$, $p = .013$) and health orientation ($r = .110$, $p = .021$). Sessions per week of anaerobic training was only correlated with health orientation ($r = .165$, $p = .048$).

The regression solutions for males indicated total sessions per week were predicted by goal achievement step 1 and affiliation step 2 ($R = .338$, $R^2 = .114$, effect size $f2 = .13$, $p < .001$). Resistance, aerobic, and anaerobic training sessions per week were not predicted by any of the participant motivation factors.

The regression solutions for females indicated total sessions per week were predicted by goal achievement step 1, affiliation step 2, health orientation step 3, and psychological coping step 4 ($R = .422$, $R^2 = .178$, effect size $f2 = .22$, $p < .001$). Resistance training session per week were marginally predicted by health orientation ($R = .187$, $R^2 = .035$, effect size $f2 = .04$, $p = .023$). Aerobic training session per week were marginally predicted by affiliation step 1 and goal achievement step 2 ($R = .185$, $R^2 = .034$, effect size $f2 = .035$, $p = .003$). Anaerobic training session per week were marginally predicted by health orientation step 1 ($R = .194$, $R^2 = .038$, effect size $f2 = .035$, $p = .039$). Cohen's $f2$ effect size for multiple regression are considered small at 0.02, medium at 0.15, and large at values greater than 0.35. The values for total training sessions per week represent moderate values and some explanatory power for female athletes and which was not the case for male athletes where most relationships displayed small and essentially nonexplanatory values (Tables 10.6, 10.7).

Table 10.6 Regression solutions for males

Model	R	R^2	Adjusted R^2	Change statistics				
				R^2 change	F change	$df1$	$df2$	Sig. F change
1	.310[a]	.096	.094	.096	40.505	1	382	.000
2	.338[b]	.114	.109	.018	7.758	1	381	.006

[a]Predictors: (constant), goal achievement
[b]Predictors: (constant), goal achievement, affiliation

Table 10.7 Regression solutions for females

Model	R	R^2	Adjusted R^2	Change statistics				
				R^2 change	F change	$df1$	$df2$	Sig. F change
1	.295[a]	.087	.085	.087	43.216	1	452	.000
2	.395[b]	.156	.152	.068	36.542	1	451	.000
3	.406[c]	.165	.159	.009	4.924	1	450	.027
4	.422[d]	.178	.171	.013	7.274	1	449	.007

[a]Predictors: (constant), goal achievement
[b]Predictors: (constant), goal achievement, affiliation
[c]Predictors: (constant), goal achievement, affiliation, health orientation
[d]Predictors: (constant), goal achievement, affiliation, health orient, psychological coping

10.4 Discussion

Total training session per week based on gender were not statistically different; however, participant motivation factors predicting the weekly sessions based on gender were different. The total weekly session in males were predicted by goal achievement and affiliation, whereas in females the predictor set was goal achievement, affiliation, health orientation, and psychological coping. It is important to highlight the first two factors in the models were goal achievement and affiliation. Cohen's *f2* effect sizes were moderate and indicated some participant motivation factors were partially predictive of training session behavior.

With male athletes' type of training session frequencies as resistance, aerobic, and anaerobic training were not predicted by participant motivation factors, suggesting minimal causation. Females displayed different responses where training type session frequency where resistance and anaerobic training were predicted by health orientation and aerobic training by affiliation then goal achievement. These results suggest at the level of total training sessions per week male and female master's athletes were influenced similarly by goal achievement and affiliation, whereas at the level of individual training type females were more influenced by participant motivation factors than males.

Multiple theories have been presented to promote physical activity such a learning theory, decision making theory, behavioral choice theory, social cognitive theory, ecological models, and relapse prevention models; motivational readiness and stages of change theory (Marcus and Forsyth 2009) and the degree of overlap of these theories with participant motivation may provide some insights into engaging masters athletes with physical training.

Learning theory and social cognitive theory emphasis goal setting which aligns with goal achievement in this study, whereas affiliation aligns with social support constructs in social cognitive theory. Decisional balance theory aligns with health orientation and psychological coping redecisional balance sheet outcomes, enhancing benefits such as better health outcomes. This indicates that learning theory and social cognitive theory are relevant to both male and female athletes as indicate and partial predictors of training frequency and in the case of female athletes training type. The additional predictors of health orientation and psychological coping in female athletes represent added dimensions when attempting to promote participation in sport with this international level cohort.

10.5 Conclusion

These links of training with participant motivation factors in male and female international competing masters athletes may serve as an important areas of applied sport psychological focus to enhance the quantity of and type physical activity to achieve health and performance related physical activity levels in this cohort.

References

Heazlewood, I. T., Walsh, J., Climstein, M., Burke, S., Kettunen, J., Adams, K. J., et al. (2011a). Motivation to participate in sport at the Sydney 2009 World Masters Games. *Medicine and Science in Sports and Exercise, 43*(5), S655.

Heazlewood, I. T., Walsh, J., Climstein, M., Burke, S., Kettunen, J., Adams, K. J., et al. (2011b). Sport psychological constructs related to participation in the 2009 World Masters Games. *World Academy of Science, Engineering and Technology, 7*, 2027–2032.

Heazlewood, I. T., Walsh, J., Climstein, M., Burke, S., Kettunen, J., Adams, K. J., & DeBeliso, M. (2012). Athlete motivations to participate in the 2010 Pan Pacific Masters Games. In *ICSEMIS 2012 Pre-Olympic Conference: Sport Inspiring a Learning Legacy*, vol. 4. 19–24 July, 2012 Glasgow, UK.

Heazlewood, I. T., Walsh, J., Climstein, M., Burke, S., Kettunen, J., Adams, K. J., & DeBeliso, M. (2015). Participant motivation: A comparison of male and female athletes competing at the 2009 World Masters Games. In *Conference Proceedings of the 2015 Asian Congress of Applied Psychology (ACAP 2015): Applied Psychology* 19 and 20 May 2015, Holiday Inn-Concorde Hotel, Singapore. Applied Psychology: 291–297. doi:10.1142/9789814723398_0016.

Marcus, B. H., & Forsyth, L. A. (2009). *Motivating people to be physically active* (2nd ed.). Champaign, IL: Human Kinetics.

Masters, K. S., Ogles, B. M., & Jolton, J. A. (1993). The development of an instrument to measure motivation for marathon running: The Motivations of Marathoners Scale (MOMS). *Research Quarterly for Exercise and Sport, 64*, 134–143.

Ogles, B. M., & Masters, K. S. (2000). Older versus younger adult male marathon runners: Participative motives and training habits. *Journal of Sport Behavior, 23*(3), 1–14.

Weinberg, R. S., & Gould, D. (2011). *Foundations of sport and exercise psychology*. Leeds: Human Kinetics.

Chapter 11
The Structural Relationships Between Foreign Language Speaking Anxiety, Perceived English Competence, English Learning Motivation, Willingness to Communicate, English Learning Engagement and Motivational Intensity in Hong Kong Secondary Students

Wai Sum Chung and Man-Tak Leung

Abstract This study recruited 305 participants (237 females and 68 males) to complete a survey consisting of six scales in examining the structural relationships among English learning motivation, foreign language speaking anxiety, perceived English competence, willingness to communicate, English learning engagement, and motivational intensity in Hong Kong secondary students. First, English learning motivation (integrative, instrumental) negatively predicts foreign language speaking anxiety, which acts as a mediator between learning motivation and willingness to communicate (speak, read, write, and listen). Second, perceived English competence, which is also a significant mediator between learning motivation and willingness to communicate (speak, read, write, listen), could be predicted positively by learning motivation. This paper might be the first to investigate on the relationships between these constructs within the context of Hong Kong. It serves as a preliminary study to explore the casual relationships of HK secondary students' psychological aspects in second language acquisition, while validating the instruments to be used in HK. On the pedagogical level, educators could understand the effects of students' motivational orientations and eventually facilitate English learning through altering students' affective factors.

W.S. Chung (✉) · M.-T. Leung
Department of Counselling of Psychology, Shue Yan University, Hong Kong, North Point, Hong Kong
e-mail: wilsonchung1@yahoo.com.hk
URL: http://www.hksyu.edu

M.-T. Leung
e-mail: mtleung@hksyu.edu

M.-T. Leung and L.-M. Tan (eds.), *Applied Psychology Readings*,
DOI 10.1007/978-981-10-2796-3_11

Keywords L2 acquisition · ESL/EFL · English learning motivation · Foreign language anxiety · Perceived competence · Willingness to communicate

11.1 Introduction

Due to globalization, people are depending more on English as a medium for communication (Montgomery and Spalding 2005; Tsai 2012). The amount of people learning English as a second or foreign language (ESL/EFL) far exceeds native speakers (Zheng 2010). Also there is an increasing trend to teach younger students English worldwide (Butler 2014; Knell and Chi 2012). In Hong Kong, English has been a compulsory subject since primary school and the use of English spans across government, business, academic sectors, and daily lives. To better prepare students in adapting to the highly competitive society, a thorough understanding of factors influencing English acquisition is necessary.

11.2 Literature Review

11.2.1 Foreign Language Anxiety

Horwitz et al. (1986) noticed that about one-third of students experience significant anxiety when studying foreign languages (Luo 2012). Campbell and Ortiz (1991) also found that half of the L2 learners in university exhibit intense language anxiety. The apprehension is not limited to English but also other foreign languages; and it is found among secondary schools, colleges, and universities (Montgomery and Spalding 2005). It may seem obvious that foreign language anxiety (FLA) encumbers L2 acquisition;, but intriguingly, positive, negative, and neutral relationships could be found (Sultan 2012; Onwuegbuzie et al. 1999). Also FLA leads to or is provoked by poor L2 acquisition depending on individual characteristics, and the degree varies across different cultures (Horwitz 2001).

However, dominant researches do agree that FLA leads to negative language performance (Liu 2013). Saito et al. (1999) also revealed that students learning Japanese as a second language exhibit highest levels of anxiety, followed by French and Russian. Recently, the study of FLA has grown even more precise and systematic, as Marcos-Llinás and Garau (2009) identified behavioral, cognitive, psycholinguistic, physical, and sociolinguistic variables as the five types of factors in relation with FLA.

Besides learning outcome, FLA is found to be related with perceived English competence (Sultan 2012), learning motivation (MacIntyre and Gardner 1991), and even perseverance (Montgomery and Spalding 2005), risk-taking behavior (Sultan 2012), learning strategies (Onwuegbuzie et al. 1999), and self-concept (Krashen 1980; Sultan 2012; Xu and Gao 2014). Sultan (2012), for example, stated that there is a negative connection between FLA, motivation, goals, perceived competence besides achievement.

11.2.2 Foreign Language Speaking Anxiety

Woodrow (2006) pointed out that communicating with teachers and reading in front of the class both contribute to speaking anxiety. In specific, activities such as oral-presentations, role-play, formal discussions, and answering questions in English are main factors for students to be anxious (Kayaoglu and Saglamel 2013). Horwitz (2000) noticed that while some students experience anxiety in any foreign language classes, other students may be prone to feeling anxious in situations, where only one particular language skill (speaking, for instance) is emphasized. In China, students found self-expression (speaking and writing) much harder than comprehension (listening and reading); while speaking is considered the most difficult English skill (Peng 2014). Mak (2011) mentioned that Western education stresses on self-expression while Chinese students tend to be inhibiting, especially in L2 lessons. On the other hand, Peng (2014) argued that the fear of speaking English is more related with skill deficiency, rather than cultural factors. In the context of Hong Kong, students' insufficient opportunity to practice speaking English constitutes to their speaking anxiety, which is further intensified by the pressure of public oral exams (Mak 2011).

Among the various aspects of foreign language anxiety, communication apprehension is most anxiety-provoking (Kriangkrai and Siriluck 2012). For example, Kim (2009) found that speaking classes induce higher anxiety than reading classes. Horwitz (2000) assumed that in various aspects of L2 acquisition, speaking provokes the most anxiety and is reflected on anxiety scales dominated by items concerning the speaking situation. As a major component of foreign language anxiety, FLSA is found to significantly hinder L2 performance. Gai and Yang (2010) pointed out that when students have high speaking anxiety, their performance on spoken English will be weaker.

11.2.3 Perceived English Competence

Students' perceived competence has been recognized as a key in predicting academic roles, achievement, and particularly fluency in L2 acquisition (Sultan 2012). As Cocks and Watt (2004) stated, students' beliefs of their values are the most proximal predictors of achievement, especially for Maths and English (Marsh and Yeung 1998). Daley et al. (1997) pointed out that students whose expectations for their language abilities are low usually perform worse. Also Harter (1999) stated that perceived competence influences affective domains, which then affects students' motivational orientation. To illustrate, a student will be more willing to learn English if he likes it because of his high perceived competence in English (Cocks and Watt 2004). On the other hand, a student who has low perceived competence is less likely to perform satisfactorily, as well as to seek ways in improving his weakness (Machr 1984). Keying on this point, Liu (2013) found that perceived competence is stronger than actual competence in predicting language proficiency.

11.2.4 Perceived English Competence and Foreign Language Speaking Anxiety

PEC is strongly related with FLA (Capan and Simsek 2012; Sultan 2012). According to Maclntyre (1994), language anxiety might be caused by low perceived communication competence. Similarly, Sultan (2012) stated that students' low perceived language competence escalates anxiety. MacIntyre et al. (1997) found that anxious students tend to underestimate their language abilities, where the reverse situation is also true. Thus, PEC and FLA are negatively related in L2 acquisition (Knell and Chi 2012; Sultan 2012). Congruent to these studies, Liu (2013) stated that perceived competence plays a significant role in influencing FLA and language achievement.

It is observed that the significance of FLA grows in time and becomes rigid, when students keep experiencing anxiety in foreign language classrooms (Kim 2009). Keying on this argument, researchers point out that it is students' sense of uncontrollability towards foreign language classrooms that results in FLA (Capan and Simsek 2012). In other words, FLA is correlated with students' perceived competence. A student believing that his English ability is not up to standard within an English classroom (whether at beginning or advanced level) will experience high anxiety (Horwitz 2001).

Bailey et al. (2000) established the Anxiety-Expectation Mediation (AEM) model, which examines the roles anxiety and perceived competence play in determining foreign language achievement. Both variables mediated the relationships between achievement and other demographic variables. To be precise, the relationships between achievement and variables such as gender and perceived self-identity are mediated by FLA, while the relationships between achievement and other variables such as age and perceived self-identity are moderated by perceived competence (Montgomery and Spalding 2005). Sultan (2012) stated that students' perceived competence determines learning strategies while influencing language anxiety. Liu (2013) took this point further and stated that perceived competence is more predictive than anxiety in determining learning strategies.

Furthermore, PEC has a significant relationship with willingness to communicate, as explained below.

11.2.5 English Learning Motivation

Among various models of second language motivation, Gardner's integrative/instrumental motivation is the most influential theory, despite debates and challenges have never ceased in examining the accuracy and applicability of such motivational theory (Zheng 2010). Dörnyei (1994), for example, believed that instrumental motivation is more practical for foreign language learners. Put it simply, students in China may not have the opportunity to encounter and develop interest (which is the rationale of integrative motivation) in the English culture (Zheng 2010). Also if the difference in students' attitudes regarding public exams is considered, it is not difficult to understand why Chinese students' motivation is so different from western students. As such, another stream of analyzing Gardner's motivation theory is to examine motivation under the scope of English as a foreign language (EFL) and English as a second language (ESL), respectively (Li 2014). However, these so-called "micro-perspectives of L2 motivation" (Zheng 2010) are beyond the scope of this research.

It is worth mentioning that viewing Gardner's motivation theory as integrative and instrumental, respectively, might be over-simplistic. In fact, they are dynamic constructs that change over time (Gardner and MacIntyre 1993). To be precise, Gardner (2001) clarified that both motivational orientations are not independent; rather, they are interactive and even correlated. It is possible for an integratively motivated student to possess and exhibit instrumental motivation in learning foreign language (Zheng 2010).

11.2.6 English Learning Motivation, Foreign Language Speaking Anxiety and Perceived English Competence

Motivation is found to be negatively related with FLA in dominant researches (Capan and Simsek 2012). As aforementioned, researchers confirmed that FLA sabotages ELM after they have recognized FLA as a unique form of anxiety and used unified measuring tools (Horwitz 2001). Besides FLA, it has been argued that the most important determinant of a child's motivation for learning is "the self-as-perceived." In their expectancy value theory of achievement motivation, Eccles and Wigfield (2002) stated that perceived competence influences intrinsic motivation (Cocks and Watt 2004). Perception of competence leads to students' different motivational orientation, hence linguistic confidence has been identified as an important factor (Zheng 2010) in interacting with variables in motivation and anxiety in L2 studies (Clément et al. 1994; Csizer and Dörnyei 2005).

11.2.7 Willingness to Communicate

Recent studies concerning L2 acquisition has been paying attention to students' willingness to communicate (Baker and MacIntyre 2003; Donovan and MacIntyre 2004; MacIntyre et al. 2001), yet willingness to communicate (WTC) is a factor that, untill today, still requires further examination (Wu and Lin 2014). Students who are reluctant to initiate communication (or give responses) in English have negative language outcomes (Knell and Chi 2012). According to MacIntyre (1994), anxiety and perceived competence are both key constructs of predicting willingness to communicate.

11.2.8 Willingness to Communicate, Foreign Language Speaking Anxiety, Perceived English Competence and English Learning Motivation

Available literatures point out that WTC is negatively related to FLA (Baker and Maclntyre 2003; Capan and Simsek 2012). Yashima (2000, 2002) found that FLA leads to lower WTC; while Onwuegbuzie et al. (1999) stated that students are less likely to answer and participate in foreign language classrooms when they experience high FLA. It is clear that students with high FLA tend to avoid expressing themselves in the foreign language (Horwitz et al. 1986), and the reason behind might be due to students' self-defeating thoughts (low perceived competence) that serves as distractions (Knell and Chi 2012; Sultan 2012).

On the other hand, WTC is found to be positively related to motivation and PEC (Hashimoto 2002; Yashima 2002; Wu and Lin 2014). Knell and Chi (2012) stated that Chinese students' WTC and PEC are the strongest predictors of English language proficiency.

Note that students' perceived competence exert a greater effect than actual competence in affecting willingness to communicate (Liu 2013). Those who possesses only average language skills but perceive themselves as more competent might be more willing to initiate conversations than those who own better skills but tend to underestimate themselves. Furthermore, Butler (2007) found that English learners' perceived competence to read English influences their motivation. Interestingly, Maclntyre et al. (2003) found that as students grow older, language learning motivation decreases but willingness to communicate and perceived competence increases.

In MacIntyre and Charos' (1996) study, they proved that WTC is significantly related to success in L2 acquisition, motivation and perceived L2 communication competence. Similar results were found in Baker and MacIntyre's study (2000), which stated that FLA and perceived competence are main predictors of WTC in a foreign language. In other words, students with high motivation in L2 learning are more willing to communicate in the foreign language (Wu and Lin 2014).

11.2.9 English Learning Motivation, Learning Engagement and Motivational Intensity

Motivation is closely associated with engagement (Chen and Kraklow 2015). Learners' engagement has been a focus of numerous educational theories, especially in language learning. Vygotsky, for example, pointed out in his theory of zone of proximal development (ZPD) that when appropriate level of opportunities and support are provided, students will engage in learning activities (Miller 2010). In language learning, studies conducted in elementary schools concerning children's comprehension stated that reading motivation is related to engagement (reading amount and frequency) (De Naeghel et al. 2012). In their study, Becker et al. (2010) found that reading engagement mediated the relationship between reading motivation and literacy. Also studying adult learners' engagement, Beder et al. (2006) noted that engaged learners have both motivation and competence to participate in and achieve targets in class. Furthermore, not only motivation but even persistence in English classes may also be related to engagement, as Schalge and Soga (2008) stated.

Moreover, motivational intensity and instrumental motivation are recognized as significant predictors of English proficiency (Biggs and Telfer 1987). Inspired by Gardner's classical model, Zhou (1996) proposed a motivation model, which is especially designed for Chinese students. He stated that motivation equals the sum of goal, effort and non-English related activities (Gao et al. 2007). Similarly, Wu et al. (1993) highlighted the significance of motivational intensity in language learning, by stating that motivational intensity exerted the most significant influence on L2 proficiency.

11.3 Methods and Designs

11.3.1 Participants

In this study, a total of 350 students will be recruited from 4 secondary schools in Hong Kong. They will be chosen by convenient sampling and each will be distributed a questionnaire composing six instruments. The questionnaire will be distributed by their teachers during class.

11.3.2 Instruments

Public Speaking Class Anxiety Scale The scale is to measure anxiety experienced by students during foreign language speaking classes and is developed by Kriangkrai and Siriluck (2012). It combines and modifies items adapted from earlier foreign language anxiety scales, such as Horwitz et al.'s Foreign Language Classroom Anxiety Scale (1986) and McCroskey's Personal Report of Public Speaking Anxiety (1970).

The PSCAS consists of 17 items and answers are on a five-point Likert scale. The internal reliability of the PSCAS was .84 Cronbach's alpha. The items are translated to Chinese through backward-translation. The sample items are: "I start to panic when I have to speak English without a preparation in advance" and "I am afraid that other students will laugh at me while I am speaking English". Four items (items 4, 8, 10, 12) are negatively coded so their responses are recoded after collection.

Perceived English Competence Scale The scale is adopted from Knell and Chi's (2012) study and 10 items are extracted to measure students' perceived English competence. It is to predict foreign language learners' belief of their communication skills in reading, writing, speaking and listening. Answers are on a four-point Likert scale; and the internal consistency of Cronbach's alpha was .90. The items are translated to Chinese through backward-translation. The sample items are: "I understand most of what my teacher says in English" and "I speak English well for someone my age."

English Learning Motivation Scale The scale is adopted from Zhang and Kim (2013) study and 19 items in Chinese are adopted to measure instrumental and integrative motivation. Answers are on a five-point Likert scale; and internal consistency shows a Cronbach's alpha of .926. Sample items are "I learn English because I want to study abroad" and "I learn English because English is an important tool for communication."

Willingness to Communicate Scale The scale is adopted from Knell and Chi's (2012) study and 25 items are extracted to measure students' willingness to communicate in English. Answers are on a four-point Likert scale; and the internal consistency shows a Cronbach's alpha of .90. The items are translated to Chinese through backward-translation. Sample items are: "how willing are you to speak English to other students in group activities" and "how willing are you to write a story in English."

English Learning Engagement Scale The scale is adopted from Chen and Kraklow's (2015) study and four items are extracted to measure how foreign language students perceive their amount of attention in learning English within and outside the classroom. Answers are on a six-point Likert scale and internal consistency shows a Cronbach's alpha of .83. The items are translated to Chinese through backward-translation. Sample items are: "I am always very attentive in English classes" and "I take notes on important content during English classes."

Motivational Intensity Scale The scale is adopted from Xu and Gao's (2014) study and nine items in Chinese are extracted to measure student's actual effort devoted in learning English. Answers are on a five-point Likert scale; and internal consistency shows a Cronbach's alpha of above .75. Sample items are: "I make conscious efforts to enlarge my English vocabulary" and "I make conscious efforts to watch English movies and videos." Five items (items 1, 3, 5, 6 and 7) are negatively coded so their responses are recoded after collection.

11.4 Results

11.4.1 Descriptive Statistics

The mean, standard deviations, and the correlations between the variables are listed in Table 11.1. All observed variables (45 pairs) are significantly correlated. The mean age is 15. The number of male and female is 68 and 237, respectively.

Table 11.1 Descriptive statistics and zero-order correlation between different variables ($N = 305$)

	1	2	3	4	5	6	7	8	9	10
1. Speak_anxiety	–									
2. Perc_competence	–.807***	–								
3. Integrative_motiv	–.511***	.541***	–							
4. Instrumental_motiv	–.550***	.576***	.738***	–						
5. Will_to_speak	–.764***	.811***	.556***	.579***	–					
6. Will_to_read	–.650***	.699***	.518***	.484***	.762***	–				
7. Will_to_write	–.688***	.757***	.559***	.531***	.816***	.759***	–			
8. Will_to_listen	–.643***	.730***	.495***	.507***	.755***	.749***	.766***	–		
9. Engagement	–.530***	.613***	.469***	.474***	.619***	.513***	.578***	.521***	–	
10. Motiv_intensity	–.739***	.758***	.587***	.607***	.729***	.613***	.632***	.621***	.635***	–
M	2.86	2.64	3.45	3.79	2.48	2.69	2.50	2.89	3.81	3.24
SD	.78	.62	.90	.91	.722	.76	.78	.72	.85	.65

Speak_anxiety = foreign language speaking anxiety, Perc_competence = perceived English competence, Integrative_motiv = integrative motivation, Instrumental_motiv = instrumental motivation, Will_to_speak = willingness to speak, Will_to_read = willingness to read, Will_to_write = willingness to write, Will_to_listen = willingness to listen, Engagement = English learning engagement, Motiv_intensity = motivational intensity

* $p < .05$; ** $p < .01$; *** $p < .00$

11.4.2 Reliability

Concerning foreign language speaking anxiety, the α of the Public Classroom Speaking Anxiety Scale is .95. Concerning perceived English competence, the α of the perceived English competence Scale is .93. Concerning English Learning Motivation, the α for the English Learning Motivation Scale is .96. The α for the subscales concerning integrative and instrumental motivation is .87 and .96, respectively.

Concerning Willingness to Communicate, the α for the Willingness to Communicate Scale is .98. The α for the subscales concerning willingness to speak, read, write and listen is .95, .93, .93, and .94, respectively.

Concerning English learning engagement, the α of the English learning motivation scale is .83. Concerning motivational intensity, the α of the motivational intensity scale is .83 (Table 11.2).

11.4.3 Validity

Confirmatory factor analysis was conducted for this study. The technique of item parceling was adapted to enhance the fitness of the model (Wong and Leung 2013). Table 11.3 presents the most commonly reported fit indices (McDonald and Ho 2002), namely CFI, GFI, RMSEA and the model chi-square of the factors examined in this study. All the CFI and GFI indices exceed .90, which indicate a good fit (Hu and Bentler 1995).

Table 11.2 Cronbach's alphas of the instruments in the main study

Scale	Cronbach's alpha (α)
1. Foreign language speaking anxiety	.95
2. Perceived English competence	.93
English learning motivation	.96
3. Integrative motivation	.87
4. Instrumental motivation	.96
Willingness to communicate	.98
5. Willingness to speak	.95
6. Willingness to read	.93
7. Willingness to write	.93
8. Willingness to listen	.94
9. English learning engagement	.83
10. Motivational intensity	.83

Table 11.3 List of goodness of fit indices

Instruments	*df*	χ^2	CFI	GFI	RMSEA
FLSA	27	61.52	.98	.95	.07
PEC	5	15.72	.99	.98	.08
ELM	13	108.34	.94	.90	.16
WTC	71	144.13	.98	.93	.06
ELE	2	9.67	.98	.98	.11
MI	5	10.40	.99	.98	.06

FLSA foreign language speaking anxiety, *PEC* perceived English competence, *ELM* English learning motivation, *WTC* willingness to communicate, *ELE* English learning engagement, *MI* motivational intensity, *df* degree of freedom, χ^2 minimum fit function chi-square, *CFI* comparative fit index, *GFI* goodness of fit index, *RMSEA* root mean square error of approximation

11.4.4 Path Analysis

Multiple regression was conducted in order to specify the predictors of foreign language speaking anxiety, perceived English competence, English learning motivation, willingness to communicate, English learning engagement and motivational intensity. Two significant path diagrams are drawn.

11.4.4.1 Path 1: English Learning Motivation, Foreign Language Speaking Anxiety, Willingness to Communicate, English Learning Engagement and Motivational Intensity

Figure 11.1 shows the path diagram concerning motivation, speaking anxiety, willingness to communicate, engagement and motivational intensity. On the first layer, both integrative ($\beta = -.23$, $t(289) = -3.28$, $p < .01$) and instrumental ($\beta = -.38$, $t(289) = -5.29$, $p < .001$) motivation are significant predictors of foreign language speaking anxiety ($F(2,287) = 69.76$, $p < .001$, $R^2 = .33$). On the second layer, willingness to communicate could be significantly predicted by foreign language speaking anxiety (FLSA). For willingness to speak ($\beta = -.76$, $t(291) = -20.18$, $p < .001$), FLSA is a significant negative predictor ($F(1,290) = 407.08$, $p < .001$, $R^2 = .58$). For willingness to read ($\beta = -.65$, $t(291) = -14.58$, $p < .001$), FLSA was a significant negative predictor ($F(1,290) = 212.51$, $p < .001$, $R^2 = .42$). For willingness to write ($\beta = -.69$, $t(291) = -16.13$, $p < .001$), FLSA was a significant negative predictor ($F(1,290) = 260.15$, $p < .001$, $R^2 = .47$). For willingness to listen ($\beta = -.64$, $t(291) = -14.29$, $p < .001$), FLSA was a significant negative predictor ($F(1,290) = 204.15$, $p < .001$, $R^2 = .41$). Also FLSA ($F(1,287) = 112.28$, $p < .001$, $R^2 = .28$) could negatively predict English learning engagement ($\beta = -.53$, $t(288) = -10.60$, $p < .001$). Lastly, motivational intensity ($\beta = -.74$, $t(266) = -17.85$, $p < .001$) could be negatively predicted by FLSA ($F(1,265) = 318.49$, $p < .001$, $R^2 = .55$).

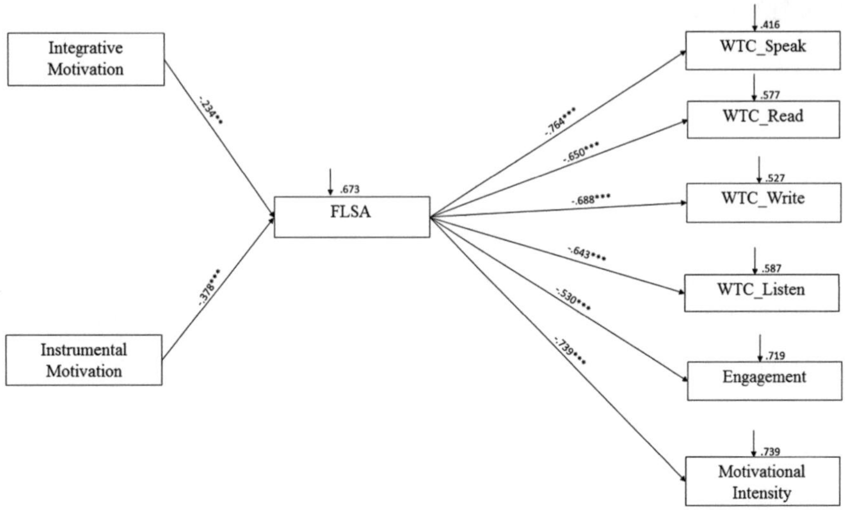

Fig. 11.1 The path diagram showing the predictive power of English learning motivation, foreign language speaking anxiety, willingness to communicate, English learning engagement and motivational intensity. *FLSA* foreign language speaking anxiety, *WTC_Speak* willingness to speak, *WTC_Read* willingness to read, *WTC_Write* willingness to write, *WTC_Listen* willingness to listen, *Engagement* English learning engagement. $^{*}p < .05$; $^{**}p < .01$; $^{***}p < .001$

11.4.4.2 Path 2: English Learning Motivation, Perceived English Competence, Willingness to Communicate, English Learning Engagement and Motivational Intensity

Figure 11.2 shows the path diagram concerning motivation, perceived competence, willingness to communicate, engagement and motivational intensity. On the first layer, both integrative ($\beta = .26$, $t(299) = 3.71$, $p < .001$) and instrumental ($\beta = .39$, $t(299) = 5.64$, $p < .001$) motivation are significant predictors of perceived English competence ($F(2{,}297) = 83.93$, $p < .001$, $R^2 = .36$). On the second layer, willingness to communicate could be significantly predicted by perceived English competence (PEC). For willingness to speak ($\beta = .81$, $t(300) = 23.96$, $p < .001$), PEC is a significant positive predictor ($F(1{,}299) = 573.85$, $p < .001$, $R^2 = .66$). For willingness to read ($\beta = .70$, $t(300) = 16.90$, $p < .001$), PEC was a significant positive predictor ($F(1{,}299) = 285.49$, $p < .001$, $R^2 = .49$). For willingness to write ($\beta = .76$, $t(300) = 20.04$, $p < .001$), PEC was a significant positive predictor ($F(1{,}299) = 401.66$, $p < .001$, $R^2 = .57$). For willingness to listen ($\beta = .73$, $t(299) = 18.48$, $p < .001$), PEC was a significant positive predictor ($F(1{,}299) = 341.42$, $p < .001$, $R^2 = .53$). Also, PEC ($F(1{,}296) = 177.88$, $p < .001$, $R^2 = .38$) could positively predict English learning engagement ($\beta = .61$, $t(297) = 13.34$, $p < .001$). Lastly, motivational intensity ($\beta = .76$, $t(274) = 19.22$, $p < .001$) could be positively predicted by PEC ($F(1{,}273) = 369.55$, $p < .001$, $R^2 = .58$).

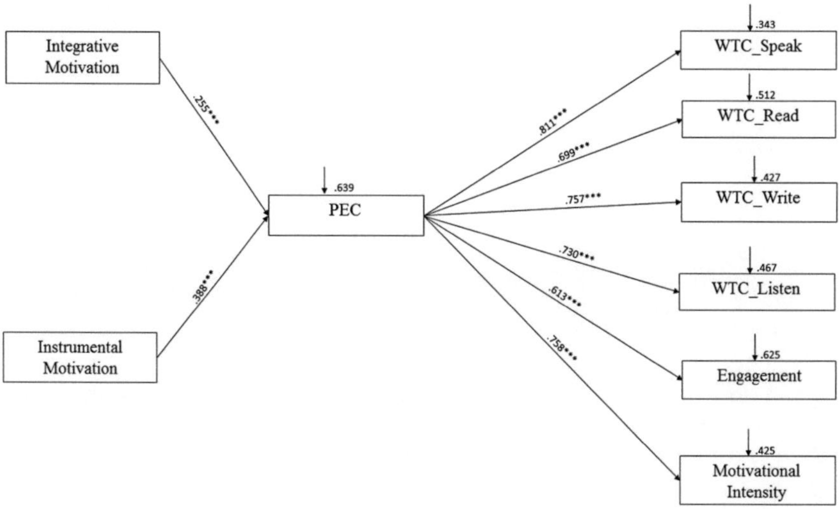

Fig. 11.2 The path diagram showing the predictive power of English learning motivation, perceived English competence, willingness to communicate, English learning engagement and motivational intensity. *PEC* perceived English competence, *WTC_Speak* willingness to speak, *WTC_Read* willingness to read, *WTC_Write* willingness to write, *WTC_Listen* willingness to listen, *Engagement* English learning engagement. $*p < .05$; $**p < .01$; $***p < .001$

11.4.5 Structural Equation Modelling (SEM)

Based on the results of the multiple regression, structural equation modelling was conducted to further estimate the direct and indirect effects among the factors, as well as measuring the relationship between the observed and latent variables (Wong and Leung 2013). Two significant SEM models are established.

11.4.5.1 Model 1: English Learning Motivation, Foreign Language Speaking Anxiety and Willingness to Communicate

Figure 11.3 shows the SEM model concerning motivation, speaking anxiety, and willingness to communicate. The indices for this model indicated a satisfying goodness of fit, as $\chi^2(12) = 17.11$, RESEA = .04, CFI = 1, GFI = .98.

There are two indicator for English Learning Motivation, namely Integrative Motivation ($\beta = .82$, $p < .001$) and Instrumental Motivation ($\beta = .78$, $p < .001$). For foreign language speaking anxiety, an indicator 'Anxiety' ($\beta = .79$, $p < .001$) was labelled. The four indicators for Willingness to Communicate are: Speak ($\beta = .88, p < .001$); Read ($\beta = .82, p < .001$), Write ($\beta = .88, p < .001$) and Listen ($\beta = .80, p < .001$).

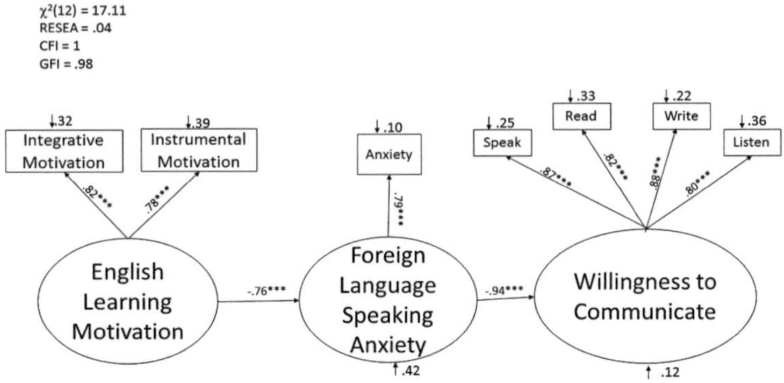

Fig. 11.3 The structural equation model for English learning motivation, foreign language speaking anxiety and willingness to communicate. *RMSEA* root mean square error of approximation, *GFI* goodness of fit index, *CFI* comparative fit index. *$p < .05$; **$p < .01$; ***$p < .001$

There are significant relationships between the three latent variables. English learning motivation is negatively related with foreign language speaking anxiety ($\beta = -.76$, $p < .001$). Foreign language speaking anxiety was also negatively related with Willingness to Communicate ($\beta = -.94$, $p < .001$).

11.4.5.2 Model 2: English Learning Motivation, Perceived English Competence and Willingness to Communicate

Figure 11.4 shows the SEM model concerning motivation, perceived competence, and willingness to communicate. The indices for this model indicated a satisfying goodness of fit, as χ^2 (12) = 21.59, RESEA = .05, CFI = .99, GFI = .98.

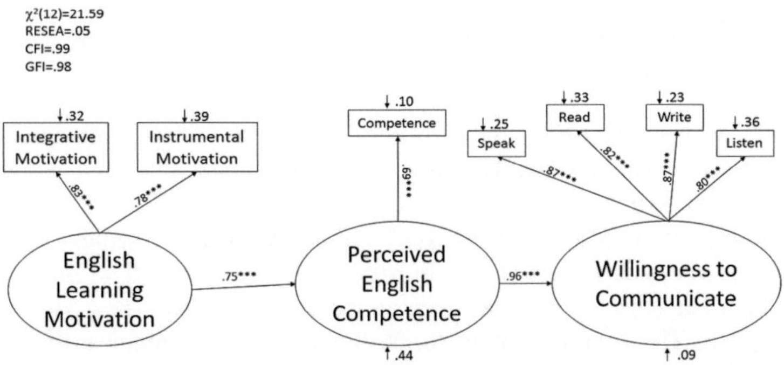

Fig. 11.4 The structural equation model for English learning motivation, perceived English competence and willingness to communicate. *RMSEA* root mean square error of approximation, *GFI* goodness of fit index, *CFI* comparative fit index. *$p < .05$; **$p < .01$, ***$p < .001$

There are two indicator for English learning motivation, namely integrative motivation ($\beta = .83$, $p < .001$) and instrumental motivation ($\beta = .78$, $p < .001$). For perceived English competence, an indicator "Competence" ($\beta = .69, p < .001$) was labelled. The four indicators for willingness to communicate are: speak ($\beta = .87$, $p < .001$); read ($\beta = .82$, $p < .001$), write ($\beta = .87$, $p < .001$), and listen ($\beta = .80, p < .001$).

There are significant relationships between the three latent variables. English learning motivation is positively related with perceived English competence ($\beta = .75, p < .001$). Perceived English competence was also positively related with willingness to communicate ($\beta = .96, p < .001$).

11.5 Discussion

11.5.1 The Relationship Between English Learning Motivation, Foreign Language Speaking Anxiety and Perceived English Competence

The findings of the present study that ELM is negatively correlated with FLSA while positively correlated with PEC are consistent with previous researches (Liu and Huang 2011). By examining the path analysis, it is observed that both integrative and instrumental motivation negatively correlate with foreign language speaking anxiety. On the other hand, both indicators of motivation correlate with perceived competence positively. The mechanism behind might be explained by looking into the nature of English learning motivation. To analyze the negative relationship between motivation and anxiety, a careful examination of motivation is needed. As motivation in the proposed model consists of two indicators, namely integrative and instrumental motivation, they might exert their effects on speaking anxiety in a different way, regarding their direction as well as their relative predictive power.

To explain, this study supports that both integrative and instrumental motivation negatively relate with speaking anxiety. Although Liu and Huang (2011) argued that pressure and anxiety could arise when teachers accentuate too much on the pragmatic purpose (instrumental motivation), it is more commonly agreed (Liu and Huang 2011; Onwuegbuzie et al. 1999) that enhancing intrinsic interest/appreciation toward the second language (L2) culture (integrative motivation) could significantly decrease foreign language anxiety and even boost performance (Liu 2012). For example, Onwuegbuzie et al. (1999) noticed that exposure to different cultures (such as traveling to the L2 country) reduces the anxiety towards that foreign language. Dominant researches hence point out that both integrative and instrumental motivation have negative relationships with foreign language anxiety (Wu and Lin 2014), which is consistent with the present study.

Furthermore, the path analysis shows difference in the relative predictive power of integrative and instrumental motivation. To illustrate the phenomenon among Hong Kong secondary students, consider the educational atmosphere of secondary schools in Hong Kong where entering university is a dominating reason for studying English. Such pragmatic purpose is commonly acknowledged, accepted and internalized by teachers, parents, and students themselves; hence, leading to a relatively lower anxiety level. It explains the reason that integrative motivation has a slightly weaker predictive power (when compared to instrumental motivation) according to the path analysis of the present study.

Second, Wigfield and Eccles' expectancy value model (2000) could be borrowed to explain the positive relationship between motivation and perceived competence. A construct within the expectancy value model, termed "utility value," concerns the student's cognitive measurement of whether a decision will benefit his future plans (Cocks and Watt 2004). This construct is highly similar to instrumental motivation, which concerns the pragmatic profit of learning. On the other hand, "intrinsic value" within the expectancy value model has common meanings with integrative motivation, which shares characteristics of intrinsic motivation (Wigfield and Eccles 2000). The finding of this research is congruent with previous researches, which confirmed the relationship between motivation and perceived competence (Cocks and Watt 2004).

11.5.2 The Relationship Between Foreign Language Speaking Anxiety, Perceived English Competence and Willingness to Communicate

First, this study found significant relationships between speaking anxiety and willingness to communicate. FLSA is negatively correlated with WTC, which is consistent with Liu and Jackson's (2008) study. On the other hand, PEC is positively correlated with WTC, mirroring Donovan and MacIntyre's (2004) study. It is indeed reasonable to postulate that a student who is terrified of speaking English refuses using it to communicate. While the reversed case is that a student who holds high confidence regarding his own language skills tend to actively seeks opportunity to initiate communication (Knell and Chi 2012).

After clarifying the opposing effects of anxiety and perceived competence, one might follow in questioning their comparative influences on WTC. Liu and Jackson (2008) pointed out in their study that anxiety is more powerful in predicting willingness to communicate, compared to perceived English competence (termed "self-rated overall proficiency in English"). In fact, others (McCroskey and Richmond 1987) also agreed that apprehension is the most significant predictor of WTC. The findings of these researchers all point to a possible path of casual relationship: perceived competence is affected by one's anxiety level, which in turns determines his willingness to communicate. Yet, MacIntyre et al. (1999)

found that apprehension has no significant effect on WTC. In their SEM model, surprisingly, the path between communication anxiety and WTC was found non-significant. The authors thus admit that perceived competence exerts stronger influences on WTC than anxiety (MacIntyre and Charos 1996; MacIntyre 1994). In short, there exist controversies regarding whether language anxiety or perceived competence has larger effects on willingness to communicate.

11.5.3 SEM Models

11.5.3.1 Model 1: English Learning Motivation, Foreign Language Speaking Anxiety and Willingness to Communicate

The fit indices for this model is satisfying, where χ^2 (12) = 17.11, RMSEA = .04, CFI = 1, GFI = .98. The β between ELM and FLSA is −.76, while the β between FLSA and WTC is −.94. It implies that anxiety has a mediating effect between motivation and willingness to communicate. Foreign language speaking anxiety exerts a significant influence on the relationship between English learning motivation and willingness to communicate through its negative predictive power.

11.5.3.2 Model 2: English Learning Motivation, Perceived English Competence and Willingness to Communicate

The fit indices for this model is satisfactory, where $\chi^2(12) = 21.59$, RMSEA = .05, CFI = .99, and GFI = .98. The β between ELM and PEC is .75, while the β between PEC and WTC is .96. It implies that perceived competence has a mediating effect between motivation and willingness to communicate. Perceived English competence exerts a significant influence on the relationship between English learning motivation and willingness to communicate through its positive predictive power.

To sum up, two significant SEM models are derived in this study. Model 1 recognizes foreign language speaking anxiety as a mediator between English learning motivation and willingness to communicate, while Model 2 recognizes perceived English competence as the mediator. As mentioned, the models in the present study support some researchers (Hashimoto 2002) as well as alienate with some other studies (Zheng 2010).

An example of diversity could be observed from Zheng's (2010) study, which identified motivation as a mediator between attitude and confidence (identical to perceived competence). Although willingness to communicate is not included in his model, the outcome is different with the present study. Hence, an interesting phenomenon was raised: just as the relationship among motivation and foreign language anxiety (Yu 2011), the reciprocal nature between motivation and perceived competence was also observed in the present study.

11.5.4 Pedagogical Implications

Summarizing the findings of this study, a few conclusions could be drawn regarding the pedagogical implications. Although this study could not definitely confirm any causal relationships, the goodness of fit indices of the structural equation models suggest that motivation is more possibly a predictor, instead of a mediator for anxiety and perceived competence. Such findings contradict with other researchers such as Dörnyei (2001). It is indeed worthwhile emphasizing since resources are limited in secondary schools and English teachers have to be precise in investing effort in different aspects to facilitate students' language outcome.

According to this research, strategies that aim at fostering students' motivation would result in a higher willingness to communicate in English. To boost integrative motivation, teachers are suggested to develop students' interest in English culture (Liu and Huang 2011). Materials such as English novels and movies are excellent tools to induce students' enthusiasm. This is to diminish students' sense of English as a 'foreign' language, and hence making them feel less strange and anxious toward learning and speaking English. Also teachers could enhance instrumental motivation by raising students' awareness toward the importance of English. As Liu and Huang (2011) believe, attempts in cultivating motivation would result in a lower anxiety. The authors suggest that the very first lessons are critical and teachers should inform students that English is challenging for many other people, particularly in the oral aspect. Teachers could then proceed in explaining to students that it is of utmost important to practice and master speaking skills due to its instrumental value. Through this sequence, students would develop instrumental motivation themselves and be less prone to anxiety.

On the other hand, measures that alter anxiety levels and perceived competence should be taken to facilitate the direct effect of motivation on willingness to communicate. Since perceived competence is found significantly correlated with speaking anxiety in this study, students who are anxious about speaking English generally have lower perceived competence. According to Knell and Chi (2012), a vicious cycle is hence created, where anxious students perceive themselves negatively and avoid communication. Thus, students are deprived of opportunities to practice speaking English and their actual competence is unlikely to improve, which in turn further devastate their perceived competence. To prevent such unconstructive self-fulfilling prophecy, teachers are suggested to promote students' perceived competence through providing positive feedbacks, analyzing, and reinforcing commendable achievements, and even provide opportunities for students to conduct positive self-evaluations (Liu and Huang 2011; Liu 2013). Once the cycle is reversed, students would feel more competent about their oral skills and be less anxious to communicate in English. They might even be motivated to initiate conversation (Knell and Chi 2012), actualizing their potentials to achieve better in foreign language.

Last but not least, the benefits of modifying anxiety levels and perceived competence might be extended to improve student's performance. Cocks and

Watt (2004), for example, found that students with higher perceived competence are more likely to invest effort and hence perform better in learning foreign language. Bailey et al. (2000) developed the Anxiety-Expectation Mediation (AEM) Model as aforementioned which highlights low anxiety levels and high expectation (generated from perceived competence) as crucial factors in advancing language performance. Although the relationship might be mediated by factors such as motivation (Montgomery and Spalding 2005), it is clear that these procedures of desensitizing students' anxiety as well as encouraging students' perceived competence yield favorable pedagogical outcomes in foreign language learning.

All in all, motivation, anxiety, perceived competence and willingness to communicate are all correlated and through direct and indirect relationships, these affective factors eventually determine the acquisition of a foreign language. For students to devote themselves into the long-term process of English learning, teachers might adapt different strategies to holistically endow students with constructive psychological factors as well as encourage in/out-of-classroom communications in order to facilitate students in acquiring distinctive language learning outcome.

11.6 Conclusion

This study contributes to prove the relationships between English learning motivation, foreign language speaking anxiety, perceived English competence and willingness to communicate. From a theoretical perspective, this study established two significant structural equation models, revealing the mediating effect of speaking anxiety and perceived competence between motivation and willingness to communicate. Suggestions for further studies are also provided.

From a practical perspective, the effects of motivation anxiety and perceived competence on willingness to communicate are clarified. Integrative motivation has a slightly weaker influence on speaking anxiety, while both motivation orientations strongly strength perceived competence. Therefore, the implication lies in identifying educators with operative channels to facilitate students' English learning. For instance, English teachers might introduce materials that could elicit students' personal interest toward English culture. However, as this study observes the context of Hong Kong secondary schools, instrumental motivation has stronger influence on speaking anxiety, and hence Hong Kong teachers should regard it as more compelling in alleviating anxiety, promoting perceived competence, and encouraging willingness to communicate.

Acknowledgments I would like to deliver my most sincere gratitude to my supervisor, Dr. Leung Man-Tak, for all his time and effort in educating me. Throughout the year, he did not merely teach me skills and steps to finish the study, instead, Dr. Leung has always been kind and encouraging in guiding and reminding me his advises on the essences of conducting research: effort, persistence, and circumspection. It is both my honour and fortune to have become his supervisee and have learnt so much from this wise professor. I would also like to say thank you to all the scholars who generously grant me their permission to use their instruments. Without their generosity, this study could not be conducted well. Lastly, I would like to express my acknowledgement to my dearest friend, Lau, who distributed the questionnaires for me. Without her aid and connection, I would never be able to obtain such a pleasant subject size. Please accept my deepest gratefulness and blessings for those who have provided me support.

References

Bailey, P., Onwuegbuzie, A. J., & Daley, C. (2000). Correlates of anxiety at three stages of the foreign language learning process. *Journal of Language and Social Psychology, 19*, 474–492.

Baker, S. C., & MacIntyre, P. D. (2000). The role of gender and immersion in communication and second language orientations. *Language Learning, 53*(1), 65–96.

Baker, S. C., & MacIntyre, P. D. (2003). The role of gender and immersion in communication and second language orientations. *Language Learning*, *53*(1), 65–96.

Becker, M., McElvany, N., & Kortenbruck, M. (2010). Intrinsic and extrinsic reading motivation as predictors of reading literacy: A longitudinal study. *Journal of Educational Psychology, 102*, 773–785.

Beder, H., Tomkins, J., Medina, P., Riccioni, R., & Deng, W. (2006). *Learners' engagement in adult literacy education* (NCSALL Reports No. 28). Cambridge, MA: National Center for the Study of Adult Learning and Literacy.

Biggs, J. B., & Telfer, R. (1987). *The process of learning* (2nd ed.). Sydney: Prentice Hall.

Butler, Y. G. (2007). Children's reading attitudes in L1 and F1. *Academic Exchange, 11*(1), 183–187.

Butler, Y. G. (2014). Parental factors in children's motivation for learning English: A case in China. *Research Papers in Education, 30*(2), 164–191.

Campbell, C. M., & Ortiz, J. (1991). Helping students overcome foreign language anxiety: A foreign language anxiety workshop. In E. K. Horwitz & D. J. Young (Eds.), *Language anxiety: From theory and research to classroom implications* (pp. 153–168). Englewood Cliffs, NJ: Prentice Hall.

Capan, S. A., & Simsek, H. (2012). General foreign language anxiety among EFL learners: A survey study. *Frontiers of Language and Teaching, 3*, 116–124.

Chen, Y. L. E., & Kraklow, D. (2015). Taiwanese college students' motivation and engagement for English learning in the context of internationalization at home: A comparison of students in EMI and Non-EMI programs. *Journal of Studies in International Education, 19*(1), 46–64.

Clément, R., Dörnyei, Z., & Noels, K. A. (1994). Motivation, self-confidence, and group cohesion in the foreign language classroom. *Language Learning, 33*, 273–291.

Cocks, R. J., & Watt, H. M. G. (2004). Relationships among perceived competence, intrinsic value and mastery goal orientation in English and Maths. *The Australian Educational Researcher, 31*, 81–111.

Csizer, K., & Dörnyei, Z. (2005). The internal structure of language learning motivation and its relationship with language choice and learning effort. *The Modern Language Journal, 89*, 19–36.

Daley, C. E., Onwuegbuzie, A. J. & Bailey, P. (1997). *Predicting achievement in college-level foreign language courses.* Poster session presented at the annual conference of the Mid-South Educational Research Association, Memphis, TN.

De Naeghel, J., Van Keer, H., Vansteenkiste, M., & Rosseel, Y. (2012). The relation between elementary students' recreational and academic reading motivation, reading frequency, engagement, and comprehension: A self-determination theory perspective. *Journal of Educational Psychology, 29*, 761–775.

Donovan, L. A., & Maclntyre, P. D. (2004). Age and sex differences in willingness to communicate, communication apprehension, and self-perceived competence. *Communication Research Reports, 21*(4), 420–427.

Dörnyei, Z. (1994). Motivation and motivating in the foreign language classroom. *The Modern Language Journal, 78*, 273–274.

Dörnyei, Z. (2001). *Teaching and researching motivation*. Harlow, UK: Longman.

Eccles, J. S., & Wigfield, A. (2002). Motivational beliefs, values, and goals. *Annual Reviews, 50*, 109–132.

Gai, F., & Yang, D. (2010). A study on college students' anxiety to spoken English. *Canadian Social Science, 6*(2), 95–101.

Gao, Y., Zhou, Y., Cheng, Y., & Zhou, Y. (2007). Relationship between English learning motivation types and self-identity changes among Chinese students. *TESOL Quarterly, 41*(1), 133–155.

Gardner, R. C. (2001). Integrative motivation and second language acquisition. In Z. Dörnyei & R. W. Schmidt (Eds.), *Motivation and second language acquisition* (pp. 1–19). Honolulu: University of Hawaii.

Gardner, R. C., & MacIntyre, P. D. (1993). On the measurement of affective variation in second language learning. *Language Learning, 43*, 157–194.

Harter, S. (1999). *The construction of the self*. New York, NY: The Guildford Press.

Hashimoto, Y. (2002). Motivation and willingness to communicate as predictors of L2 use. *Second Language Studies, 20*, 29–70.

Horwitz, E. K. (2000). It ain't over 'til it's over: On foreign language anxiety, first language deficits, d the confounding of variables. *The Modern Language Journal*, *84*, 256–259.

Horwitz, E. K. (2001). Language anxiety and achievement. *Annual Review of Applied Linguistics, 21*, 112–126.

Horwitz, E. K., Horwitz, M. B., & Cope, J. (1986). Foreign language classroom anxiety. *The Modern Language Journal, 70*(2), 125–132.

Hu, L. T., & Bentler, P. M. (1995). Evaluating model fit. In R. H. Hoyle (Ed.), *Structural equation modeling: Concepts, issues, and applications*. London: Sage Publications.

Kayaoglu, M. C., & Saglamel, H. (2013). Students' perceptions of language anxiety in speaking classes. *Journal of History Culture and Art Research, 2*(2), 142–160.

Kim, S. Y. (2009). Questioning the stability of foreign language classroom anxiety and motivation across different classroom contexts. *Foreign Language Annals, 42*(1), 138–157.

Knell, E., & Chi, Y. (2012). The roles of motivation, affective attitudes, and willingness to communicate among Chinese students in early English immersion programs. *International Education, 41*(2), 66–87.

Krashen, S. D. (1980). The input hypothesis. In J. E. Alatis (Ed.), *Current issues in bilingual education: Georgetown University round table on language and linguistics* (pp. 168–180). Washington, DC: Georgetown University Press.

Kriangkrai, Y., & Siriluck, U. (2012). A measure of EFL Public Speaking Anxiety Scale: Scale development and preliminary validation and reliability. *English Language Teaching, 5*(12), 23–35.

Li, Q. (2014). Differences in the motivation of Chinese learners of English in a foreign and second language context. *System, 42*, 451–461.

Liu, M. (2012). Motivation in Chinese university EFL learners in varying learning contexts. *TESL Reporter, 45*(2), 17–39.

Liu, H. J. (2013). Effects of foreign language anxiety and perceived competence on learning strategy use. *International Journal of English Linguistics, 3*(3), 76–87.

Liu, M., & Huang, W. (2011). An exploration of foreign language anxiety and English learning motivation. *Education Research International, 2011*, 1–8.

Liu, M., & Jackson, J. (2008). An exploration of Chinese EFL learners' unwillingness to communicate and foreign language anxiety. *The Modern Language Journal, 92*, 71–86.

Luo, M. L. (2012). The problems of senior three students' "Mute-Crux" in English learning in China. *Sino-US English Teaching, 9*(5), 1139–1144.

MacIntyre, P. D., Babin, P. A., & Clément, R. (1999). Willingness to communicate: Antecedents & consequences. *Communication Quarterly, 47*(2), 215–229.

MacIntyre, P. D., & Charos, C. (1996). Personality, attitudes, and affect as predictors of second language communication. *Journal of Language and Social Psychology, 15*, 3–26.
MacIntyre, P. D., & Gardner, R. C. (1991). Methods and results in the study of anxiety and language learning: a review of the literature. *Language Learning, 41*, 85–117.
MacIntyre, P. D., Noels, K. A., & Clément, R. (1997). Biases in self-ratings of second language proficiency: The role of language anxiety. *Language Learning, 47*, 265–287.
Maclntyre, P. D. (1994). Variables underlying willingness to communicate: A causal analysis. *Communication Research Reports, 11*(2), 135–142.
Maclntyre, P. D., Baker, S. C., Clément, R., & Conrod, S. (2001). Willingness to communicate, social support, and language-learning orientations of immersion students. *Studies in Second Language Acquisition, 23*, 369–388.
Maclntyre, P. D., Baker, S. C., Clément, R., & Donovan, L. A. (2003). Talking in order to learn: Willingness to communicate and intensive language programs. *The Canadian Modem Language Review, 59*(4), 589–607.
Maehr, M. L. (1984). Meaning and motivation: toward a theory of personal investment. In R. E. Ames & C. Ames (Eds.), *Research on Motivation in Education*. Orlando, FA: Academic Press.
Mak, B. (2011). An exploration of speaking-in-class anxiety with Chinese EFL learners. *System, 39*, 202–214.
Marcos-Llinás, M., & Garau, M. J. (2009). Effects of language anxiety on three proficiency-level courses of Spanish as a foreign language. *Foreign Language Annals, 42*(1), 94–111.
Marsh, H. W., & Yeung, A. S. (1998). Longitudinal structural equation models of academic self-concept and achievement: Gender differences in the development of math and English constructs. *American Educational Research Journal, 35*, 705–738.
McCroskey, J. C. (1970). Measures of communication-bound anxiety. *Speech Monograph, 37*, 269–277.
McCroskey, J. C., & Richmond, V. P. (1987). Willingness to communicate. In J. C. McCroskey & J. A. Daly (Eds.), *Personality and interpersonal communication*. Newbury Park, CA: Sage.
McDonald, R. P., & Ho, M. H. R. (2002). Principles and practice in reporting statistical equation analyses. *Psychological Method, 7*(1), 64–82.
Miller, S. F. (2010). *Promoting learner engagement when working with adult English language learners*. Retrieved from www.cal.org/caelanetwork
Montgomery, C., & Spalding, T. (2005). Anxiety and perceived English and French language competence of education students. *The Canadian Journal of Higher Education, 35*(4), 1–26.
Onwuegbuzie, A. J., Bailey, P., & Daley, C. (1999). Factors associated with foreign language anxiety. *Applied Psycholinguistics, 20*, 217–239.
Peng, S. (2014). Analysis of perceived difficulty rank of English skills of college students in China. *Studies in Literature and Language, 8*(3), 2014.
Saito, Y., Horwitz, E. H., & Garza, T. J. (1999). Foreign language reading anxiety. *Modern Language Journal, 83*, 202–218.
Schalge, S., & Soga, K. (2008). "Then I stop coming to school": Understanding absenteeism in an adult English as a second language program. *Adult Basic Education and Literacy Journal, 2*(3), 151–161.
Sultan, S. (2012). Students' perceived competence affecting level of anxiety in learning English as a foreign language. *Pakistan Journal of Psychological Research, 27*(2), 225–239.
Tsai, R. Y. (2012). Investigating the relationships among cognitive learning styles: Motivation and strategy use in reading English as a foreign language. *International Journal of Business and Social Science, 3*(13), 188–197.
Wigfield, A., & Eccles, J. S. (2000). Expectancy-value theory of achievement motivation. *Contemporary Educational Psychology, 25*, 68–81.
Wong, K. Y., & Leung, M. T. (2013). *The structural model on the roles of achievement emotions between action control and learning strategies of undergraduates in Hong Kong*. Paper presented at the AARE annual conference, Adelaide, Australia. Retrieved from http://www.aare.edu.au/publications-database.php/8563/the-structural-model-on-the-roles-of-achievement-emotions-between-action-control-and-learning-strate

Woodrow, L. (2006). Anxiety and speaking English as a second language. *RELC Journal, 37*, 308–328.

Wu, C. P., & Lin, H. J. (2014). Anxiety about speaking a foreign language as a mediator of the relationship between motivation and willingness to communicate. *Perceptual and Motor Skills, 119*(3), 785–798.

Wu, Y. A., Liu, R. Q., & Jeffrey, P. (1993). Learner factors and language learning achievement: A survey. *Foreign Language Teaching and Research, 1993*(1), 36–46.

Xu, H., & Gao, Y. (2014). The development of English learning motivation and learners' identities: A structural equation modeling analysis of longitudinal data from Chinese universities. *System, 47*, 102–115.

Yashima, T. (2000). Orientations and motivations in foreign language learning: A study of Japanese college students. *JACET Bulletin, 31*, 121–133.

Yashima, T. (2002). Willingness to communicate in a second language: The Japanese EFL context. *The Modem Language Journal, 86*(1), 54–66.

Yu, M. (2011). Effect of communication variables, affective variables, and teacher immediacy on willingness to communicate of foreign language learners. *Chinese Journal of Communication, 4*(2), 218–236.

Zhang, Q. M., & Kim, T. Y. (2013). Cross-grade analysis of Chinese students' English learning motivation: A mixed-methods study. *Asia Pacific Education Review, 2013*(14), 615–627.

Zheng, Y. (2010). *Chinese university students' motivation, anxiety, global awareness, linguistic confidence, and English test performance: A casual and correlational investigation.* Unpublished doctoral dissertation, Queens University, Canada.

Zhou, Y. (1996). Social-psychological factors and language learning. In G. Xu (Ed.), *ELT in China 1992* (pp. 49–83). Beijing: Foreign Language Teaching and Research Press.

Chapter 12
The Structural Model of Perceived Parenting Style as Antecedent on Achievement Emotion, Self-regulated Learning and Academic Procrastination of Undergraduates in Hong Kong

Ka-Yu Yip and Man-Tak Leung

Abstract The present study is conducted to investigate the impact of perceived parenting style on self-regulated learning and academic procrastination with mediating effect of achievement emotion. The sample of this study consisted of 218 undergraduates through convenient sampling from universities in Hong Kong. Parenting Authority Questionnaire, Academic Emotion Questionnaire, Motivated Strategies for Learning Questionnaire, and Procrastination Scale were used to collect the data. To analyze the data, reliability was investigated by Cronbach's alpha. Correlation, path analysis, and structural equation modeling were also conducted. Result found that perceived parenting style is significantly associated with achievement emotion. And achievement emotion is significantly associated with self-regulated learning and academic procrastination. Result of the structural equation modeling also found that perceived authoritative parenting style show an impact on positive achievement emotion (enjoyment, hope and pride) and in succession affect the self-regulated learning and academic procrastination. The present study concerns mainly on the complex relationship among perceived parenting style, achievement emotion, self-regulated learning, and academic procrastination. It may bring the practical significance to Hong Kong parent to aware the effect of their parenting style on children's learning strategies and procrastination style. It may also bring some insight on enhancing student's self-regulated learning behaviors and reduce student's academic procrastination.

K.-Y. Yip · M.-T. Leung (✉)
Department of Counselling and Psychology, Hong Kong Shue Yan University,
North Point, Hong Kong
e-mail: mtleung@hksyu.edu
URL: http://www.hksyu.edu

M.-T. Leung and L.-M. Tan (eds.), *Applied Psychology Readings*,
DOI 10.1007/978-981-10-2796-3_12

Keywords Perceived parenting style · Academic procrastination · Achievement emotion · Self-regulated learning

12.1 Introduction

Academic procrastination is commonly appearing among students, either in Western countries or in Asia. From several Western studies published had stated that over 60–70 % of the college students would procrastinate in study (Steel 2007; Vahedi et al. 2009; Rabin et al. 2011; Zakeri et al. 2013), and over half of the college students present constant academic procrastination (Steel 2007; Vahedi et al. 2009; Soysa and Weiss 2014). This showed academic procrastination a continuous and common problem in college setting in Western.

Not only in Western culture, procrastination among college students also occurred in Asia. In Mainland China, several news had reported that over 40 % of the college students in Mainland would habitually procrastinate which result in increasing stress and nervous feeling ("Around 40 % of college student," 2015). The situation in Hong Kong seemed more serious. News ("65 % students", 2006) and survey conducted by Oriental Daily (2014) had found that nearly 65 % of college students had tried to be late in school or skip classes. The above data showed the seriousness of procrastination among Hong Kong college students. Study of the factors causing procrastination is valued in improving the situation.

Academic procrastination had been proved to be linked with students' learning strategies, self-regulated learning and their performance (Steel 2007; Klassen et al. 2008; Senecal et al. 1995). However, there is an uncertainty whether academic procrastination would be affected by perceived parenting style under the raising concern of "Hong Kong Child" and the overly caring Hong Kong parenting style. This research aimed to investigate how perceived parenting style affect the achievement emotion, and in turn affect self-regulated learning and academic procrastination of undergraduates in Hong Kong.

12.2 Literature Review

12.2.1 Academic Procrastination

Researcher studying procrastination suggested that procrastination is related to several aspects (Popoola 2005). Several definitions had been given to it.

From behavioral aspect, Solomon and Rothblum (1984) had defined procrastination as a kind of unnecessary delay until the individual feels uneasy or discomfort. Ellis and Knaus (1977) described procrastination as avoiding doing something and being blame by making reasonable excuse. Noran (2000) described procrastination as the behavior of avoiding finishing work that should have been finished. Ferrari et al. (1995) suggested that procrastination is behavior result from failure in effective time management. There are also some other researcher agreed that procrastination is the behavior to complete the work late or postpone making decision (Milgram et al. 1998; Haycock et al. 1998; Kachgal et al. 2001). In general, procrastination seemed to be an intentional behavior.

For emotional aspect, some researchers described procrastination as the way to release from anxiety (Tice et al. 2001; Popoola 2005), and a result from low confidence of self-competence (Ferrari and Emmons 1995), which may also referred to low self-esteem (Effert and Ferrari 1989).

For cognitive aspect, some researcher suggested that procrastination is the failure of or low level of self-regulation (Steel 2007; Klassen et al. 2008; Senecal et al. 1995). Wolters (2003) found that metacognitive self-regulation was one of the strongest predictor of procrastination.

Other than the above, Lay (1986) defined procrastination is one' motive or character to avoid the fear of failure or success. Blatt and Quinlan (1967) and McCown et al. (1987) describe procrastination of students is the behavior against their parents who are either too demanding or conniving, or a denial to the anxiety.

Among different type of procrastination, academic procrastination is highly prevailing among college students for long time. It was defined by current study as a kind of intention to delay or postpone starting or completing academic activities, even with the awareness of a lower grading in academic performance (Senecal et al. 1995; Brownlow and Reasinger 2000; Klassen et al. 2008; Rabin et al. 2011; Azar 2013; Zakeri et al. 2013). For example, delay in doing and finishing the assignments or task, or delay in studying for the test.

12.2.2 Perceived Parenting Style

Parenting style refers to the attitude or teaching style of parents given or showing to their children, involving verbal language, nonverbal behaviors, or emotions climate created by parents (Zakeri et al. 2013). Baumrind (1967) was the first one who had conceptualized the parenting style into three categories, including authoritarian, authoritative, and permissive style. Parents with authoritarian style were usually highly controlling and demanding (Baumrind 1967; Gonzalez and Wolters 2006). Parents with authoritative style were less demanding and controlling, but they were more supportive and communicative to their children (Baumrind 1967; Gonzalez and Wolters 2006) and would provide warmth family climate to their children as well. In the relation with learning, Nyarko (2011) pointed that authoritative style had positive relationship with children's academic result. Parents with permissive style were totally not demanding and controlling, but were given high autonomy to their children. (Baumrind 1967; Gonzalez and Wolters 2006). They do not concern much on children's rules and obedience, but highly accepted to children's behaviors and decision. In learning, permissive parents usually being less directive to children compared with other two kinds of parenting.

12.2.3 Perceived Parenting Style and Academic Procrastination

The direct relationship between perceived parenting style and academic procrastination was still not very clear. But still, some studies had indicated the correlation and causal relationship between them.

Ferrari and Emmons in two of their studies published in 1993 and 1994 provided evidence for the linking between parental influence and procrastination. The studies implied that high parental expectation may have indirect positive relationship with procrastination, parenting with low flexibility and high control was also correlated to decisional procrastination. But these results were only from female. Flett et al. (1995) suggested that procrastination was students' response to the expectation of harsh and controlling parenting style. Ferrari et al. (1999) examined the relationship between procrastinator and their parents, and significant relationship was found between procrastination and conflictive parents–child relationship.

From recent study, Pychyl et al. study in 2002 examine the relationship between parenting style, procrastination, and self-worth among adolescences. The study indicated that only authoritative and authoritarian styles were found to have significant relationship with procrastination. Maternal-authoritative parenting was significantly negatively related to procrastination for both male and female adolescences. Paternal authoritative parenting was significantly negatively related to procrastination for only female adolescences. Also, paternal authoritarian parenting was significantly positively related to procrastination.

Vahedi et al. study in 2009 found that supportive parenting style predicting lower level of procrastination, while harsh or unsupportive parenting style predicting higher level of procrastination.

Zakeri et al. study in 2013 found that parenting style was a significant predictor of academic procrastination. In the research, "behavioral strictness-supervision," "acceptance-involvement," and "psychological autonomy-granting" styles were examined. Behavioral strictness-supervision style referred to overcontrolling parenting style that similar to authoritarian style. Acceptance-involvement style referred to a warm and involved parenting that similar authoritative style. Psychological autonomy-granting style referred to the democratic parenting style that similar to permissive style. The result of the study found that "behavioral strictness-supervision" style was significantly positively correlated with academic procrastination. Also, "acceptance-involvement" and "psychological autonomy-granting" style can significantly negatively predicting academic procrastination.

Also, Hong et al. study in 2014 examined the relationship among helicopter parenting, self-regulated learning, and procrastination. The study defined helicopter parenting as highly involving, supportive with low autonomy, which is similar to the authoritative or authoritarian parenting. The result found that perceived helicopter parenting was a positive predictor of procrastination. Soysa and Weiss (2014) also indicated that academic procrastination was a mediator between perceived authoritarian parenting style and test anxiety in vocational high school students.

From the above article, there is evidence that perceived parenting style is significantly related to academic procrastination.

12.2.4 Achievement Emotions and Academic Procrastination

The relationship between achievement emotions and academic procrastination was still largely uninvestigated. No Western study had found the direct relationship between them. However, from other study, indirect relationship between them can be predicted. Also, some Chinese articles had examined the direct relationship between them.

For Western study, study of Pekrun related to achievement emotions (Pekrun et al. 2002, 2011) had mentioned that positive achievement emotions had positive relationship with self-regulation of learning and academic result. In converse, negative achievement emotions had negative relationship with self-regulation of learning and academic result. As mentioned, self-regulated learning was proved to be strong negative predictor of procrastination. It may predict an indirect relationship between achievement emotions and academic procrastination.

For Chinese study, Li (2012) had examined the relationship between achievement emotion and academic procrastination. The result indicated that positive achievement emotions showed negative relationship with academic procrastination, while negative achievement emotions showed positive relationship with academic procrastination. Study by Zhang et al. (2012) also indicated significant founding on relationship between achievement emotion and academic procrastination. Also, it indicated a mediating effect of achievement motivation on relationship between achievement emotion and academic procrastination.

12.2.5 Self-regulated Learning, Academic Procrastination, and Academic Performance

For the relationship between self-regulated learning and academic procrastination, a lot of study had been done which give strong evidence to prove that self-regulated learning had strong relationship with academic performance.

As mentioned, some studies had defined academic procrastination as the result of failure of or low level of self-regulated learning (Steel 2007; Klassen et al. 2008; Senecal et al. 1995). These studies gave a consistent finding that self-regulated learning was negatively predicting academic procrastination. It implied that self-regulated learning was a significant predictor of academic procrastination.

12.3 Research Hypotheses

Referred to the literature review, two hypotheses are formed in this study, hypothesis are listed below.

(1) Perceived parenting style is significantly associated with academic procrastination mediated by achievement emotion.
(2) Perceived parenting style is significantly associated with self-regulated learning mediated by achievement emotion.

12.4 Methodology

12.4.1 Participants and Sampling Method

Two hundreds and eighteen students (63 males, 155 females) studying in universities in Hong Kong aging from 17 to 24 were invited to participate in this research study. Convenient sampling had been used to select the participants. A consent form would be distributed to them first, followed with a set of self-reported questionnaire. They needed to finish the set of questionnaire following the instructions given after the consent form was signed. A simple debriefing was given to them after the questionnaire was finished.

12.4.2 Measures

12.4.2.1 Parenting Authority Questionnaire (PAQ)

The Parenting Authority Questionnaire (PAQ) was proposed by Buri (1991). The PAQ had reported high test–retest reliability varied from .77 to .92, and high-internal consistency reliability varied from .74 to .87. PAQ consisted of two forms, one each for investigating the maternal and paternal parenting style. It composed of three subscales of 10 items each with a 5-point Likert scale from 1 (strongly disagree) to 5 (strongly agree).

12.4.2.2 Self-regulated Learning Scale

The self-regulated learning of students was assessed by using MSLQ. Part three related to learning strategies of MSLQ was used. This part contained five parts in total 31 items, including rehearsal (4 items), elaboration (6 items), organization (4 items), critical thinking (5 items), and metacognitive self-regulation (12 items). It was a 7-point Likert scale ranging from 1 (not at all true of me) to 7 (very true of me). This part of questionnaire reported a satisfied reliability varied from .74 to .83.

12.4.2.3 Achievement Emotions Scale

The Academic Emotions Scale proposed by Huang (2010) was used. This scale was translated and adjusted based on the Achievement Emotions Questionnaire (AEQ) developed by Pekrun in 2005.

This scale had reported a high reliability varied from .85 to .94 and satisfied validity for both the positive academic emotions, RMSEA = .07, NFI = .98, NNFI = .98, CFI = .98, IFI = .98, GFI = .99, and AGFI = .98, and the negative academic emotions, RMSEA = .00, NFI = .96, NNFI = 1.01, CFI = 1.00, IFI = 1.01, GFI = .82, and AGFI = .79.

This scale contains eight types of academic emotions, in total 46 items in a 5-point Likert scale from 1 (strongly disagree) to 5 (strongly agree). The eight type of academic emotions including enjoyment (6 items), pride (6 items), hope (5 items), anger (6 items), anxiety (6 items), hopelessness (6 items), boredom (6 items), and shame (5 items).

As the scale is originally used to measure the academic emotions of students in English lesson, so the scale was modified to measure the general academic emotions in this research. And the adjusted questionnaire found high reliability in pilot test varied from .865 to .925.

12.4.2.4 Academic Procrastination Scale

The academic procrastination scale was proposed by Lay (1986). This scale reported a high reliability of .82. This scale was originally consisted of 20 items in a 5-point Likert scale ranging from 1 (strongly disagree) to 5 (strongly agree). However, five of the items that are unrelated to academic setting were canceled and only 15-items related to academic setting left to measure student's academic procrastination.

12.5 Results

12.5.1 Reliability Analysis

The reliabilities of all the variables in this research were shown in Table 12.1. For the perceived parenting style, the scale had been divided into two set, one each for maternal and paternal parenting style. And each parenting style consisted of three types, including permissive, authoritative, and authoritarian. For maternal parenting style, the internal consistency was .64, which is an acceptable reliability. The three subscales also report satisfactory reliabilities ranging from .65 to .86. Among the three subscales, the permissive maternal parenting style reported the lowest reliability, $\alpha = .65$, and the authoritative style report the highest reliability, $\alpha = .86$. For paternal parenting style, the internal consistency was .69, which is

Table 12.1 Reliability analysis ($N = 218$)

Scales	Means	Cronbach's alpha (α)
Perceived parenting style (mother)	3.134	.641
Permissive	3.037	.652
Authoritarian	3.106	.808
Authoritative	3.267	.858
Perceived parenting style (father)	3.153	.691
Permissive	3.219	.626
Authoritarian	3.040	.834
Authoritative	3.180	.866
Self-regulated learning	4.245	.923
Rehearsal	4.553	.776
Elaboration	4.448	.825
Organization	4.531	.731
Critical thinking	4.245	.733
Metacognitive self-regulation	4.201	.775
Achievement emotions	2.767	.874
Enjoyment	2.973	.838
Hope	3.282	.804
Pride	3.296	.816
Anger	2.255	.831
Anxiety	2.644	.782
Shame	2.721	.785
Hopelessness	2.216	.835
Boredom	2.890	.870
Academic procrastination	3.158	.778

satisfactory. The three subscales also report satisfactory reliabilities ranging from .63 to .87. Among the three subscales, the permissive style reported the lowest but acceptable reliability, $\alpha = .63$, while the authoritative style report the highest reliability, $\alpha = .87$.

For the self-regulated learning, the reliability of the whole scale was .92, which indicated a high-internal consistency among the five subscales. For the five subscales of self-regulated learning, all of them reported a good reliability ranging from .73 to .83. Elaboration report the highest reliability, $\alpha = .83$.

For the achievement emotion scale, the reliability of it was .87, which indicated a high-internal consistency among the eight subscales. For the eight subscales, all of them report good reliability ranging from .78 to .87.

For academic procrastination scale, the reliability of it was .78, which indicated a good reliability.

12.5.2 Correlation Analysis

The mean, standard deviations and correlations of perceived parenting style, achievement emotion, self-regulated learning, and academic procrastination are indicated in Table 12.2 shown below. There are total 20 variables, 95 out of 190 correlations were found significant.

In general, some perceived parenting style is positively associated with some achievement emotions, and negatively associated with academic procrastination. For self-regulated learning, it had moderate positive association with positive achievement emotions, and moderate negative association with negative association with academic procrastination. For achievement emotion, positive shown negative association with academic procrastination, while negative achievement emotions shown the opposite association.

12.5.3 Path Analysis

12.5.3.1 Perceived Parenting Style, Achievement Emotions, and Academic Procrastination

In Fig. 12.1 shown below, a multiple regression was considered predicting the academic procrastination by perceived maternal and paternal parenting style mediated by achievement emotions. From the figure, paternal permissive style, paternal authoritative style, and maternal-authoritative style, were significant predictors of hope, $F(6, 191) = 3.34$, $p < .01$, $R^2 = .095$. Paternal authoritarian style was a significant predictor of shame, $F(6, 190) = 2.75$, $p < .05$, $R^2 = .080$. Maternal permissive style and maternal authoritarian style were a significant predictors of hopelessness, $F(6, 190) = 3.31$, $p < .01$, $R^2 = .095$. However, compared the paternal and maternal parenting style, perceived maternal parenting style was stronger predictors than perceived paternal parenting style.

Also, both hope, $\beta = -.22$, $t(206) = -2.31$, $p < .05$, and hopelessness, $\beta = -.23$, $t(206) = -2.38$, $p < .05$, were significant negative predictors of academic procrastination, while shame was significant positive predictors of academic procrastination, $\beta = -.23$, $t(206) = -2.60$, $p = .01$.

From the result, it can found that the perceived parenting style from both mother and father were significant predictors of academic procrastination mediated by some achievement emotions, including hope, hopelessness, and shame. This result supports the hypothesis (1).

However, there is a conflict that both hope and hopelessness were negative predictors of academic procrastination, which violate with the information from the literature. Detailed may discussed in the discussion part.

Table 12.2 Correlation analysis ($N = 218$)

	1	2	3	4	5	6	7	8	9	10	11	12	13	14	15	16	17	18	19	20
Mpermiss	1																			
Mautarian	−.484**	1																		
Mautative	.416**	−.294**	1																	
Fpermiss	.310**	−.082	.169*	1																
Fautarian	−.107	.506**	−.003	−.396**	1															
Fautative	.233**	−.094	.451**	.370**	−.179**	1														
Rehearsal	−.087	−.019	.124	−.043	.020	.067	1													
Elabora	−.058	.022	.089	−.011	.030	.073	.693**	1												
Organ	.030	.039	.113	.021	.094	.119	.683**	.630**	1											
Crithink	.123	.033	.138*	.150*	.051	.139*	.431**	.582**	.447**	1										
Metacog	.011	.030	.064	.008	.090	.137*	.631**	.709**	.657**	.550**	1									
Enjoy	−.018	.113	.055	−.060	.156*	.136*	.361**	.311**	.358**	.243**	.481**	1								
Hope	.035	.015	.215**	−.118	.108	.171*	.403**	.447**	.370**	.411**	.579**	.638**	1							
Pride	.001	.069	.130	.033	.114	.050	.311**	.348**	.271**	.310**	.408**	.566**	.633**	1						
Anger	.032	.105	−.096	.076	.045	−.158*	−.284**	−.202**	−.153*	−.025	−.192**	−.294**	−.291**	−.098	1					
Anxiety	.037	.182**	−.055	−.058	.192**	−.024	.080	.058	.147*	.009	.116	.168*	−.016	.223**	.425**	1				
Shame	−.038	.192**	−.108	−.110	.241**	−.117	.048	.002	.131	−.084	−.001	.120	−.055	.264**	.344**	.650**	1			
Hopeless	.188**	.115	.032	.026	.101	.021	−.205**	−.211**	−.149*	−.061	−.243**	−.284**	−.352**	−.258**	.603**	.439**	.324**	1		
Boredom	.062	.055	.089	.026	.044	−.037	−.151*	−.114	−.176**	−.055	−.332**	−.434**	−.335**	−.130	.519**	.257**	.338**	.590**	1	
Aprocast	−.025	.018	−.088	.006	.059	−.231**	−.184**	−.150*	−.181**	−.169*	−.384**	−.196**	−.264**	−.101	.133	.010	.196**	.085	.332**	1

*$p < .05$, **$p < .01$

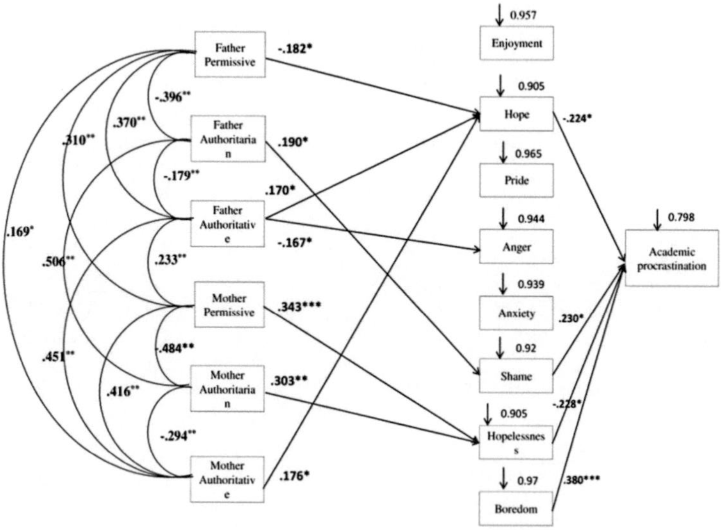

Fig. 12.1 Path analysis of the relationship among perceived parenting style, achievement emotions, and academic procrastination. *$p < .05$, **$p < .01$, ***$p < .001$

12.5.3.2 Perceived Parenting Style, Achievement Emotions, and Self-regulated Learning

In Fig. 12.2, Hope was significant positive predictors of rehearsal, $\beta = .27$, $t(199) = 2.75$, $p < .01$, while anger was significant negative predictors of rehearsal, $\beta = -.29$, $t(199) = -3.40$, $p = .001$. Hope was also strong significant positive predictors of elaboration ($\beta = .36$, $t(204) = 3.77$, $p = .00$), organization ($\beta = .29$, $t(205) = 2.99$, $p < .01$), critical thinking ($\beta = .36$, $t(206) = 3.79$, $p = .00$), and metacognitive self-regulation ($\beta = .44$, $t(203) = 5.29$, $p = .00$). Shame was significant negative predictors of critical thinking, $\beta = -.20$, $t(206) = -2.29$, $p < .05$. Anxiety was significant positive predictors of metacognitive self-regulation, $\beta = .202$, $t(203) = 2.47$, $p < .05$.

From the result, it can found that the perceived parenting style from both mother and father were significant predictors of self-regulated learning mediated by some achievement emotions, including hope, anger, anxiety, and shame. This result supports the hypothesis (2).

12.5.4 Confirmatory Factor Analysis (CFA)

A confirmatory factor analysis (CFA) was conducted using LISREL to examine the validity of several scales. Before conducting the CFA, exploratory

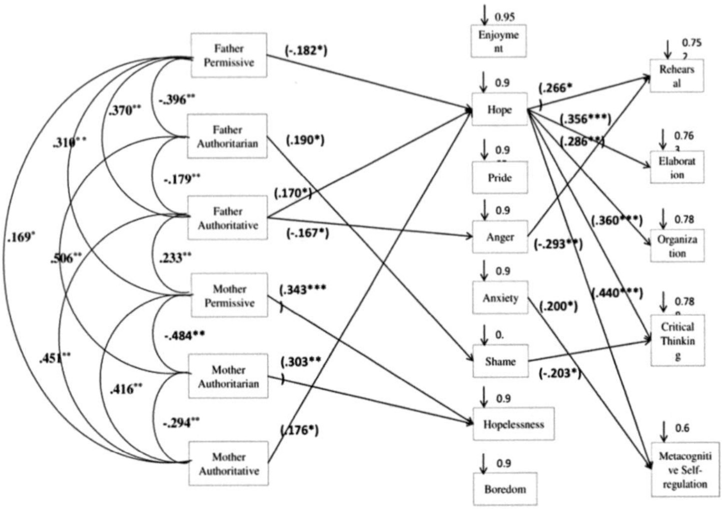

Fig. 12.2 Path analysis of the relationship among perceived parenting style, achievement emotions, and self-regulated learning. **p* < .05, ***p* < .01, ****p* < .001

factor analyses (EFA) was also conducted using SPSS for items parceling and deletion. For the scale of procrastination, it CFA result was $\chi^2(20) = 71.519$, RMSEA = .11, NNFI = .89, CFI = .92, GFI = .91. All factors loadings were significant, and the average loading was .54. For the self-efficacy scale, the CFA result of it was $\chi^2(20) = 92.36$, RMSEA = .13, NNFI = .94, CFI = .96, GFI = .92. All factors loadings were significant, and the average loading was .73.

12.5.5 Structural Equation Modeling (SEM)

12.5.5.1 Perceived Paternal Parenting Style, Positive Achievement Emotions and Self-regulated Learning

The model of perceived paternal parenting style, positive achievement emotions, and self-regulated learning was examined conducted by structural equation modeling using LISREL. Results from LISREL revealed that the model fit the data, χ^2 (26) = 47.931, $\chi^2/df = 1.84$, RMSEA = .0663, CFI = .98, NNFI = .98, GFI = .95. The SEM model was shown in Fig. 12.3.

In this SEM model, authoritative was the only indicator of the perceived paternal parenting style that fit the model. It was significantly positively associated with positive achievement emotions ($\beta = .19$, $p < .05$). The other two types of perceived paternal parenting style, including permissive and authoritarian had also been tried to add into the SEM model. However, the model failed to fit the data.

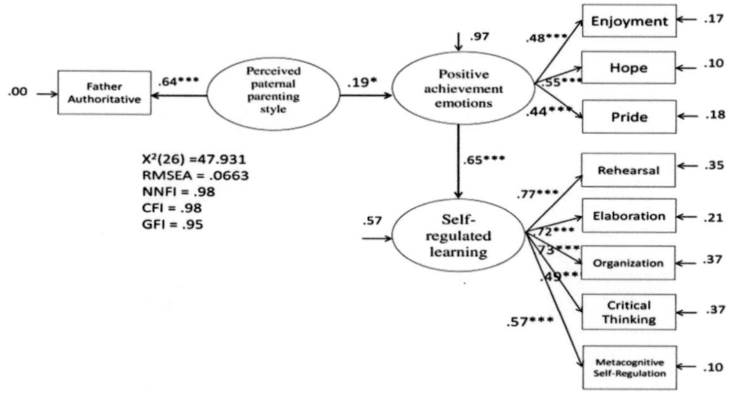

Fig. 12.3 The structural equation modeling of interrelationships among perceived paternal parenting style, positive achievement emotions, and self-regulated learning. *Note RMSEA* Root mean square error of approximation, *NNFI* Non-normed fit index, *CFI* Comparative fit index, *GFI* Goodness of fit index. $^{*}p < .05$, $^{**}p < .01$, $^{***}p < .001$

It could imply that authoritative was the strongest predictor of perceived paternal parenting style on positive achievement emotions.

Moreover, it was also found that positive achievement emotions was significantly positively associated with self-regulated learning ($\beta = .65$, $p < .001$). In positive achievement emotions, all the three indicators were positively associated with it, including enjoyment ($\beta = .48$, $p < .001$), hope ($\beta = .55$, $p < .001$) and pride ($\beta = .44$, $p < .001$). In self-regulated learning, all the five indicators were also positively associated with it, including rehearsal ($\beta = .77$, $p < .001$), elaboration ($\beta = .72$, $p < .001$), organization ($\beta = .73$, $p < .001$), critical thinking ($\beta = .49$, $p < .001$) and metacognitive self-regulation ($\beta = .57$, $p < .001$). Also, rehearsal, elaboration and organization were the stronger indicators of self-regulated learning among the five indicators.

In addition, the SEM model revealed that the perceived paternal parenting style was an indirect positive predictor of self-regulated learning ($\beta = .12$, $p < .05$) with positive achievement emotions as the mediator.

12.5.5.2 Perceived Maternal Parenting Style, Positive Achievement Emotions, and Self-regulated Learning

The model of perceived maternal parenting style, positive achievement emotions, and self-regulated learning was examined conducted by structural equation modeling using LISREL. Results from LISREL revealed that the model fit the data, $\chi^2(26) = 51.059$, $\chi^2/df = 1.96$, RMSEA = .0701, CFI = .98, NNFI = .98, GFI = .94. The SEM model was shown in Fig. 12.4.

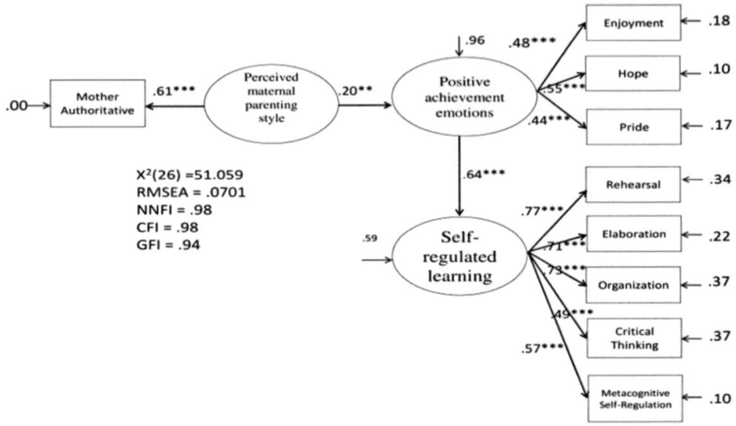

Fig. 12.4 The structural equation modeling of interrelationships among perceived maternal parenting style, positive achievement emotions, and self-regulated learning. *NoteRMSEA* Root mean square error of approximation, *NNFI* Non-normed fit index, *CFI* Comparative fit index, *GFI* Goodness of fit index. *$p < .05$, **$p < .01$, ***$p < .001$

In this SEM model, authoritative was the only indicator of the perceived maternal parenting style that fit the model. It was significantly positively associated with positive achievement emotions ($\beta = .19$, $p < .05$). It could imply that authoritative was a moderate predictor of perceived maternal parenting style on positive achievement emotions.

Moreover, it was also found that positive achievement emotions was significantly positively associated with self-regulated learning ($\beta = .64$, $p < .001$). In positive achievement emotions, all the three indicators were positively associated with it, including enjoyment ($\beta = .48$, $p < .001$), hope ($\beta = .55$, $p < .001$) and pride ($\beta = .44$, $p < .001$). In self-regulated learning, all the five indicators were also positively associated with it, including rehearsal ($\beta = .77$, $p < .001$), elaboration ($\beta = .71$, $p < .001$), organization ($\beta = .73$, $p < .001$), critical thinking ($\beta = .49$, $p < .001$), and metacognitive self-regulation ($\beta = .57$, $p < .001$). Also, rehearsal, elaboration, and organization were the stronger indicators of self-regulated learning among the five indicators.

In addition, the SEM model revealed that the perceived maternal parenting style was an indirect positive predictor of self-regulated learning ($\beta = .13$, $p < .05$) with positive achievement emotions act as the mediator.

12.5.5.3 Perceived Paternal Parenting Style, Positive Achievement Emotions, and Academic Procrastination

The model of perceived paternal parenting style, positive achievement emotions, and academic procrastination was examined conducted by structural equation modeling using LISREL. Results from LISREL revealed that the model fit

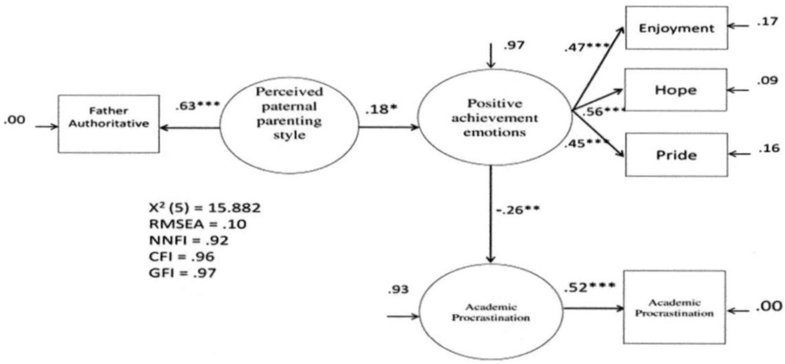

Fig. 12.5 The structural equation modeling of interrelationships among perceived paternal parenting style, positive achievement emotions, and academic procrastination. *Note RMSEA* Root mean square error of approximation, *NNFI* Non-normed fit index, *CFI* Comparative fit index, *GFI* Goodness of fit index. $^{*}p < .05$, $^{**}p < .01$, $^{***}p < .001$

the data, $\chi^2(5) = 15.882$, $\chi^2/df = 3.18$, RMSEA = .10, CFI = .92, NNFI = .96, GFI = .97. The SEM model was shown in Fig. 12.5.

In this SEM model, authoritative was the only indicator of the perceived paternal parenting style that fit the model. It was significantly positively associated with positive achievement emotions ($\beta = .18$, $p < .05$). The other two types of perceived paternal parenting style, including permissive and authoritarian had also been tried to add into the SEM model. However, the model failed to fit the data. It implied that authoritative was the strongest predictor of perceived paternal parenting style on positive achievement emotions.

Moreover, it was also found that positive achievement emotions was significantly negatively associated with academic procrastination ($\beta = -.26$, $p < .01$). The result implied that positive achievement emotions were strong negative predictors on academic procrastination. Also, in positive achievement emotions, all the three indicators were positively associated with it, including enjoyment ($\beta = .47, p < .001$), hope ($\beta = .56, p < .001$) and pride ($\beta = .45, p < .001$).

In addition, the SEM model revealed that the perceived paternal parenting style was an indirect negative predictor on academic procrastination ($\beta = -.046$, $p < .05$) with positive achievement emotions act as the mediator.

12.5.5.4 Perceived Maternal Parenting Style, Positive Achievement Emotions, and Academic Procrastination

The model of perceived maternal parenting style, positive achievement emotions, and academic procrastination was examined conducted by structural equation modeling using LISREL. Results from LISREL revealed that the model fit the data, $\chi^2(5) = 11.08$, $\chi^2/df = 2.22$, RMSEA = .076, CFI = .96, NNFI = .98, GFI = .98. The SEM model was shown in Fig. 12.6.

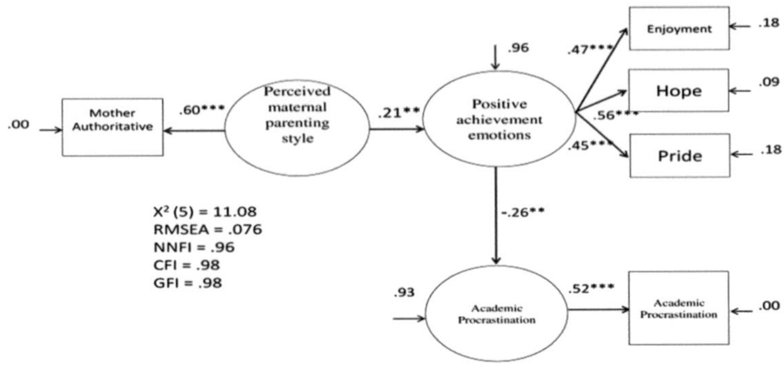

Fig. 12.6 The structural equation modeling of interrelationships among perceived maternal parenting style, positive achievement emotions and academic procrastination. *Note RMSEA* Root mean square error of approximation, *NNFI* Non-normed fit index, *CFI* Comparative fit index, *GFI* Goodness of fit index. $^{*}p < .05$, $^{**}p < .01$, $^{***}p < .001$

In this SEM model, authoritative was the only indicator of the perceived maternal parenting style that fit the model. It was significantly positively associated with positive achievement emotions ($\beta = .21$, $p < .01$). It could imply that authoritative was a moderate predictor of perceived maternal parenting style on positive achievement emotions.

Moreover, it was also found that positive achievement emotions was significantly positively associated with academic procrastination ($\beta = -.26$, $p < .01$). The result implied that positive achievement emotions were negative predictor of academic procrastination. Also, in positive achievement emotions, all the three indicators were positively associated with it, including enjoyment ($\beta = .47$, $p < .001$), hope ($\beta = .56$, $p < .001$), and pride ($\beta = .45$, $p < .001$). All the three subscales were strong indicators of positive achievement emotions.

In addition, the SEM model revealed that the perceived maternal parenting style was an indirect negative predictor of academic procrastination ($\beta = -.05$, $p < .05$) with positive achievement emotions act as the mediator.

12.6 Discussion

12.6.1 Mediating Effect of Positive Achievement Emotions Between Perceived Parenting Style and Academic Procrastination

Referred to the path model (Fig. 12.4), it was found that all types of maternal and paternal parenting style were correlated with academic procrastination. However, referred to the structural equation model (Figs. 12.5, 12.6), it was found that only perceived parental authoritative style was found to be negatively significantly associated with academic procrastination. The result implied that among the three types of parenting style, including authoritarian, authoritative and permissive parenting style, the perceived authoritative style was the only and the strongest predictor of academic procrastination. However, some researches mentioned in the above part had suggested that both permissive style and authoritarian style should also be the predictor of academic procrastination (Vahedi et al. 2009; Pychyl et al. 2002; Zakeri et al. 2013), where as permissive parenting style was negative predictor of academic procrastination and authoritarian style was positive predictor of academic procrastination. So, discrepancy found between the result of the present study and the previous findings.

To evaluate, the discrepancy may be the difference between Western parenting style and the Chinese parenting style. In Western culture, authoritarian was defined as a cold and distant parenting style. In other word, authoritarian parenting style was labeled in a negative way. Among the three parenting styles, Western parent may prefer more on authoritarian style. However, in Chinese culture, authoritarian parenting style was not viewed as negative as Western culture. Also, Chinese parenting style seemed much more complex than Western view of point.

Traditionally, Chinese parenting style was described by study or Western parents as overcontrolling, demanding, and authoritarian, in which they set high goals and rules to children. However, according to Chao's study (1994, 1996), it pointed out that authoritative and authoritarian were not appropriate in describing Chinese parenting style, as Chinese parents were high controlling at the same time with high involvement in direct parent–child interaction and high physical proximity. Chao described it as the notion of "guan." Chinese parenting style was not as cold and distant as mentioned. Rather, they would show their closeness and warmth to the children even though they had high expectation on children. They would also emphasize children's effort on work and achievement (Stevenson and Lee 1990). Also, in view of Chinese children, they would not felt distanced by parents as Western studies predict, but they also felt connected with parents (Chao 2001). So, Chinese parents had close connection with their children even with high control. This may be the reason why the linkage between authoritarian style and academic procrastination fail to be shown.

12.6.2 Achievement Emotion and Academic Procrastination

Referred to the path model (Fig. 12.4), it was found that both hope and hopelessness reported negative relationship with academic procrastination, whereas hope was defined as positive emotion and hopelessness was defined as negative emotion. Conflict found as previous studies indicated that positive emotion should be negatively related to academic procrastination, while negative emotion should be positively related to academic procrastination (Li 2012a, b; Zhang et al. 2012). The conflict can be explained as followed.

First, the conflict may because of the unclear definition of academic procrastination. According to Chu and Choi (2005) study, academic procrastination can be further divided into two categories, active and passive procrastination. Passive procrastination referred to the traditional type of procrastination, which the tendency of procrastination may increase when hope decrease. Active procrastinator referred to those who make deliberate decision on procrastination, so there may be increase in the tendency of procrastination when they feel hopelessness. However, the scale used in this research is adjusted from a general scale of procrastination, no subscale were used to divide academic procrastination into these two categories. Therefore, the conflict result occurred.

Secondly, the conflict may due to the different in academic attitude of the participants. Flett et al. (1995) indicated that students who have perfectionism may actively procrastinate because of the needs of perfection of their performance on work. Also, the study pointed that perfectionism can produce work inhibition and is one of the factors to the lack of striving for achievement. In this study, the result may affected by two types of student, those who have perfectionism and those who have not. So, conflict occurred.

12.7 Conclusion

This research study had examined the relationship between perceived parenting style, self-efficacy, achievement emotion, self-regulated learning, and academic procrastination. The result from the correlation and path analysis found that self-efficacy is a stringer predictor in predicting both the self-regulated learning and academic procrastination mediated mainly by hope. In addition, both perceived maternal and paternal parenting style are week to moderate predictors of self-regulated learning and academic procrastination mediated hope, anger, and shame.

References

Azar, F. S. (2013). *Self-efficacy, achievement motivation and academic procrastination as predictors of academic achievement in pre-college students*. Proceeding of the Global Summit on Education, pp 173–178.

Baumrind, D. (1967). Child care practices anteceding three patterns of preschool behavior. *Genetic Psychology Monographs, 75*(5), 43–88.

Blatt, S. J., & Quinlan, P. (1967). Punctual and procrastinating students: A study of temporal parameters. *Journal of Consulting Psychology, 31*(2), 169–174.

Buri, J. R. (1991). Parental authority questionnaire. *Journal of Personality Assessment, 57*(1), 110–119.

Brownlow, S., & Reasinger, R. D. (2000). Putting off until tomorrow what is better done today: Academic procrastination as a function of motivation toward college work. *Journal of Social Behavior & Personality, 15*(5), 15–34.

Chao, R. (1994). Beyond parental control; authoritarian parenting style: Understanding Chinese parenting through the cultural notion of training. *Child Development 45*, 1111–1119. http://www.parentingscience.com/chinese-parenting.html#sthash.F8CieorZ.dpuf

Chao, R. (1996). Chinese and European American mother's belief about the role of parenting in children's school success. *Journal of Cross-Culture Psychology, 27*, 403–423.

Chao, R. (2001). Extending research on the consequences of parenting style for Chinese Americans and European Americans. *Child Development 72*, 1832–1843. http://www.parentingscience.com/chinese-parenting.html#sthash.F8CieorZ.dpuf

Chu, C. H., & Choi, J. N. (2005). Rethinking procrastination: Positive effects of "Active" procrastination behavior on attitudes and performance. *Journal of Educational Psychology, 145*(3), 245–264.

Da xue sheung jin si cheng huan shang tuo yan zheng wu cheng bu yuan wei zuo ye fei shen. (大學生近四成患上"拖延症" 五成不願為作業費神) [Around 40 % of college students had procrastination and 50 % of them are unwilling to spent time in doing homework]. (2015, Dec 14). Chinese News. Retrieved from http://www.chinanews.com/life/2015/12-14/7670139.shtml

Da xue sheung lan san, kuang ke shi deng xian. (大學生懶散曠課視等閒) [Lazy College Students Regarded Truancy as Minor Problem]. (2014, Feb 26). Oriental Daily. Retrieved from http://orientaldaily.on.cc/cnt/news/20140226/00176_097.html

Effert, B. R., & Ferrari, J. R. (1989). Decisional procrastination, examining personality correlates. *Journal of Social Behaviour and Personality, 4*, 151–156.

Ellis, A., & Knaus, W. J. (1977). Overcoming Procrastination. *Institute for Rational Living*. New York.

Ferrari, J. R., & Emmons, R. A. (1995). Methods of procrastination and their relation to self-control and self-reinforcement: An exploratory study. *Journal of Social Behaviour and Personality, 10*, 135–142.

Ferrari, J. R., & Olivette, M. J. (1993). Perceptions of parental control and the development of indecision among late adolescent females. *Adolescence, 28*, 963–970.

Ferrari, J. R., & Olivette, M. J. (1994). Parental authority and the development of female dysfunctional procrastination. *Journal of Research in Personality, 28*, 87–100.

Ferrari, J. R., Harriott, J. S., & Zimmerman, M. (1999). The social support networks of procrastinators: Friends or family in times of trouble? *Personality & Individual Differences, 26*(2), 321–331.

Ferrari, J. R., Jonhson, J. L., & McCown, W. G. (1995). *Procrastination and task avoidance: Theory, research and treatment*. New York: Plenum.

Flett, G. L., Hewitt, P. L., & Martin, T. R. (1995). Dimensions of perfectionism and procrastination. In J. R. Ferrari, J. L. Johnson, & W. G. McCown (Eds.), *Procrastination and task avoidance: Theory, research and treatment*. New York: Plenum Press.

Gonzalez, A. L., & Wolters, C. A. (2006). The relation between perceived parenting practices and achievement motivation in mathematics. *Journal of Research in Childhood Education, 21*(2), 203–217.

Haycock, L. A., McCarthy, P., & Skay, C. L. (1998). Procrastination in college students: The role of self-efficacy and anxiety. *Journal of Counselling Development, 76*, 317–323.

Hong, J. C., Hwang, M. Y., Kuo, Y. C., & Hsu, W. Y. (2014). Parental monitoring and helicopter parenting relevant to vocational student's procrastination and self-regulated learning. *Learning and Individual Differences, 42*, 139–146.

Huang, L. C. (2010). *Examination of the effect of emotion regulation strategies on academic emotions process model.* Unpublished Journal.

Kachgal, M. M., Hansen, L. S., & Nutter, K. J. (2001). Academic procrastination prevention/intervention: Strategies and recommendations. *Journal of Development and Education, 25*, 14–21.

Klassen, R. M., Krawchuk, L. L., & Rajani, S. (2008). Academic procrastination of undergraduates: Low self-efficacy to self-regulate predicts higher levels of procrastination. *Contemporary Educational Psychology, 33*, 915–931.

Lay, C. H. (1986). At last, my research article on procrastination. *Journal of Research in Personality, 20*, 479–495.

Li, C. (2012). Examining 'active' procrastination from a self-regulated learning perspective. *Educational Psychology,* 1–31.

Li da xue sheung liu cheng bam zeng zou tang. (理大學生六成半曾走堂) [65 % students of Polytechnic University had skip classes]. (2006, Jan 17). Apple Daily. Retrieved from http://hk.apple.nextmedia.com/news/art/20060117/5580333

Li, G. (2012b). *A study of the correlation between academic procrastination and academic emotions and group intervention*. Shanghai: Shanghai Normal University.

McCown, W., Petzel, T., & Rupert, P. (1987). An Experimental study of some hypothesized behaviors and personality variables of college student procrastinators. *Personality and Individual Differences, 8*(6), 781–786.

Milgram, N., Mey-Tal, G., & Levison, Y. (1998). Procrastination, generalized or specific, in college students and their parents. *Personality and Individual Differences, 25*(2), 297–316.

Noran, F.Y. (2000). *Procrastination among students in institutes of higher learning: Challenges for K-Economy*. Retrieved from http://www.mahdzan.com/papers/Procrastinate/

Nyarko, K. (2011). The influence of authoritative parenting style on adolescents' academic achievement. *American Journal of Social and Management Sciences, 2*(3), 278–282.

Pekrun, R., Goetz, T., Titz, T., & Perry, R. P. (2002). Academic emotions in students' self-regulated learning and achievement: A program of qualitative and quantitative research. *Educational Psychologist, 37*(2), 91–106.

Pekrun, R., Goetz, T., Frenzel, A. C., Barchfeld, P., & Perry, R. P. (2011). Measuring emotions in students' learning and performance: The Achievement Emotions Questionnaire (AEQ). *Contemporary Educational Psychology, 36*(1), 36–48.

Popoola, B. I. (2005). A study of the relationship between procrastinatory behaviour and academic performance of undergraduate students in a Nigerian University. *African Symposium*. Retrieved from http://www.ncsu.edu/ncsu/aern/TAS5.1.htm

Pychyl, T. A., Coplan, R. J., & Reid, P. A. M. (2002). Parenting and procrastination: Gender differences in the relations between procrastination, parenting style and self-worth in early adolescence. *Personality and Individual Differences 33*, 271–285. Retrieved from http://users.ugent.be/wbeyers/scripties2012/artikels/Pychyl%20et%20al._2002.pdf

Rabin, L. A., Fogel, J., & Nutter-Upham, K. E. (2011). Academic procrastination in college students: The role of self-reported executive function. *Journal of Clinical and Experimental Neuropsychology, 33*(3), 344–357.

Senecal, C., Koestner, R., & Vallerand, R. J. (1995). *The Journal Social Psychology, 135*(5), 607–619.

Solomon, L. J., & Rothblum, E. D. (1984). Academic procrastination: Frequency and cognitive-behavioral correlates. *Journal of Counseling Psychology, 31*(4), 503–509.

Soysa, C. K., & Weiss, A. (2014). Mediating perceived parenting styles–test anxiety relationships: Academic procrastination and maladaptive perfectionism. *Learning and Individual Differences, 34*, 77–85.

Steel, P. (2007). The nature of procrastination: A meta-analytic and theoretical review of quintessential self-regulatory failure. *Psychological Bulletin, 133*(1), 65–94.

Stevenson, H. W., & Lee, S. Y. (1990). Contexts of achievement: A study of American, Chinese, and Japanese children. *Monograph of the Society for Research in Child Development, 55*(221), 1–2.

Tice, D. M., Bratslavsky, E., & Baumeister, R. F. (2001). Emotional distress regulation takes precedence over impulse control: If you feel bad, do it! *Journal of Personality and Social Psychology, 80*, 53–67.

Vahedi, S., Mostafafi, F., & Mortazanajad, H. (2009). Self-regulation and dimensions of parenting styles predict psychological procrastination of undergraduate students. *Iranian Journal of Psychiatry, 4*, 147–154.

Wolters, C. A. (2003). Understanding procrastination from a self-regulated learning perspective. *Journal of Educational Psychology, 95*, 179–187.

Zakeri, H., Esfahanib, B. N., & Razmjoeec, M. (2013). Parenting styles and academic procrastination. *Procedia Social and Behavioral Sciences, 84*, 57–60.

Zhang, X. X., Xiong, J. M., & Li, J. (2012). The mediated effect of achievement motivation between the relationship of achievement emotions and academic procrastination. *Journal of Southwest Agricultural University (Social Science Edition), 10*(9), 249–252.

Zimmerman, B. J. (1990). Self-regulated learning and academic achievement: An overview. *Educational Psychologist, 25*(1), 3–17.

Chapter 13
Pathways to Bullying and Victimization—Psychological Perspectives

Ann Joma Job and Sherin P. Antony

Abstract *Background* Previous researches have explained pathways leading to victimization and bullying. However, the origin of the process and link between the factors leading to bullying behaviour and victimization is less known knowledge. *Objective* The current study aimed to understand the personal experiences of bullies and victims using qualitative approach. The study focused on the experiences in different dimensions of Family dynamics; Defence mechanism; Coping; Perception of school; Life events; and Role of peers, teachers, and parents. *Method* The study undertaken utilizes a qualitative research design. Semi-structured interviews were used to collect data from 10 bullies and 6 victims from different CBSE schools of Kerala. Purposive sampling technique was used to collect data. The data from the interviews were analyzed using qualitative methods of content analysis and Interpretative Phenomenological Analysis. *Results* The bullies displaced the anger while the victims tried to repress the emotions turning the anger inward. The bullies and victims experienced insecure attachment styles. However, bullies got disengaged from their families and victims got enmeshed with their parents. Bullies tend to describe bullying as "fun" and victims on the other hand restrict themselves from expressing their feelings of hurt and laugh when targeted. The contradictory meanings created by bullies and victims influenced their perception of school and their worldview. This also makes one group become responsible while make another group feel helpless. *Conclusions* The social implications and scope of further research suggestions will be discussed.

A.J. Job (✉) · S.P. Antony
Department of Psychology, Jain University, Bengaluru, Karnataka 560027, India
e-mail: annjjob@gmail.com

S.P. Antony
Department of Psychology, Acharya Institute of Graduate Studies,
Bengaluru, Karnataka 560107, India
e-mail: sherin.anil@yahoo.com

M.-T. Leung and L.-M Tan (eds.), *Applied Psychology Readings*,
DOI 10.1007/978-981-10-2796-3_13

Keywords Bullying victimization pathways · Family dynamics · Defence mechanisms

13.1 Introduction

An act of bullying is defined as one that is persisted against those who are weaker than the bullies either psychologically, emotionally, or physically. There are various factors that work together interlinking with each other in the prevalence of bullying in schools. The impact of bullying on children is yet to be looked into in Indian researches. Below are mentioned certain reasons for bullying to occur along with the negative impact that each of the behaviour has on the bullies and victims in the bullying scenarios on the basis of the previous studies conducted in the area.

13.1.1 Family Dynamics

13.1.1.1 Parenting Styles and Peer Relations

Family structures play a role in behavioural, cognitive, and emotional development of children. These familial structures are formed on the basis of the interaction patterns engaged by the parents. Baumrind (1991) explains three approaches of parenting that impacts behaviours of children. Children raised in an authoritative setting are highly warm and nurturing in their method of communication with peers. This is because parents demonstrating authoritative style provide a conducive environment that encourages children to reflect high self-esteem and self-reliance along with behaviours that are self-controlled. Children raised in authoritarian backgrounds are more likely to be aggressive, have lower self-esteem and are also low in peer competence. Lastly, children hailed in permissive households which indulge in lesser structure and higher warmth fail at being responsible and self-control is depreciated.

Attachment Styles and Peer Relations

The cognitive representations of stimuli that individuals possess are largely influenced from childhood experiences. Subsequent relationships, as individuals grow, is strongly impacted by the attachment styles experienced with primary caregivers. This is also consistent with the kind of interaction that these individuals share with their peers. Bowlby (1969) explained attachment styles via an experiment called Strange Situation Classification (SSC). There are three types of insecure attachment styles that are prevalent among children. Children experiencing insecure–avoidant attachment style are independent physically as well as emotionally. They would explore a new environment without any positive reinforcement from the caregiver. Due to lack of trust these children perceive most situations as hostile are therefore more likely to be aggressive towards their peers (Renken et al. 1989; Shaver et al. 1996). Insecure–disorganized attachment style is where the children are not sure as to how to act in a new situation even in the presence of their primary caregiver. Children who engage in insecure disorganized attachment style have expressed elevated levels of aggression (Lyons-Ruth 1996). Insecure ambivalent attachment is both clingy as well as avoidant because of the inconsistency in the way help was provided to them by the caregiver. They are prone to have low self-esteem and are unstable in their relationships as they express considerable amount of temper while interacting with others. They are highly vulnerable and victimized and exhibit anxiety and negative attitudes in expressing their peer relationships (Elicker et al. 1992). Secure attachment style are adaptive in their relationships with their peers and enjoy peer acceptance (Elicker et al. 1992; Thompson 2008). They also have been observed to be empathetic and express low negative affect (LaFreniere and Sroufe 1985; Shaver et al. 1996). Secure children have positive communication system in social situations while children who are insecure have poor peer relations (Berlin et al. 2008; Kerns 2008).

13.1.2 Defence Mechanisms v/s Coping

Defence mechanisms are unconscious tools exercised used in times of anxiety and stress. Successful adaptation depends on engaging in these moderately. However, excessive use of the same could lead to maladjustments. The strategies used in times of stress are repression, suppression, fantasy, displacement, denial, regression and humour (Cramer 2008).

Coping are cognitive as well as behavioural methods engaged consciously by individuals when elicited due to a stressor. Engaging in a particular coping is beneficial irrespective of it being unsuccessful. In a bullying scenario, children firstly evaluate if it is a high large group or small group or a dyad. Secondly they consider their options of coping by walking away, ignoring, and problem-solving. Lastly, the coping strategy is implemented.

13.1.2.1 Internalizing

There have been longitudinal studies indicating internalizing behaviours among victims. These individuals have greater risks of loneliness (Juvonen et al. 2000; Kochenderfer and Ladd 1996), emotional issues, somatization, negative affect (Dill et al. 2004), and withdrawal (Bond et al. 2001; Goldbaum et al. 2007).

13.1.2.2 Externalizing

Parental maltreatment has been linked to externalizing behaviours among bullies (Sontag and Graber 2010). They have a better ability to reason and rationalize the aggressive behaviour that they engage in (Hymel and Bonanno 2014). Bullies are less capable of understanding others feelings and are prone to dominate others motivated by the desire to disempower others (Rigby and Smith 2011a, b).

13.1.3 Frustration and Anger

The lack of attachment shared with parents leads to anger and frustration. The inability to gain the attention of the primary caregivers induces the feeling of anger, which is reinforced by the attention and comfort that they receive following anger outburst. The inability to maintain relationships in the case of children who share insecure attachment styles have an increased level of frustration and aggression (Dutton 2011). Such children focus on themselves as a result of lack of attention from primary caregivers, which when cumulated with negative affect made tendencies of prosocial behaviours rare (Graziano et al. 2007). Anger has been explained as a result of perceiving a stimuli as frustrating, and the goal is to protect oneself or harm others (Berkowitz 1983). Therefore, any individual who perceives to be the victim of intentional harm would experience anger and act on it (Berkowitz 1983, 1989).

There have been many studies validating the relationship between anger and bullying (Bosworth et al. 1999; Mahady et al. 2000). In some studies only bullies have been explained as experiencing anger (Rieffe et al. 2012) while other studies have reflected that those children with anger are targeted (Dodge 1991). There are other studies which have explained anger as being higher among bullies and victims rather than those not involved, however, to be comparatively higher among bullies (Marsh et al. 2011). Bullies externalize their anger while victims internalize.

13.1.4 Perception of School

13.1.4.1 Academic

There is a complex relationship between victimization and academic achievement and adjustment. These experiences have been explored in longitudinal studies. Children who are chronically victimized in elementary school are observed to be less happy in school (Arseneault et al. 2006). The academic scores of these children keep decreasing through elementary school (Schwartz et al. 2005) and intermediate school (Esbensen and Carson 2009; Juvonen et al. 2011). By the time the children reach high school the perception of school as a negative place and the thought of school being a place exposed to risk is heightened (Smith et al. 2004a, b).

13.1.4.2 Social Relationships/Hierarchy

Peer victimization decreases popularity (Hanish and Guerra 2002). The feeling of rejection (Hodges and Perry 1999) as well as peer dislike (Scholte et al. 2007) increases from elementary school through high school. Longer the victimization experience, higher the problems faced in social relationships (Kumpulainen and Räsänen 2000; Smith et al. 2004a, b) due to loss of friends in school (Smith et al. 2004a, b).

13.1.5 Social Information Processing

Social Information Processing theory reformulated by Crick and Dodge (1994) is a process occurring in five mental steps in a circular fashion. The first step is when the recipients select the information to be given attention out of all the stimuli the individual is exposed to. The second would be to analyze that, what they would want to attain from the stimuli so as to abstract particular outcomes. In order to do this they search information from their long-term memory, which is coloured by the attributions that they have created in order to achieve the goals created by the individuals. Then one of the responses is chosen by the recipient of the stimuli on the basis of the matter of the response, the expected outcome and their ability to perform. The last loop involves the recipient's capability of parallel processing and of feedback loops.

Crick and Dodge used the steps to explain the adaptive and maladaptive ways of expressing behaviour. Bullying–victimization process can be explained in terms of this theory. Children who are aggressive in nature, tend to pay attention to cues that are aggressive. The interpretation of stimuli is largely dependent on the attribution that the children make, the analysis of the situation, the way they evaluate their self-efficacy, and the cues that they associate from their memory. Therefore, these processes are influenced by the schemata and the internal processes or models. The aggressive children are likely to attribute stimuli as hostile (Dodge 1985; Dodge and Frame 1982; Steinberg and Dodge 1983). Therefore, these children are more likely to choose and act upon a goal that is inappropriate in the particular situation. Thereby damaging their relationships, while those who are more adjusted with the situation tend to form positive relationships (Renshaw and Asher 1983; Slaby and Guerra 1988). The children respond to situations on the basis of their memory or something novel if the situation is new. Studies show that children who are rejected are less prosocial and not very friendly (Asher et al. 1980; Asarnow and Callan 1985). They are also likely to make poor choices (Asher et al. 1980; Rubin et al. 1982) as they are not aware on how to make positive choices. Further research results portray that children who are aggressive do not associate positive consequences to adaptive behaviours (Crick and Dodge 1994; Dodge et al. 1986; Quiggle et al. 1992).

13.1.6 Attachment, Anger, and Social Information Processing on Bullying and Victimization

The interlinking of the Social Information Processing with Lemerise and Arsenio's (2000), elaborates the influence of anger on the way stimuli is processed is related to the insecure attachment style experienced with parents in childhood (Nigg et al. 2010). Children's internal model of unreliability, lack of trustworthiness, and inconsistency has a higher likelihood of getting angry. This internal working model thereby influences their social information processing in the future. This explains the vicious cycle of poor social skills as being rooted on negative relationship with primary caregivers. Consequently, aggressive behaviour emerges (Dodge et al. 1990).

The study aimed at exploring the lived experiences of bullying and victimization, and conceptualization of the pathways. In addition, the factors that contributed to the bullying process were analyzed. Lastly, this bullying cycle was conceptualized to examine the adaptive or maladaptive ways.

13.2 Methodology

13.2.1 Research Design

An exploratory research design was implemented. The pathway leading to bullying and victimization was analyzed using Interpretative Phenomenological Analysis as a qualitative method.

13.2.2 Procedure

There were three stages to the data collection and analysis.

13.2.2.1 Description of the Psychological Perspectives in Explaining the Pathways to Bullying and Victimization

In the first stage of the study, review of literature was prepared to analyze the existing research on school bullying. This helped in conceptualizing the pathways to bullying and victimization on the basis of the existing literature. The aim of the study was to examine the experiences of both bullies and victims, and increase the knowledge into the pathway that leads them into bullying and victimization.

13.2.2.2 Collection of Participants' Description of the Psychological Perspectives of the Pathways Leading to Bullying and Victimization

Purposive sampling method was employed to collect data from CBSE schools of Kerala in India. Firstly, checklists were distributed among the high school teachers of these schools which helped in identifying the bullies and victims. The selection of the students was on the basis of the ratings that the teachers provided. Thereby, reliability of the ratings provided by the teachers in identifying school bullies and victims was established.

Sixteen high school students were selected to conduct the semi-structured interview. Out of the 16, 10 were bullies and 6 were victims within the age range of 13–16 years. Since, the participants had substantial amount of experience in bullying and victimization at the time of interview, as they were exposed to it since middle school. This presented with greater insight into the family dynamics, perception of school, coping, defence mechanism, frustration and anger, and social information processing as underpinnings of the pathways, during the interview process. The participants who were selected had volunteered themselves and confidentiality was maintained throughout. The extensive review of literature and the objectives of the study were the foundation in developing the format of the semi-structured interview (Tables 13.1, 13.2).

The exploration of the personal experiences throws light on the individual stories of the participant helping in the understanding of the pathways leading to bullying and victimization

Table 13.1 The interview topics incorporated

The family dynamics
Perception of school
Coping
Defence mechanism
Frustration and anger
Social Information Processing

Table 13.2 The probing questions in the interview process

Could you share the experiences that you have with your parents since childhood?
How would you explain the pleasant and unpleasant experiences that you have faced in this school with teachers?
How would you explain the pleasant and unpleasant experiences that you have faced in this school with peers?
What are the ways that you chose to respond in the situations that hurt you?
How did you feel emotionally and physically during those times? What did you o do make yourself feel better?
What were your thoughts when you experienced the hurt feelings? Could you describe
Could you share any moments of anger felt in school or at home?

In order to facilitate the direction of the interview to ascertain the factors leading to the pathways of bullying and victimization open-ended were used. The researchers incorporating Phenomenological method do not include leading questions in their interviews to explore the lived experience

13.2.2.3 Reading and Analysis of all the Participant Descriptions of Psychological Perspectives in Explaining the Pathways Leading to Bullying and Victimization

Data analysis involved deep and repeated reading of all the data (transcripts and field notes) and use analysis procedures as described below. The researcher transcribed each of the interview tapes. Consequently, after reading each transcript multiple times and then coding them manually Thereafter, each transcript was read multiple times and the transcript was manually coded for themes that emerged, explored the participant's experiences from different dimensions. Major themes identified were (i) family dysfunction (ii) social relationships (iii) coping, and (iv) frustration and anger. The sub-headings were:

(i) Family dysfunction

(a) Bullies

- Emotional distance
- Parental conflict
- Difference in parenting

(b) Victims

- Perception of warmth
- Enmeshment

(c) Bullies and Victims

- Punitive parenting

(ii) Social relationships

(a) Perception of school

- Bullies
- Enjoys school
- Negative intention
- Need for power
- Victims
- Victims
- Injustice

(b) Self-perception

- Bullies
- Ideal self-image

- Victims
- Body image

(c) Role of teachers

- Bullies
- Perception of partiality
- Victims
- Negative intention

(iii) Coping

(a) Internalization

a. Bullies
- Internalization
- Psychosomatization

b. Victims
- Isolation

(b) Externalization

- Bullies
- Aggression

(c) Defence mechanism

a. Victims
- Rationalization
- Repression
- Displacement

(iv) Frustraion and anger

(a) Bullies

a. Acting outward
- Physical bullying
- Verbal bullying
- Nonverbal bullying

(b) Victims

a. Acting inward

These emerged themes have been analyzed and discussed the basis of their personal experiences, context of psychological theories and previous empirical researchers.

13.2.3 Ethical Conduct

The school principals were approached to obtain approval to conduct the study. They were provided with a brief description before gaining permission. After this, informed consent was received from the teachers to volunteer in the study. The privacy and confidentiality of the school, teachers, and students were maintained. Pseudonyms were used to maintain anonymity of the students. They were also made aware of the possibility to withdraw any time from the study.

13.3 Results and Discussion

13.3.1 Family Dynamics

Family characteristics of both bullies and victims have been linked with underlying family dysfunctions. The path where family dysfunction diverges is in kind of turmoil that persists among the members. The themes were parental conflict, emotional distance from family and difference in parenting among bullies. Among victims it was perception of lack of warmth and enmeshment (Table 13.3). However, both had been exposed to punitive parenting (Bowes et al. 2009; Cook et al. 2010).

13.3.2 Social Relationships

Beyond family, peers and teachers have a crucial role in the socialization process. The social skills of the children are influenced by the interaction patterns with peers and teachers. These engagements have an association with the prevalence of bullying and victimization in schools. The present study has explored the perception of school, role of teachers, and self-perception (Table 13.4).

Bullies and victims had viewed teachers in a negative light. The former attributed their dislike to the partiality exhibited by the teachers, whereas the latter elucidated it as being targeted by them (Richard et al. 2011) In spite of having negative experiences with teachers, bullies perceive school as a place of enjoyment with peers through making fun of others and thereby gaining power. Victims reported being in the midst of unpleasant situations, which have been associated with injustice received from both teachers and peers (Pepler et al. 2010; Barboza et al. 2009).

Feeling of inadequacy is prevalent among bullies and victims. It is on this framework that bullies try to create and project ideal self-image while victims have a lower body image which is induced by others thereby reducing their self-esteem (Esbensen and Carson 2009).

Table 13.3 Themes emerged in the family dynamics experienced by bullies and victims

Family dynamics	
Bullies	Victims
Parental conflict	*Perception of lack of warmth*
"I like it when people respect each other. If my mother does something to my father or vice versa, I get totally irritated and feel insufficient. I use abusive words. I just blurtthem out but only when I am alone."	"Mother will start scolding me if I don't wake up early. She will just keep ion and on. So to avoid that I just wake up. I just wish she could stop chattering."
Punitive parenting	
"They will only show (scoffs)…. Show only…. (scoffs)…. Beating… ea(scoffs)….. they hit … very hard…. It pains"	"My mother hits me if I get hurt. Usually all mother's make sure that their child is okay and takes care of the child when he is hurt. I don't understand why is my mother like that."
Emotional distance from family	*Enmeshment*
"I don't talk to my parents a lot, I just share those that were funny especially I do that when I'm taking a break from studies and all that. I feel like increasing their trust in everything that I do."	"I don't feel like telling my parents about all this. Why make them sad. They are already upset about many things. I don't want to make it a reason to add on the problem."
	Insecure attachment style "I am scared of telling my mother anything. She is very moody. Sometimes, she is angry or sad or in a jovial mood."
Difference in parenting	*Parentification*
My mother wants to send me. Father wants me to be here and take over his business	"I have lots of responsibilities. After father passed away I need to take care of the family. I need to get a job, get my sisters married, need to make a nice house."

13.3.3 Coping V/S Defence Mechanism

The participants had adopted internalization as a coping strategy to deal with the personal encounters. Bullies had used both internalization and externalization as coping strategies. The former was observed in the form of psychosomatization whereas the latter was under the framework of aggression (Camodeca et al. 2002; Pepler et al. 2008). The internalization feeling of loneliness (McDougall and Vailliancourt 2015) and defence mechanisms such as displacement, rationalization, and repression were also explored in the study (Table 13.5).

13.3.4 Frustration and Anger

From the results it is reflected that bullies and victims express anger differently. The bullies express anger outwardly and act on it which leads to aggression. There

Table 13.4 Themes emerged as the similarities and differences in the social relationships of bullies and victims

Social relationships	
Bullies	Victims
Perception of school	
Enjoys school	*Injustice*
"School is the best place.... I always interact with my friends..." *Negative intention* "We make fun of those who study really well by calling them nerds and all that. They show off a lot because they study. They don't help if we ask anything. If we ask for something they won't tell, they wouldn't talk to us only in the first place." *Need for power* "I'm the house captain. I like this power"	*Unpleasant situation* "This boy went and told in his class that I hit him. People from three classes came to hit me. They went and told sir all kind of lies and these boys told me that I don't need to show off. They made their part clear in front of sir"
Role of teachers	
Perception of partiality	*Negative intention of teachers*
"She does a lot of partiality... so many of us have told her even I have told that "miss, I think you have partiality"	"Everyone came to hit me and I told sir that I did not do anything. Even if I don't go and create any issues they come and create problem"
Self-perception	
Ideal self-image	*Body image*
"I created a different face for myself. Basically everybody knows the problems of being a single child. I hate sympathies like he is just an only child."	"What can I do if God create me like this. He is the one who didn't make me tall. That's how I think when they make fun of me. They call me names 'stouty' because of my height"

are three forms of aggression explored in this study: physical bullying, verbal bullying, and nonverbal bullying (Table 13.6). The link between childhood experiences with primary caregivers have been studied (Mikulincer et al. 1993; Berlin and Cassidy 2003).

13.3.5 Pathways—Social Information Processing

Although the experience of bullies and victims is similar, the expression is different. This divergence in expression of experience could be in the difference in the way social stimuli is processed. There is unpleasantness experienced by both bullies and victims at school as well as at home with parents, teachers, and peers. Maladaptive ways were chosen by both bullies and victims to the unpleasantness experienced. Although their response was maladaptive, the pathways they had taken were poles apart, leading to roles of bullying and victimization. These

Table 13.5 Themes emerged as the similarities and differences in the type of coping mechanisms that bullies and victims engaged in along with the defence mechanisms that victims incorporate

Coping	
Bullies	Victims
Internalization	
Psychosomatization	*Isolation*
"I think I have gastric problems, when my ears were waxed I considered myself partially deaf for at least a week or so. But when I consulted the doctor he said everything was fine."	"They make me the liar and say that I say lies but I am the one who is saying the truth."
Externalization	Defence mechanisms
Aggression	*Rationalization*
"I hit others for no reason but otherwise nothing….."	"It's okay. Its like learning to ride a cycle. Its difficult in the beginning but then we get used to it later. When they make fun I felt sad in the beginning but now I am used to it." *Repression* "I didn't really do anything about it. After sometime it would just pass away. The sorrow I felt about the just kept it aside." *Displacement* "The sadness does not but I just feel good that I have hit something."

Table 13.6 Themes emerged as the differences in way anger and frustration experienced by bullies and victims

Frustration and anger	
Bullies	Victims
Acting outward	*Acting inward*
"When we in 9th grade I was getting down the stairs he just grabbed me by the tie and asked me to stand up in front. I pushed him when the tie caught tighter around my neck." *Physical bullying* "We physically hit each other when it becomes too much." *Verbal bullying* "We just say things about those who write our names because we talk." *Nonverbal bullying* "When he is around we do similar actions, like use our hands a lot."	"Sometimes when I give answers in class it would be funny because it would be a mistake. I take it lightly initially. Then when people go on saying it and repeatedly making and gossip about it I get really angry. I feel like hitting them and making sure that blood oozes out. However, I try controlling and punching my hand against the wall."

pathways are mediated by the way social stimuli are processed. The negative experiences of anger and frustration aroused within, due to family and school, is externalized and expressed outward as aggression by bullies while victims internalize and turn it inward making them feel isolated.

13.4 Conclusion

Bullying is a process and there are various factors that are interconnected which are involved in the incidence of bullying. The interaction of parents with their children affects the way the children interact at school. Those with better social support group gain higher status among the peers. It was seen that the victims had fewer friends while bullies had more. Thus, schools need to incorporate methods to help students create a peer support system by helping them in social skills that would make school a happier place for everyone.

References

Arseneault, L., Walsh, E., Trzesniewski, K., Newcombe, R., Caspi, A., & Moffitt, T. E. (2006). Bullying victimization uniquely contributes to adjustment problems in young children: A nationally representative cohort study. *Pediatrics, 118*, 130–138. doi:10.1542/peds.2005-2388.

Asarnow, J. R., & Callan, J. W. (1985). Boys with peer adjustment problems: Social cognitive processes. *Journal of Consulting and Clinical Psychology, 53*, 80–87. doi:10.1037/0022-006X.53.1.80.

Asher, S. R., Renshaw, P. D., & Geraci, R. L. (1980). Children's friendships and social competence. *International Journal of Psycholinguistics, 7*, 27–39.

Barboza, G. E., Schiamberg, L. B., Oehmke, J., Korzeniewski, S. J., Post, L. A., & Heraux, C. G. (2009). Individual characteristics and the multiple contexts of adolescent bullying: An ecological perspective. *Journal of Youth and Adolescence, 38*, 101–121. doi:10.1007/s10964-008-9271-1.

Baumrind, D. (1991). The influences of parenting style on adolescent competence and substance use. *Journal of Early Adolescence, 11*, 56–95.

Berkowitz, L. (1983). Aversively stimulated aggression: Some parallels and differences in research with animals and humans. *American Psychologist, 38*, 1135–1144. doi:10.1037/0003-066X.38.11.1135.

Berkowitz, L. (1989). Frustration Aggression Hypothesis: Examination and Reformulation. *Psychological Bulletin, 106*, 59–73.

Berlin, L. J., & Cassidy, J. (2003). Mothers' self-reported control of their preschool children's emotional expressiveness: A longitudinal study of associations with infant-mother attachment and children's emotion regulation. *Social Development, 12*, 477–495. doi:10.1111/1467-9507.00244.

Berlin, L. J., Cassidy, J., & Appleyard, K. (2008). The influence of early attachments on other relationships. In J. Cassidy & P. R. Shaver (Eds.), *Handbook of attachment: Theory, research, and clinical applications* (2nd ed., pp. 348–365). New York, NY: Guilford Press.

Bond, L., Carlin, J. B., Thomas, L., Rubin, K., & Patton, G. (2001). Does bullying cause emotional problems? A prospective study of young teenagers. *British Medical Journal, 323*, 480–484. doi:10.1136/bmj.323.7311.480.

Bosworth, K., Espelage, D. L., & Simon, T. R. (1999). Factors associated with bullying behavior in middle school students. *Journal of Early Adolescence, 19*, 341–362. doi:10.1177/0272431699019003003.

Bowes, L., Arseneault, L., Maughan, B., Taylor, A., Caspi, A., & Moffitt, T. E. (2009). School, neighborhood, and family factors are associated with children's bullying involvement: A nationally representative longitudinal study. *Journal of the American Academy of Child and Adolescent Psychiatry, 48*, 545–553. doi:10.1097/CHI.0b013e31819cb017.

Bowlby, J. (1969). *Attachment and loss,* (Vol. 1) New York: Basic Books, 2009.

Camodeca, M., Goossens, F. A., MeerumTerwogt, M., & Schuengel, C. (2002). Bullying and victimization among school-age children: Stability and links to proactive and reactive aggression. *Social Development, 11*, 332–345. doi:10.1111/1467-9507.00203.

Cook, C. R., Williams, K. R., Guerra, N. G., Kim, T. E., & Sadek, S. (2010). Predictors of bullying and victimization in childhood and adolescence: A meta-analytic investigation. *School Psychology Quarterly, 25*, 65–83. doi:10.1037/a0020149.

Cramer, P. (2008). Seven Pillars of defense mechanism theory. *Social and Personality Psychology Compass, 2*, 1963–1981.

Crick, N. R., & Dodge, K. A. (1994). A review and reformulation of social information processing mechanisms in children's social adjustment. *Psychological Bulletin, 115*, 74–101.

Dill, E. J., Vernberg, E. M., Fonagy, P., Twemlow, S. W., & Gamm, B. K. (2004). Negative affect in victimized children: The roles of social withdrawal, peer rejection, and attitudes toward bullying. *Journal of Abnormal Child Psychology, 32*, 159–173. doi:10.1023/B:JACP.0000019768.31348.81.

Dodge, K. A. (1985). Attributional bias in aggressive children. In P. C. Kendall (Ed.), *Advances in cognitive-behavioral research and therapy. Advances in cognitive-behavioral research and therapy* (Vol. 4, pp. 73–110). San Diego, CA, US: Academic Press.

Dodge, K. A. (1991). The structure and function of reactive and proactive aggression. In D. J. Pepler & K. H. Rubin (Eds.), *The development and treatment of childhood aggression* (pp. 201–218). Hillsdale: Lawrence Erlbaum Associates Inc.

Dodge, K. A., & Frame, C. L. (1982). Social cognitive biases and deficits in aggressive boys. *Child Development, 53*, 620–635. doi:10.2307/1129373.

Dodge, K. A., Bates, J. E., & Pettit, G. S. (1990). Mechanisms in the cycle of violence. *Science, 250*, 1678–1683. doi:10.1126/science.2270481.

Dodge, K. A., Pettit, G. S., McClaskey, C. L., & Brown, M. M. (1986). Social competence in children. *Monographs of the Society for Research in Child Development, 51*, 1–85. doi:10.2307/1165906.

Dutton, D. G. (2011). Attachment and violence An anger born of fear. In P. R. Shaver & M. Mikulincer (Eds.), *Human aggression and violence Causes, manifestations, and consequences. Herzilya Series on Personality and Social Psychology* (pp. 259–275). Washington, DC: American Psychological Association. doi:10.1037/12346-014.

Elicker, J., Englund, M., & Sroufe, L. A. (1992). Predicting peer competence and peer relationships in childhood from early parent-child relationships. In R. Parke & G. Ladd (Eds.), *Family-peer relations: Models of linkage* (pp. 77–106). Hillsdale, NJ: Erlbaum.

Esbensen, F., & Carson, D. C. (2009). Consequences of being bullied: Results from a longitudinal assessment of bullying victimization in a multisite sample of American students. *Youth & Society, 41*, 209–233. doi:10.1177/0044118X09351067.

Goldbaum, S., Craig, W. M., Pepler, D., & Connolly, J. (2007). Developmental trajectories of victimization: Identifying risk and protective factors. In J. E. Zins, M. J. Elias, & C. A. Maher (Eds.), *Bullying, victimization, and peer harassment: A handbook of prevention and intervention* (pp. 143–160). New York, NY: Haworth Press.

Graziano, W. G., Habashi, M. M., Sheese, B. E., & Tobin, R. M. (2007). Agreeableness, empathy, and helping: A person X situation perspective. *Journal of Personality and Social Psychology, 93*, 583–599. doi:10.1037/0022-3514.93.4.583.

Hanish, L. D., & Guerra, N. G. (2002). A longitudinal analysis of patterns of adjustment following peer victimization. *Development and Psychopathology, 14*, 69–89. doi:10.1017/S0954579402001049.

Hodges, E. V. E., & Perry, D. G. (1999). Personal and interpersonal antecedents and consequences of victimization by peers. *Journal of Personality and Social Psychology, 76*, 677–685. doi:10.1037/0022-3514.76.4.677.

Hymel, S., & Bonanno, R. (2014). Moral disengagement processes in bullying. *Theory into Practice, 53*, 278–285. doi:10.1080/00405841.2014.947219.

Kerns, K. A. (2008). Attachment in middle childhood. In J. Cassidy & P. R. Shaver (Eds.), *Handbook of attachment: Theory, research, and clinical applications* (2nd ed., pp. 366–382). New York, NY: Guilford Press.

Kumpulainen, K., & Räsänen, E. (2000). Children involved in bullying at elementary school age: Their psychiatric symptoms and deviance in adolescence. An epidemiological sample. *Child Abuse and Neglect, 24*, 1567–1577. doi:10.1016/S0145-2134(00)00210-6.

LaFreniere, P. J., & Sroufe, L. A. (1985). Profiles of peer competence in the preschool: Interrelations between measures, influence of social ecology, and relation to attachment history. *Developmental Psychology, 21*, 56–69. doi:10.1037/0012-1649.21.1.56.

Lemerise, E. A., & Arsenio, W. F. (2000). An integrated model of emotion processes and cognition in social information processing. *Child Development, 71*, 107–118. doi:10.1111/1467-8624.00124.

Lyons-Ruth, K. (1996). Attachment relationships among children with aggressive behavior problems: The role of disorganized early attachment patterns. *Journal of Consulting and Clinical Psychology, 64*, 64–73. doi:10.1037/0022-006X.64.1.64.

Mahady W. M. M., Craig, W. M., & Pepler, D. J. (2000). Emotional regulation and display in classroom victims of bullying: Characteristic expressions of affect, coping styles, and relevant contextual factors. *Social Development, 9*, 226–245.

Marsh, H. W., Nagengast, B., Morin, A. J. S., Parada, R. H., Craven, R. G., & Hamilton, L. R. (2011). Construct validity of the multidimensional structure of bullying and victimization: An application of exploratory structural equation modeling. *Journal of Educational Psychology, 103*, 701–732.

McDougall, P., & Vailliancourt, T. (2015). Long-term adult outcomes of peer victimization in childhood and adolescence: Pathways to adjustment and maladjustment. *American Psychologist, 70*, 300–310. doi:10.1037/a0039174.

Mikulincer, M., Florian, V., & Weller, A. (1993). Attachment styles, coping strategies, and posttraumatic psychological distress: The impact of the Gulf War in Israel. *Journal of Personality and Social Psychology, 64*, 817–826. doi:10.1037/0022-3514.64.5.817.

Nigg, J., Martel, M. M., Nikolas, M., & Casey, B. J. (2010). Intersection of emotion and cognition in developmental psychopathology. In S. D. Calkins & M. A. Bell (Eds.), *Child development and the intersection of emotion and cognition* (pp. 225–245). Washington, D.C.: American Psychological Association.

Pepler, D., Craig, W., & O'Connell, P. (2010). Peer processes in bullying: Informing prevention and intervention strategies. In S. R. Jimerson, S. M. Swearer, & D. L. Espelage (Eds.), *Handbook of bullying in schools: An international perspective New York* (pp. 469–479). NY: Routledge.

Pepler, D., Jiang, D., Craig, W., & Connolly, J. (2008). Developmental trajectories of bullying and associated factors. *Child Development, 79*, 325–338.

Quiggle, N. L., Garber, J., Panak, W. F., & Dodge, K. A. (1992). Social information processing in aggressive and depressed children. *Child Development, 63*, 1305–1320. doi:10.2307/1131557.

Renshaw, P. D., & Asher, S. R. (1983). Children's goals and strategies for social interaction. *Merrill-Palmer Quarterly, 29*, 353–374.

Richard, J. F., Schneider, B. H., & Mallet, P. (2011). Revisiting the whole school approach to bullying: Really looking at the whole school. *School Psychology International, 33*, 263–284. doi:10.1177/0143034311415906.

Rigby, K., & Smith, P. K. (2011a). Is school bullying really on the rise? *Social Psychology of Education, 14*, 441–455. doi:10.1007/s11218-011-9158-y.

Rubin, K. H., Daniels-Beirness, T., & Hayvren, M. (1982). Social and social-cognitive correlates of sociometric status in preschool and kindergarten children. *Canadian Journal of Behavioral Science, 14*, 338–349. doi:10.1037/h0081268.

Slaby, R. G., & Guerra, N. G. (1988). (Cognitive mediators of aggression in adolescent offenders: I. *Assessment. Developmental Psychology, 24*, 580–588. doi:10.1037/0012-1649.24.4.580.

Smith, P. K., Talamelli, L., Cowie, H., Naylor, P., & Chauhan, P. (2004a). Profiles of non-victims, escaped victims, continuing victims and new victims of school bullying. *British Journal of Educational Psychology, 74*, 565–581. doi:10.1348/0007099042376427.

Sontag, L. M., & Graber, J. A. (2010). Coping with perceived peer stress: Gender-specific and common pathways to symptoms of psychopathology. *Developmental Psychology, 46*, 1605–1620. doi:10.1037/a0020617.

Steinberg, M. S., & Dodge, K. A. (1983). Attributional biases in aggressive adolescent boys and girls. *Journal of Social and Clinical Psychology, 1*, 312–321. doi:10.1521/jscp.1983.1.4.312.

Juvonen, J., Nishina, A., & Graham, S. (2000). Peer harassment, psychological adjustment, and school functioning in early adolescence. *Journal of Educational Psychology*, *92*, 349–359. KIDSCAPE. http://info.smkb.ac.il/home/home.exe.

Juvonen, J., Wang, Y., & Espinoza, G. (2011). Bullying experiences and compromised academic performance across middle school grades. *The Journal of Early Adolescence, 31*, 152–173. doi:10.1177/0272431610379415.

Kochenderfer, B. J., & Ladd, G. W. (1996). Peer victimization: manifestations and relations to school adjustment in kindergarten. *Journal of School Psychology, 34*(3), 267–283.

Renken, B., Egeland, B., Marvinney, D., Mangelsdorf, S., & Sroufe, L. A. (1989). Early childhood antecedents of aggression and passive-withdrawal in early elementary school. *Journal of Personality, 57*, 257–281.

Rieffe, C., Camodeca, M., Pouw, L. B. C., Lange, A. M. C., & Stockmann, L. (2012). Don't anger me! Bullying, victimization, and emotion dysregulation in young adolescents with ASD. *European Journal of Developmental Psychology, 9*, 351–370.

Rigby, K., & Smith, P. K. (2011b). Is school bullying really on the rise? *Social Psychology of Education, 14*, 441–455. doi:10.1007/s11218-011-9158-y.

Schwartz, D., Gorman, A. H., Nakamoto, J., & Toblin, R. L. (2005). Victimization in the peer group and children's academic functioning. *Journal of Educational Psychology, 97*, 425–435. doi:10.1037/0022-0663.97.3.425.

Shaver, P., Collins, N. L., & Clark, C. (1996). Attachment theory and internal working models of self and relationship partners. In G. Fletcher & J. Fitness (Eds.), *Knowledge structures in close relationships: A social psychological approach* (pp. 25–61). Hillsdale: Erlbaum.

Smith, P. K., Talamelli, L., Cowie, H., Naylor, P., & Chauhan, P. (2004b). Profiles of non-victims, escaped victims, continuing victims and new victims of school bullying. *British Journal of Educational Psychology, 74*, 565–581. doi:10.1348/0007099042376427.

Thompson, R. A. (2008). Early attachment and later development: Familiar questions, new answers. In J. Cassidy & P. R. Shaver (Eds.), *Handbook of attachment: Theory, research, and clinical applications* (2nd ed., pp. 348–363). New York, NY: Guilford Press.

Chapter 14
Adult Attachment Internal Working Model of Self and Other, Self-Esteem and Romantic Relationship Satisfaction in Chinese Culture: By Multilevel–Multigroup Structural Equation Modelling

Wing-Yip Chui and Man-Tak Leung

Abstract It was discovered that self-esteem could have a significant and positive contribution to an individual's romantic relationship satisfaction. Over decades, researches found that secure attachment could have significant and positive impacts on self-esteem as well as romantic relationship satisfaction. In the current research, internal working model of self and other, which serve as an individual's lifelong schema, was found to bear impact on self-concept and romantic relationship satisfaction. The self-model was discovered to have a significant and positive contribution to self-esteem and romantic relationship satisfaction. The findings of the current research can further extend the previous studies on the relationship between self-esteem and romantic relationship satisfaction. On top of the previous relevant research findings, the self-model was found to be the precursor influencing self-esteem and resulting in change in romantic relationship satisfaction. In consequence, mentalization-based treatment could be adopted to deal with attachment-related issues at individual levels. The conventional couple therapy could be reduced from a dyadic to an individual level which is more practical and cost-effective.

Keywords Attachment internal working model of self and other · Self-esteem · Romantic relationship satisfaction · Chinese culture · Multilevel–multigroup structural equation modelling

W.-Y. Chui (✉)
Department of Psychology and Assessment Research Centre of The Education, University of Hong Kong, Hong Kong, SAR, China
e-mail: francischui.fc@gmail.com

M.-T. Leung
Department of Counselling and Psychology, Hong Kong Shue Yan University, Hong Kong, SAR, China
e-mail: mtleung@hksyu.edu

M.-T. Leung and L.-M. Tan (eds.), *Applied Psychology Readings*,
DOI 10.1007/978-981-10-2796-3_14

14.1 Introduction

In Chui and Leung (2014), Chui and Leung discovered that self-esteem could have a significant and positive contribution to an individual's romantic relationship satisfaction. Over decades, researches found that secure attachment could have significant and positive impacts on self-esteem as well as romantic relationship satisfaction (Mikulincer and Shaver 2003, 2007). An internal working model (IWM) of self and other was validated in 2016 by Chui and Leung. The current research investigated the relationships among attachment internal working model, self-esteem and romantic relationship satisfaction.

14.2 Conceptual Overview

14.2.1 Attachment Theory

Attachment theory was devised by Bowlby (1969) to study how infant–caregiver emotional bond could be internalized. The internalized emotional bond, namely attachment, could bear a profound impact on the individual's affective, behavioural and cognitive responses in social contexts across the individual's lifetime (Fraley et al. 2011). The emotional bond of attachment was found not only to be confined to infant–caregiver dyads, but also to be generalized to those who could provide consistent support and care (Ainsworth 1979). According to Ainsworth and Bowlby (1991), an infant's proximity seeking behaviour is a basic instinct. Under threatening circumstances, the infant would experience psychological distress and the attachment system would then be activated (Bowlby 1969, 1982). Thus, the infant would demonstrate proximity seeking and protest behaviours, like crying and yelling.

Internal working model (IWM) is a hypothetical model proposed by Bowlby (1969, 1982). IWM is a schema about an individual himself/herself and others that would guide the individual's daily functioning, particularly in the interpersonal contexts (Bowlby 1973; Dykas and Cassidy 2011). Although the IWM is subject to changes, the initial framework of the IWM is stable throughout an individual's life (Bowlby 1969, 1982). Therefore, new experiences should be accommodated by the current IWM before integration (Prior and Glaser 2006).

Ainsworth and Bowlby (1991; Mikulincer and Shaver 2007) postulated the following characteristics of the attachment theory. An individual would assess and maintain "proximity" to the individual attachment figure for founding a "secure base" paving for further exploration. The individual would treat the attachment figure as a "safe haven" while psychologically distressed. The individual would experience "separation anxiety" whenever the individual perceives that attachment figure is leaving.

The attachment theory develops and follows two different trajectories (Dinero et al. 2011). One focuses on studying child–caregiver attachment and its impacts on infancy and late adolescence (Allen and Land 1999). The other studies the adult attachment and its impact on adult romantic relationship as well as marital satisfaction (Mikulincer and Shaver 2003, 2007).

14.2.2 Adult Attachment of Internal Working Model

The attachment is active not only in childhood but also in adulthood (Doherty and Feeney 2004). Similar to attachment in childhood, adult attachment functions for promoting an individual's sense of security by means of proximity seeking and protest behaviours mediated by the IWM. In presence of psychological distress, an individual's adult attachment system as well as IWM would be activated to facilitate the individual to return to the individual's psychological baseline (Mikulincer and Shaver 2003, 2007). An adult usually forms attachments to family members, romantic partner and close friends (Ainsworth 1989). However, not all relationships could activate the attachment system (Doherty and Feeney 2004). Instead, a lot of relationships, such as acquaintances and colleagues, could not trigger the system (Weiss 1993).

Extending Bowlby's definition of IWM, Bartholomew (1990) defined two underlying dimensions of IWM: (1) the self model and, (2) the other model. With the positivity and negativity of each dimension, four different attachment prototypes could be defined. High positivity of the self model would refer to an individual's internalization of a sense of own self-worth, whereas high negativity of the self model would be associated with self-blaming (Griffin and Bartholomew 1994). High positivity of the other model would be embodied by an individual's anticipation of others to be available and supportive while the negativity of the other model would indicate an individual's expectation of others to be indifferent. The conceptualization of the self model and the other model is depicted in Fig. 14.1 below.

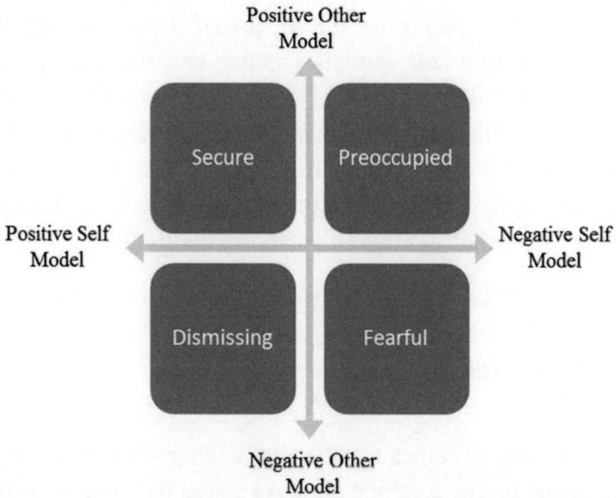

Fig. 14.1 Conceptualization of attachment internal working model of self and other

An individual possesses a positive self model and a positive other model is conceptualized to be securely attached. An individual possesses a positive self model yet a negative other model is deemed as being dismissing. An individual possesses a negative self model but a positive other model is thought to be preoccupied. An individual possesses both a negative self model and a negative other model is conceptualized to be fearful.

14.2.2.1 Cultural Differences in Adult Attachment Manifestations

Researches illustrated cultural differences between Chinese and Westerners' love attitudes and behaviours (Luo 2008). Chinese people fulfil their romantic relationship needs differently from what their Western counterparts do (Wan et al. 2000). When compared to Western cultures, Chinese people tend to focus on less passionate elements in romantic relationship (Kline et al. 2008). Chinese would also be more likely to take commitment more seriously and to involve that in romantic relationships (Gao 2001). Although Bartholomew and Horowitz (1991) and Mikulincer and Shaver (2007) espoused that a fearful-avoidant individual would tend to oscillate between preoccupied and dismissing attachment styles, when compared to the American counterparts, Hong Kong Chinese would experience a stronger linkage between "partner support and romantic attachment avoidance" (Ho et al. 2010). Furthermore, Hong Kong Chinese and Anglo-Australian demonstrated different romantic coping strategies (Leung et al. 2011). Emotional suppression is widely conceptualized to be a maladaptive coping strategy in Western culture (Chen et al. 2005). Nonetheless, Chen and colleagues found that emotional suppression could not predict the psychological well-being of the Chinese individuals. In general, the aforementioned researches imply that cultural differences are present in the elements of adult attachment patterns and romantic relationships across Chinese and Western cultures.

According to the model studies using the Attachment Style Questionnaire-Short Form (ASQ-SF; Chui and Leung 2016 ASQ), two attachment dimensions were derived from the four prototypical ratings. The self model dimension rating was acquired by summing the means of the ratings of the two attachment prototypes with positive self models (secure and dismissing) and subtracting the means of the ratings of the two prototypes with negative self models (preoccupied and fearful). The other model dimension rating was acquired by summing the means of the ratings of the two attachment prototypes with positive other models (secure and preoccupied) and subtracting the means of the ratings of the two prototypes with negative other models (dismissing and fearful).

14.2.3 Self-Esteem

According to James (1910), one's self-esteem is a derivative of one's perceived competence in one's valued area. As stated by Cooley (1902), an individual's self-esteem involves the individual's reflected self-perceptions of others, i.e. one's self-esteem entails the self-worth from the "looking glass self". An individual's self-esteem was also viewed as others' evaluation of the individual's self-worth (Baumeister 1993). Nonetheless, recent researches found that there were two domains under the construct of self-esteem: (a) "contingent self-esteem" (Neff 2003; Rosenberg 1965), and (b) "true self-esteem" (Neff 2003; Kernis 2003).

According to Neff and Rosenberg, contingent self-esteem is one's self-evaluation about competence in one's valued life domains. It is similar to James' and Cooley's definitions of self-esteem. Contingent self-esteem is relatively unstable that depends on one's capacity of successful coping with stressful life events on situation-to-situation basis (Neff 2003).

On the contrary, as espoused by Neff and Kernis, true self-esteem is relatively stable and independent of one's actions and competence of coping. Deci and Ryan (1995) evinced that true self-esteem would be conceptualized similar to the unconditional positive regards (Rogers 1961). "True self-esteem" is a concept grounded on in the self-determination theory (SDT; Deci and Ryan 2000). Ryan and Deci espoused three basic human needs for optimal psychological well-being: (a) competence, (b) autonomy, and (c) relatedness. So far as SDT, competence refers to an individual's successful interaction with the environment (Guay et al. 2003). Moreover, an individual would experience a sense of optimal functioning given that the individual achieved accomplishments with autonomy. By SDT, autonomy is conceptualized as an individual's endeavour to experience volitional initiation, sustainment, evaluation and modification of the individual's behaviours. Ryan and Deci defined relatedness as one's need to communicate with others. An individual experience a healthy self-esteem by whenever the aforementioned three basic human needs are satisfied (Moller et al. 2006). For the sake of specificity, the term "self-esteem" refers to the "contingent self-esteem" hereinafter.

14.2.4 Attachment, Self-Esteem and Romantic Relationship Satisfaction

Previous researches illustrated that attachment security would be significantly and positively associated with global self-esteem (Fass and Tubman 2002). With regard to attachment styles, it was found that individuals with secure attachment would demonstrate higher global self-esteems than those with insecure attachment styles (Meyers 1998; McCathy 1999; Huntsinger and Luecken 2004; Park et al. 2004). In summary, attachment security would be significantly and positively associated with self-esteem.

Murray and Holmes (2000) proposed a dependency regulation model and evinced that individuals of low and high self-esteems would experience various levels of emotional vulnerability. Moreover, an individual's dependency would be an over manifestation of the individual's emotional vulnerability correspondingly. In light of an individual's low self-esteem, the individual would perceive himself/herself emotionally vulnerable and experience a sense of insecurity specific to the relationship (Lemay and Clark 2008). The low self-esteem individual would overgeneralize the individual's customary self-evaluation to the partner. The individual would presume that others, including the partner, would have the same perceptions as the individual view himself/herself. In other words, a low self-esteem individual would be more susceptible to the negative "reflected appraisal" (Murray and Holmes 2000; Lemay and Clark 2008). By the dependency regulation model, an individual with low self-esteem would underestimate the partner's positive regards. Low self-esteem individuals were found to more readily experience the sense of conditional regards from their partners (Murray and Holmes 2000). According to the expression-based authenticity doubt model, with the negative reflected appraisal, an emotionally vulnerable individual would be prone to "authenticity doubt" (Lemay and Clark 2008) of the partner's positive regards. A low self-esteem individual would perceive the partner's positive regards as flattery and would consequently avoid intimate distance with the partner. The expression-based authenticity doubt model also suggested that a low self-esteem individual's relationship-specific avoidance attitude may originate from their fear of both conflict and rejection (Murray and Holmes 2000) which would in turn lead to possible disruption to the relationship. To conclude, the consequence predicted by the above-mentioned two models resemble the self-fulling prophecy (Snyder 1992), i.e. an individual with higher self-esteem would tend to selectively attend to the partner's positive behaviours whereas an individual with lower self-esteem would tend to selectively attend to the partner's negative behaviours. Besides, the expression-based authenticity doubt model models is more specific to the romantic relationships of the individuals with high perceived emotional vulnerability.

14.3 Current Study

Given the relationships among attachment, self-esteem and romantic relationship satisfaction, the authors attempted to investigated the aforementioned relationships and to establish a structural model universally across four different attachment prototypes using multilevel analysis (Muthén 1994; Byrne and van de Vijver 2014) using the statistical package LISREL 9.20. The descriptive statistics were analysed by SPSS 22.0.

14.3.1 Method

14.3.1.1 Participants

The questionnaires were done on the paper-and-pencil basis. The descriptive statistics were analysed with "SPSS 22.0". Participants were recruited ($N = 385$)

under the criteria of being (1) Chinese, and (2) 18–64 years (3) heterosexual, and (4) in a date relationship for at least 3 months at that point (Sciangula and Morry 2009) (*M* length = 5.59 years, SD = 6.23 years) since 3 months would be a sufficient period of mutual understanding between partners. The sampling strategy was purposive snowballing. There were 172 males (44.68 %) while there were 213 females (55.32 %) recruited. There were 221 samples with secure attachment style (57.40 %); 93 samples with dismissing attachment style (24.16 %); 51 samples with preoccupied attachment style (13.27 %) and 20 samples with fearful attachment style (5.19 %).

14.3.1.2 Rationale for Analyses

Multilevel–Multigroup Perspective

The current research adopted the multilevel–multigroup (Muthén 1994; Byrne and van de Vijver 2014) which could address the disaggregated individual and aggregated attachment prototype data at two different levels. The current research aimed at first validating a measurement universally adaptive the four attachment prototypes, i.e. the measurement validity of generalizations from the sample to the attachment level would be equivalent across the individual and attachment levels (Muthén 1994; Byrne and van de Vijver 2014). Unless the measurement equivalence were validated across the country levels, it would be invalid to investigate into the structural equivalence across the individual level (Muthén 1994; Byrne and van de Vijver 2014), i.e. unless the measurement were found to be universally adaptive across countries, it would be inappropriate to establish any structural models for multigroup studies with the measurement. Measurement equivalence refers to the equality of the mean of the manifest variable. On the other hand, structural equivalence means the equality of the relationships among latent variables. The latent variable approach would outperform the manifest variable approach (Selig et al. 2008). The latent variable approach would facilitate the decomposition of the total variance into within- and between-group components and enhance specifying separate structural model at each level (Byrne and van de Vijver 2014). So as to conduct the multilevel–multicultural perspective, this research would be composed of four main studies. Study 1 would be the construct validation of the studied measurement by confirmatory factor analysis (CFA). Study 2 would establish a multilevel structural equation model (MSEM) to examine the measurement and structural equivalence across the attachment and individual levels. Based on the research question, the corresponding variables would be examined by MSEM by maximum likelihood (ML) using statistical package LISREL 9.20 (Kline 2016). The criteria for good model fitness are comparative fit index (CFI) $\geq .90$, goodness of fit index (GFI) $\geq .90$, root mean square error of approximation (RMSEA) $\leq .08$ and standardized root mean square residual (SRMR) $\leq .08$ (Byrne 1998; Hu and Bentler 1999; Kline 2016).

In addition, throughout the MSEM in study 2, bootstrapping resampling technique would be adopted (Efron 1979; Ferro and Speechley 2013) as the number of samples of fearful attachment style was comparative low ($N = 20$, 5.19 %). The bootstrap is an approach of resampling with replacement from an existing dataset, generating datasets that imitate the original. In consequence, the bootstrap samples are assumed to emerge from the same underlying population as the original dataset. Parameters describing characteristics of a population, such as mean, and the relevant error, such as standard error, can be estimated for each bootstrap sample, and under most circumstances, leading to asymptotic confidence intervals for parameter estimates (Bickel and Freedman 1984), and is appropriate for regressions applications (Efron and Tibshirani 1986). As suggested by Efron and Tibshirani (1986 BS 2), 1000 bootstrap sample were drawn to acquire effect estimates with robust confidence intervals of 95 %.

14.3.1.3 Measures

Attachment internal working model was measured by the Attachment Style Questionnaire-Short Form (ASQ-SF; Chui and Leung 2016) which is a 15-item inventory using a 5-point Likert-type scale ranging from 1 (strongly disagree) to 5 (strongly agree). ASQ-SF consists of four subscales, namely secure, fearful, preoccupied and dismissing. In Chui's and Leung's study, the internal consistencies of each subscale were .731, 870, .837 and .780, respectively. The ASQ-SF exhibited appropriate construct validity: CFI = .947, GFI = .935.

Global self-esteems were measured by Rosenberg (1965) 10-item self-esteem scale (RSE) using 4-point Likert-type scale ranging from 1 (strongly disagree) to 4 (strongly agree). The scale demonstrated appropriate internal reliability. With CFA, Afari et al. (2012) derived a one-factor model for the RSE. The RSE demonstrated appropriate reliability and construct validity ($\alpha = .80$, $\chi^2 = 80.10$, CFI = .90, IFI = .91, RMSEA = .071).

Romantic relationship satisfaction was measured by Hendrick's (1988) 7-item relationship assessment scale (RAS; see appendix 8g) using 5-point Likert-type scale ranging from 1 (not satisfied) to 5 (very satisfied). Vaughn and Matyastik Baier (1999) found that internal consistency for the RAS was .86 which fitted the one-factor model proposed by Hendrick (1988).

14.4 Results

14.4.1 Study 1

The analyses were composed of two phases. First, in order to ensure the construct validity of the teaching and learning understanding items, the relationships among the items and the latent factors were evaluated by CFAs by means of ML estimation. According to Marsh et al. (1999), this step would be conducive to investigating and ameliorating the potential measurement problems. With regard to CFA, there is an assumption of normality regarding the data since violation of normality would lead to biased results. Nevertheless, the problem of skewness and kurtosis would not become a major concern provided that the sample size were larger than 200 (Tabachnick and Fidell 2001). Prior to the CFAs, multivariate and univariate data screening had been conducted involving the investigating outliers, skewness and kurtosis. All of the data were retained because the examinations of skewness and kurtosis demonstrated no outliers. The skewnesses and kurtoses of all the studied variables of the entire dataset and samples classified into four attachment styles are illustrated by Tables 14.1, 14.2, 14.3, 14.4 and 14.5 below. Referring Tables 14.1, 14.2, 14.3, 14.4 and 14.5, the skewnesses and kurtoses reflected that the data did not falsify the parametric assumptions. Hence, CFA and MSEM by maximum likelihood could be adopted, i.e. the skewnesses of all the items fell between −2 and 2 while the kurtoses of all the items fell between −7 and 7 (George and Mallery 2010). The internal consistencies of all the adopted scales and subscales are illustrated by Table 14.6 where all the adopted scales and subscales exhibited satisfying internal consistencies, i.e. Cronbach's alphas are greater than .7 (Chui and Leung 2016). The means, *SDs* and the intercorrelations of and among all the studied variables are tabulated by Table 14.7 below.

The CFA result indicated that the ASQ-SF model was sufficiently fit to the data: $\chi^2(df = 85) = 203.046$, $p = .0000$, CFI = .947, SRMR = .0522, GFI = .935, RMSEA = .0601. Hence, the result demonstrated excellent construct validity of the ASQ-SF. The aforementioned CFA model is depicted by Fig. 14.1. The CFA result indicated that the RSE model was sufficiently fit to the data: $\chi^2(df = 35) = 219.033$, $p = .0000$, CFI = .905, SRMR = .0553, GFI = .889,

Table 14.1 The skewnesses and kurtoses of the items of the ASQ-SF, the RSE and the RSA of the overall samples

ASQ	Skewness	Kurtosis	RSE	Skewness	Kurtosis	RSA	Skewness	Kurtosis
Secure 1	−.628	−.120	RSE 1	−.350	−.072	RSA 1	−.608	.085
Secure 2	−.662	.123	RSE 2	−.440	−.880	RSA 2	−.579	.098
Secure 3	−.729	.188	RSE 3	−.293	−.442	RSA 3	−.612	.050
Fearful 1	.423	−.597	RSE 4	−.355	−.158	RSA 4	−.656	−.456
Fearful 2	.252	−.872	RSE 5	−.493	−.712	RSA 5	−.490	−.237
Fearful 3	.294	−.980	RSE 6	−.534	−.839	RSA 6	−.614	−.304
Fearful 4	.350	−.976	RSE 7	−.678	−.081	RSA 7	−.130	−.507
Fearful 5	.674	−.345	RSE 8	.568	−.269			
Preoccupied 1	−.426	−.804	RSE 9	−.464	−.871			
Preoccupied 2	−.091	−1.185	RSE 10	−.598	−.646			
Preoccupied 3	−.141	−.908						
Dismissing 1	−.901	.506						
Dismissing 2	−.250	−.424						
Dismissing 3	−.526	−.480						
Dismissing 4	−.195	−.779						

Table 14.2 The skewnesses and kurtoses of the items of the ASQ-SF, the RSE and the RSA of the samples with secure attachment style

ASQ	Skewness	Kurtosis	RSE	Skewness	Kurtosis	RSA	Skewness	Kurtosis
Secure 1	−.803	.602	RSE 1	−.506	.684	RSA 1	−.826	.864
Secure 2	−.575	−.119	RSE 2	−.588	−.677	RSA 2	−.615	.476
Secure 3	−.802	.305	RSE 3	−.423	−.140	RSA 3	−.753	.509
Fearful 1	.905	.801	RSE 4	−.331	−.180	RSA 4	−.832	−.068
Fearful 2	.773	.354	RSE 5	−.759	−.238	RSA 5	−.494	−.197
Fearful 3	.780	.190	RSE 6	−.725	−.499	RSA 6	−.648	−.319
Fearful 4	.864	.288	RSE 7	−.798	.271	RSA 7	−.171	−.168
Fearful 5	.864	.288	RSE 8	.542	−.399			
Preoccupied 1	−.564	−.347	RSE 9	−.707	−.335			
Preoccupied 2	−.108	−1.087	RSE 10	−.680	−.439			
Preoccupied 3	−.268	−.704						
Dismissing 1	−.865	.729						
Dismissing 2	−.263	−.280						
Dismissing 3	−.333	−.640						
Dismissing 4	−.061	−.592						

Table 14.3 The skewnesses and kurtoses of the items of the ASQ-SF, the RSE and the RSA of the samples with dismissing attachment style

ASQ	Skewness	Kurtosis	RSE	Skewness	Kurtosis	RSA	Skewness	Kurtosis
Secure 1	−.274	−.342	RSE 1	−.166	−.665	RSA 1	−.467	−.321
Secure 2	−.511	.037	RSE 2	−.458	−.783	RSA 2	−.593	−.271
Secure 3	−.311	−.203	RSE 3	−.323	−.390	RSA 3	−.646	−.083
Fearful 1	.025	−.413	RSE 4	−.665	.550	RSA 4	−.542	−.806
Fearful 2	−.155	−.597	RSE 5	−.537	−.717	RSA 5	−.472	−.425
Fearful 3	−.032	−.963	RSE 6	−.819	−.218	RSA 6	−.561	−.184
Fearful 4	−.169	−.878	RSE 7	−.800	.348	RSA 7	−.034	−.663
Fearful 5	.135	−1.038	RSE 8	.366	−.455			
Preoccupied 1	.537	−.459	RSE 9	−.640	−.732			
Preoccupied 2	.552	−.374	RSE 10	−.978	.013			
Preoccupied 3	.402	−.019						
Dismissing 1	−.805	−.374						
Dismissing 2	−.338	−.865						
Dismissing 3	−1.062	1.461						
Dismissing 4	−.845	.485						

RMSEA = .117. Hence, the result demonstrated appropriate construct validity of the RSE. The aforementioned CFA model is depicted by Fig. 14.2. The CFA result indicated that the RAS model was sufficiently fit to the data: $\chi^2(df = 14) = 74.570$, $p = .0000$, CFI = .960, SRMR = .0430, GFI = .950, RMSEA = .106.

Hence, the result demonstrated appropriate construct validity of the RAS. The aforementioned CFA model is depicted by Fig. 14.3 (Fig. 14.4).

Table 14.4 The skewnesses and kurtoses of the items of the ASQ-SF, the RSE and the RSA of the samples with preoccupied attachment style

ASQ	Skewness	Kurtosis	RSE	Skewness	Kurtosis	RSA	Skewness	Kurtosis
Secure 1	−.350	−.648	RSE 1	.157	−.106	RSA 1	.108	−.888
Secure 2	−.221	−.727	RSE 2	.377	−.757	RSA 2	−.249	−.465
Secure 3	−.541	−.148	RSE 3	.163	−.307	RSA 3	−.101	−.413
Fearful 1	−.053	−.239	RSE 4	.261	−.570	RSA 4	−.311	−.538
Fearful 2	−.371	−.894	RSE 5	−.100	−.516	RSA 5	−.235	−.514
Fearful 3	−.811	.495	RSE 6	.353	−.448	RSA 6	−.656	−.428
Fearful 4	−.422	−.877	RSE 7	−.073	−.639	RSA 7	.403	−.804
Fearful 5	.536	−.390	RSE 8	.882	1.349			
Preoccupied 1	−1.399	3.675	RSE 9	.409	.015			
Preoccupied 2	−1.399	3.675	RSE 10	.756	.295			
Preoccupied 3	−.136	−.434						
Dismissing 1	−.072	−.719						
Dismissing 2	.108	−.509						
Dismissing 3	−.087	−.732						
Dismissing 4	.539	−.253						

Table 14.5 The skewnesses and kurtoses of the items of the ASQ-SF, the RSE and the RSA of the samples with fearful attachment style

ASQ	Skewness	Kurtosis	RSE	Skewness	Kurtosis	RSA	Skewness	Kurtosis
Secure 1	.440	.253	RSE 1	−.176	−.212	RSA 1	−1.449	1.526
Secure 2	.244	.374	RSE 2	.021	−1.310	RSA 2	−1.003	.189
Secure 3	−.676	−.347	RSE 3	.296	−1.399	RSA 3	.396	−.547
Fearful 1	−.418	−.826	RSE 4	−.151	.082	RSA 4	−.467	−.532
Fearful 2	−.396	−.547	RSE 5	.713	.154	RSA 5	−.119	−.726
Fearful 3	−1.467	2.015	RSE 6	.028	−1.528	RSA 6	−.358	−.008
Fearful 4	−.177	−.548	RSE 7	−.194	−.357	RSA 7	.000	−.279
Fearful 5	−.419	−.386	RSE 8	.292	−.734			
Preoccupied 1	−.177	−.548	RSE 9	.343	−1.210			
Preoccupied 2	−.219	−.817	RSE 10	−.249	−.999			
Preoccupied 3	.028	−.774						
Dismissing 1	−1.206	1.137						
Dismissing 2	.279	−.447						
Dismissing 3	−.555	−.080						
Dismissing 4	−.282	−.945						

14.4.2 Study 2

The MSEM result indicated that the multilevel structural model was sufficiently fit to the data: $\chi^2(df = 953) = 1958.428$, $p = .0000$, CFI = .962, SRMR = .0742, GFI = .859, RMSEA = .0524. Therefore, the multilevel structural model

Table 14.6 The internal consistencies of the ASQ, the RSE and the RSA

Scale/subscale	Cronbach's alpha
Secure	.731
Fearful	.870
Preoccupied	.837
Dismissing	.780
RSE	.893
RSA	.867

Table 14.7 The means, SDs and intercorrelations of and among all the studied variables

Variable	Mean	SD	1	2	3	4	5	6	7	8
1. Secure	3.984	.720	1.000							
2. Fearful	2.563	.951	−.334***	1.000						
3. Preoccupied	3.205	1.079	039	.246***	1.000					
4. Dismissing	3.627	.809	−.039	.098	−.272**	1.000				
5. Self model	1.843	2.099	.455***	−.655***	−.718***	.468***	1.000			
6. Other model	.999	1.976	.557***	−.507***	.553***	−.619***	−.105*	1.000		
7. Self-esteem	2.908	.616	.308***	−.443***	−.434***	.232***	.618***	−.008	1.000	
8. Relation satisfaction	3.715	.724	.214***	−.186***	−.113*	.092	.250***	.067	.236***	1.000

* $p < .05$; ** $p < .01$; *** $p < .001$

demonstrates antecedent and outcome relationships among attachment internal working model, self-esteem and romantic relationship satisfaction. The between-group model is visualized by Fig. 14.5, whereas the within group model is depicted by Fig. 14.6.

There was a significant and positive standardized indirect effect of the latent independent variable on the latent dependent variable which is illustrated by the following Table 14.8. The presence of indirect effect suggested that self-esteem served as a mediator between self-model and romantic relationship satisfaction.

14.5 Discussion

This study discovered that global self-esteem could serve as a mediator between self model and romantic relationship satisfaction. The result reflected a phenomenon stipulated by "the expression-based authenticity doubts model" (Lemay and Clark 2008). The model indicated that the individuals with lower self-esteem or "reflected appraisals of vulnerability" would be prone to "authenticity doubts", i.e. they would tend to "believe that their partners would express more positive regards than he or she truly feels and conceals". In a nutshell, the individuals with lower self-esteems would be more sceptical about their partners' positive regards but more likely to personalize their partners' negative regards. Although the

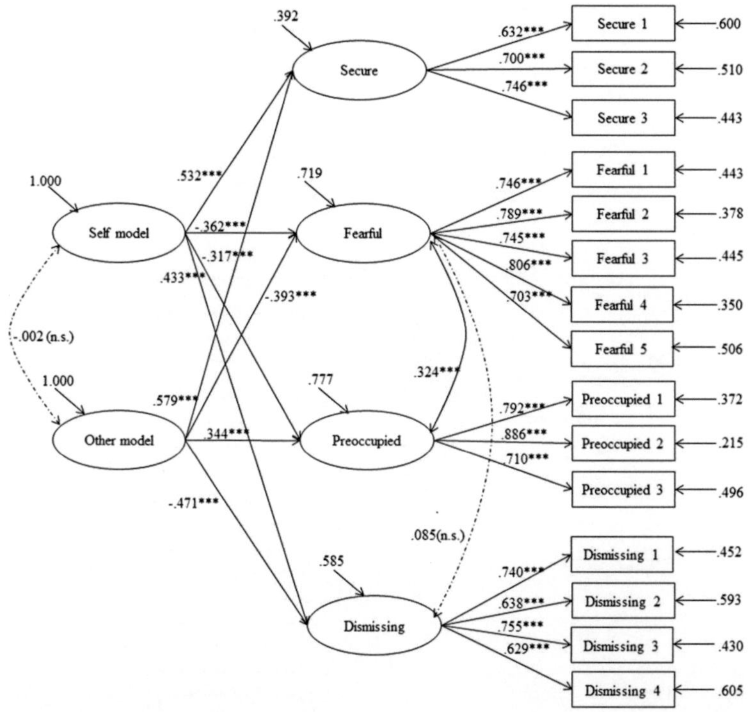

Fig. 14.2 The CFA model of the ASQ-SF

expression-based authenticity doubt model demonstrated a circular path between reflected appraisal of vulnerability, authenticity doubts and relationship satisfaction, the structural model of the current study revealed a precursor of self-esteem and perceived self-vulnerability, namely the model of self. Suggested by the model of the current study, an individual with a more positive self model would tend to have higher self-esteem while less an individual with a more negative self model would be likely to have lower self-esteem.

With respect to positive self model, it refers to secure and dismissing attachment styles. As mentioned above, securely attached individuals were found higher in self-esteem when compared to the insecurely individuals. On the other hand, a dismissing individual tends to either "idealize" himself/herself and his/her intimate partner (Mikulincer and Shaver 2003, 2007). Therefore, the current research results indicated that positive self-model had significant and positive contribution to both perceived self-esteem and romantic relationship satisfaction. In terms of mentalization which refers to (Bateman and Fonagy 2004; Fonagy et al. 2004) to an individual's capacity to understand and make sense of others' mental processes and behaviours. A dismissing individual is conceptualized to be prone to "pretend mode" (Bateman and Fonagy 2004; Fonagy et al. 2004) in which the individual's mental state is decoupled from external or physical reality, but the internal state

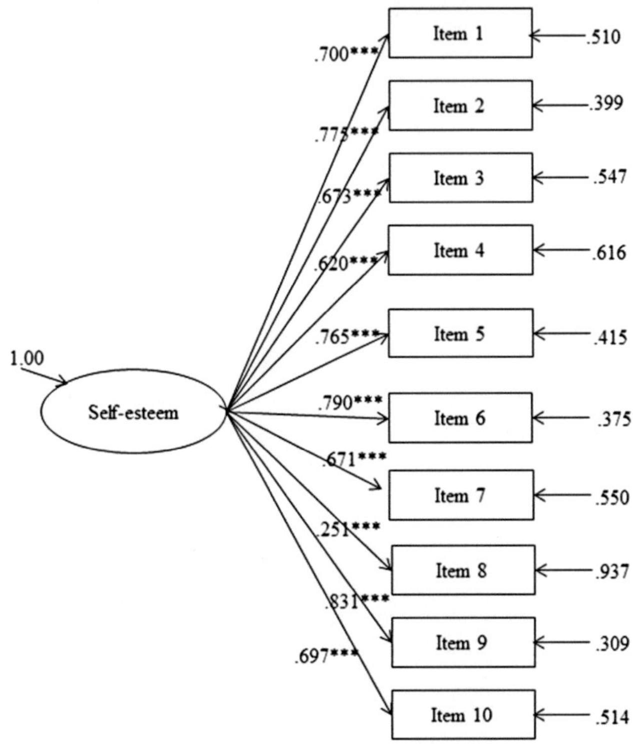

Fig. 14.3 The CFA model of the RSE

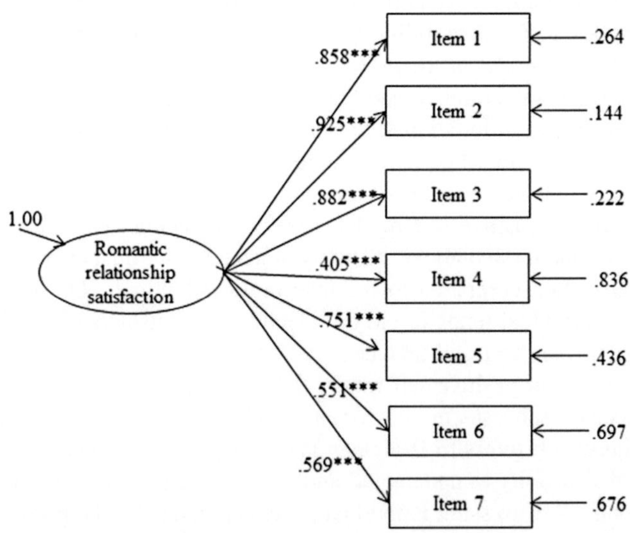

Fig. 14.4 The CFA model of the RAS

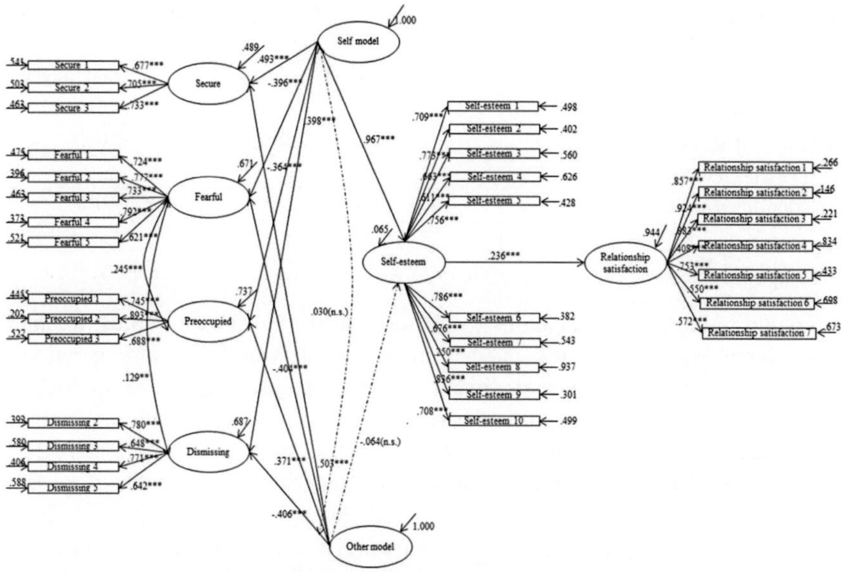

Fig. 14.5 The between-group structural model

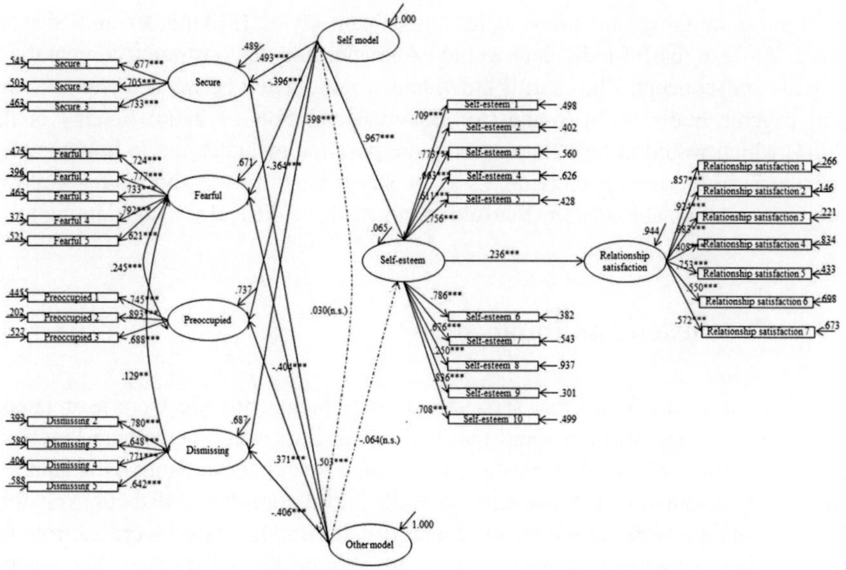

Fig. 14.6 The within group structural model

Table 14.8 The standardized indirect effects of the independent latent variables on the dependent latent variable at different levels

	Self model	Other model
The between-group model		
Relationship satisfaction	.228***	−.015
The within-group model		
Relationship satisfaction	.228***	−.015

* $p < .05$; ** $p < .01$; *** $p < .001$

is thought to have no implications for the outside world. In other words, the individual inner experience is separated from the outside world. The aforementioned conceptualization explains thein dismissing individuals' tendencies to idealize themselves as well as their intimate partners. On the contrary, negative self model entails preoccupied and fearful attachment styles. With regard to maternalization conceptualization, a preoccupied occupied individual is more likely to demonstrate "psychic equivalence" (Bateman and Fonagy 2004; Fonagy et al. 2004) which involves the projection of the fantasy to the outside world is felt to be compellingly real. Simply speaking, a preoccupied individual appears to have a relatively undifferentiated ego boundary and be influenced by the outside world readily. Psychic equivalence provides an intact explanation to the expression-based authenticity doubts model. As a fearful individual is inclined to oscillate between dismissing and preoccupied attachment styles (Mikulincer and Shaver 2003, 2007), a fearful individual would experience and demonstrate a comparative volatile self-concept. The fearful individual would switch between pretend mode and psychic equivalence to-and-fro (Bateman and Fonagy 2004; Fonagy et al. 2004) which would in turn cause even more psychological distress to him/herself. It is because the fearful individual's self-concept is so diffuse and his/her coping modes are so unstable that the fearful individuals have difficulty with adapting to.

14.6 Conclusion and Implication

Over years, it was found that self-esteem and attachment style were associated. Moreover, it was also discovered that low self-esteem would perpetuate low perceived romantic relationship satisfaction. In this research, nevertheless, the authors linked up attachment, self-esteem and romantic relationship satisfaction on the basis of internal working model and found that self-model played a critical role in determining self-esteem as well as romantic relationship satisfaction. The newly validated multilevel structural model provides different points of intervention for couple therapy. On the one hand, a therapist can enhance a couple's intimate relationship satisfaction by empowering their self-esteems. On the other hand, the therapist can also work on the clients' internal working model of self. As it is the internal working model of self that is effective in determining in self-esteem and romantic relationship satisfaction, mentalization-based treatment (MBT; Bateman and Fonagy 2004) can be adopted to deal with attachment related issues at individual levels. The conventional couple therapy could be reduced from a dyadic to an individual level which is more practical and cost-effective.

14.7 Limitations

Several limitations should be taken into account when evaluating the current study. First, the data collected in the current study were on the basis of self-report which was void of observations of behaviours. The sampling size ($N = 385$) suggested that the potential biased errors were present and generalization to other samples might be limited. The current study was fundamentally a cross-sectional survey in Chinese culture. The research design was not a longitudinal study investigating the causal effects among the variables. Hence, the causal relationships among the currently studied variables might not be valid. Further interpretations must be made carefully and modestly in the current study. In the future, a causal model of the studied phenomenon should be established which could more elaborately portray the mechanism for devising further therapeutic interventions. Furthermore, empirical researches should be conducted to investigate the effectiveness of the aforementioned interventions in terms of their impacts on the attachment internal working model, self-esteem and perceived romantic relationship satisfaction.

References

Afari, E., Ward, G., & Khine, M. S. (2012). Global self-esteem and self-efficacy correlates: Relation of academic achievement and self-esteem among Emirati students. *International Education Studies, 5*(2), 49–57. doi:10.5539/ies.v5n2p49.

Ainsworth, M. S. (1979). Infant–mother attachment. *American Psychologist, 34*(10), 932–937. doi:10.1037/0003-066X.34.10.932.

Ainsworth, M. S. (1989). Attachments beyond infancy. *American Psychologist, 44*(4), 709–716.

Ainsworth, M. S., & Bowlby, J. (1991). An ethological approach to personality development. *American Psychologist, 46*(4), 333–341. doi:10.1037/0003-066X.46.4.333.

Allen, J. P., & Land, D. (1999). Attachment in adolescence. In J. Cassidy & P. R. Shaver (Eds.), *Handbook of attachment: Theory, research and clinical applications* (pp. 319–335). New York: Guilford Press.

Bartholomew, K. (1990). Avoidance of intimacy: An attachment perspective. *Journal of Social and Personality Psychology, 61*, 226–244.

Bartholomew, K., & Horowitz, L. M. (1991). Attachment styles among young adults: A test of a four category model. *Journal of Personality and Social Psychology, 61*, 226–244.

Bateman, A., & Fonagy, P. (2004). *Psychotherapy for borderline personality disorder: Mentalization-based treatment*. UK: Oxford University Press.

Baumeister, R. (Ed.). (1993). *Self-esteem: The puzzle of low self-regard.* New York: Plenum Press.

Bickel, P., & Freedman, D. A. (1984). Asymptotic normality and the bootstrap in stratified sampling. *Annals of Statistics, 12*, 470–482.

Bowlby, J. (1969). *Attachment and loss: Vol. 1. Attachment*. London: Hogarth.

Bowlby, J. (1973). *Separation: Anxiety and anger*. New York, NY: Basic Books.

Bowlby, J. (1982). Attachment and loss: Retrospect and prospect. *American Journal of Orthopsychiatry, 52*, 664–678.

Byrne, B. M. (1998). *Structural equation modeling with LISREL, PRELIS, and SIMPLIS: Basic concepts, applications and programming*. New York: Lawrence Erlbaum Associates.

Byrne, B. M., & van de Vijver, F. J. R. (2014). Factorial structure of the family values scale from a multilevel–multicultural perspective. *International Journal of Testing, 14*, 168–192.

Chen, S. X., Cheung, F. M., Bond, M. H., & Leung, J. P. (2005). Decomposing the construct of ambivalence over emotional expression in a Chinese cultural context. *European Journal of Personality, 19*, 185–204.

Chui, W. Y., & Leung, M. T. (2014). A structural equation model (SEM) of self compassion, self-esteem, perceived partner behaviour and romantic relationship satisfaction. *International Journal of Chinese Applied Psychology, 6*(2), 20–34.

Chui, W. Y., & Leung, M. T. (2016). Adult attachment internal working model of self and other in Chinese culture: Measured by the Attachment Style Questionnaire-Short Form (ASQ-SF) by confirmatory factor analysis (CFA) and item response theory (IRT). *Personality and Individual Differences, 96*, 55–64.

Cooley, C. H. (1902). *Human nature and the social order*. New York: Scribner.

Deci, E., & Ryan, R. (1995). Human autonomy: The basis for true self esteem. In M. H. Kernis (Ed.), *Efficacy, agency, and self-esteem* (pp. 31–49). New York, NY: Plenum Press.

Deci, E. L., & Ryan, R. M. (2000). The 'what' and 'why' of goal pursuits: Human needs and the self-determination of behavior. *Psychological Inquiry, 11*, 227–268.

Dinero, R. E., Conger, R. D., Shaver, P. R., Widaman, K. F., & Larsen-Rife, D. (2011). Influence of family of origin and adult romantic partners on romantic attachment security. *Couple and Family Psychology: Research and Practice, 1*(8), 16–30. doi:10.1037/2160-4096.1.S.16.

Doherty, N. A., & Feeney, J. A. (2004). The composition of attachment networks throughout the adult years. *Personal Relationships, 11*(4), 469–488. doi:10.1111/j.1475-6811.2004.00093.x.

Dykas, M. J., & Cassidy, J. (2011). Attachment and the processing of social information across the life span: Theory and evidence. *Psychological Bulletin, 137*(1), 19–46. doi:10.1037/a0021367.

Efron, B. (1979). Bootstrap methods: Another look at the jackknife. *Annals of Statistics, 7*, 1–26.

Efron, B., & Tibshirani, R. (1986). Bootstrap methods for standard errors, confidence intervals, and other measures of statistical accuracy. *Statistical Science, 12*, 470–482.

Fass, M. E., & Tubman, J. G. (2002). The influence of parental and peer attachment on college students' academic achievement. *Psychology in the Schools, 39*, 561–574.

Ferro, M. A., & Speechley, K. N. (2013). Stability of latent classes in group-based trajectory modeling of depressive symptoms in mothers of children with epilepsy: An internal validation study using a bootstrapping procedure. *Social Psychiatry and Psychiatric Epidemiology, 48*, 1077–1086.

Fonagy, P., Gergely, G., Jurist, E. L., & Target, M. (2004). *Affect regulation, mentalization, and the development of the self*. UK: Karnac Ltd.

Fraley, R. C., Vicary, A. M., Brumbaugh, C. C., & Roisman, G. I. (2011). Patterns of stability in adult attachment: An empirical test of two models of continuity and change. *Journal of Personality and Social Psychology, 101*(5), 974–992. doi:10.1037/a0024150.

Gao, G. (2001). Intimacy, passion and commitment in Chinese and US American romantic relationships. *International Journal of Intercultural Relations, 25*, 329–342.

George, D., & Mallery, M. (2010). *SPSS for windows step by step: A simple guide and reference, 17.0 update* (10th ed.). Boston: Pearson.

Griffin, D., & Bartholomew, K. (1994). Models of the self and other: Fundamental dimensions underlying measures of adult attachment. *Journal of Personality and Social Psychology, 67*(3), 430–445.

Guay, F., Senecal, C., Gauthier, L., & Fernet, C. (2003). Predicting career indecision: A self-determination theory perspective. *Journal of Counselling Psychology, 50*(2), 165–177.

Hendrick, S. S. (1988). A generic measure of relationship satisfaction. *Journal of Marriage and the Family, 50*, 93–98.

Ho, M. Y., Zhang, H., Lin, D., Lu, A., Bond, M. H., Chan, C., et al. (2010). Saving graces: Impact of partner support and maternal attachment on partner attachments in an individualistic and a collectivist context. *Asian Journal of Social Psychology, 13*, 19–29.

Hu, L. T., & Bentler, P. M. (1999). Cutoff criteria for fit indexes in covariance structure analysis: Conventional criteria versus new alternatives. *Structural Equation Modeling, 6*(1), 1–55.

Huntsinger, E. T., & Luecken, L. J. (2004). Attachment relationships and health behaviour: The mediational role of self-esteem. *Psychology and Health, 19*, 515–526.

James, W. J. (1910). *Principles of psychology*. New York: Holt.

Kernis, M. H. (2003). Toward a conceptualization of optimal self-esteem. *Psychological Inquiry, 14*, 1–26. doi:10.1207/S15327965PLI1401_01.

Kline, R. B. (2016). *Principles and practice of structural equation modeling* (4th ed.). New York: Guilford Press.

Kline, S. L., Horton, B., & Zhang, S. (2008). Communicating love: Comparisons between American and East Asian university students. *International Journal of Intercultural Relations, 32*, 200–214.

Lemay, E. P., & Clark, M. S. (2008). "Walking on eggshells": How expressing relationship insecurities perpetuates them. *Journal of Personality and Social Psychology, 95*(2), 420–441.

Leung, C., Morre, S., Karnilowicz, W., & Lung, C. L. (2011). Romantic relationships, relationship styles, coping strategies, and psychological distress among Chinese and Australian young adults. *Social Development, 20*(4), 783–804. doi:10.1111/j.1467-9507.2011.00616.x.

Luo, B. (2008). Striving for comfort: "Positive" construction of dating cultures among second-generation Chinese American youths. *Journal of Social and Personal Relationships, 25*, 867–888.

Marsh, H. W., Byrne, B. M., & Yeung, A. A. (1999). Causal ordering of academic self-concept and achievement: Reanalysis of a pioneering study and revised recommendations. *Educational Psychologist, 34*, 155–167.

McCarthy, G. (1999). Attachment style and adult love relationships and friendships: A study of a group of women at risk of experiencing relationship difficulties. *British Journal of Medical Psychology, 72*, 305–321.

Meyers, S. A. (1998). Personality correlates of adult attachment style. *Journal of Social Psychology, 138*, 407–409.

Mikulincer, M., & Shaver, P. R. (2003). The attachment behavioral system in adulthood: Activation, psychodynamics, and interpersonal processes. In M. P. Zanna (Ed.), *Advances in experimental social psychology* (Vol. 35, pp. 53–152). New York: Academic Press.

Mikulincer, M., & Shaver, P. R. (2007). *Attachment in adulthood: Structure, dynamics, and change*. New York, NY: Guilford Press.

Moller, A. C., Friedman, R., & Deci, E. L. (2006). A self-determination theory perspective on the interpersonal and intrapersonal aspects of self-esteem. In M. H. Kernis (Ed.), *Self-esteem issues and answers: A sourcebook of current perspectives* (pp. 201–208). New York: Psychology Press.

Murray, S. L., & Holmes, J. G. (2000). Seeing the self through a partner's eyes: Why self-doubts turn into relationship insecurities. In A. Tesser, R. B. Felson, & J. M. Suls (Eds.), *Psychological perspectives on self and identity* (pp. 173–197). Washington, DC: American Psychological Association.

Muthén, B. O. (1994). Multilevel covariance structure analysis. *Sociological Methods and Research, 22*, 376–398.

Neff, K. (2003). The development and validation of a scale to measure self-compassion. *Self and Identity, 2*, 223–250. doi:10.1080/15298860309027.

Park, L. E., Corcker, J., & Mickelson, K. D. (2004). Attachment styles and contingencies of self-worth. *Personality and Social Psychology Bulletin, 30*, 1243–1254.

Prior, V., & Glaser, D. (2006). *Understanding attachment and attachment disorders: Theory, evidence and practice*. London: Jessica Kingsley.

Rogers, C. R. (1961). *On becoming a person: A therapist's view of psychotherapy*. London: Constable & Company Ltd.

Rosenberg, M. (1965). *Society and the adolescent self-image*. Princeton, NJ: Princeton University Press.

Sciangula, A., & Morry, M. M. (2009). Self-esteem and perceived regard: How I see myself affects my relationship satisfaction. *The Journal of Social Psychology, 149*(2), 143–158.

Selig, J. P., Card, N. A., & Little, T. D. (2008). Latent variable structural equation modeling in cross cultural research: Multigroup and multilevel approaches. In F. J. R. van de Vijver, D. A. van Hemert, & Y. H. Poortinga (Eds.), *Multilevel analysis of individuals and cultures* (pp. 93–119). New York, NY: Taylor & Francis.

Snyder, M. (1992). Motivational foundations of behavioral confirmation. In M. P. Zanna (Ed.), *Advances in experimental social psychology* (Vol. 25, pp. 67–114). San Diego, CA: Academic Press.

Tabachnick, B. G., & Fidell, L. S. (2001). *Using multivariate statistics*. New York: Harper Collins.

Vaughn, M. J., & Matyastik Baier, M. E. (1999). Reliability and validity of the relationship assessment scale. *The American Journal of Family Therapy, 27*(2), 137–147.

Wan, W. W. N., Luk, C. L., & Lai, J. C. L. (2000). Personality correlates of loving styles among Chinese students in Hong Kong. *Personality and Individual Difference, 29*, 169–175.

Weiss, R. S. (1993). The attachment bond in childhood and adulthood. In C. Parkes, J. Stevenson-Hinde, & P. Marris (Eds.), *Attachment across the life cycle* (pp. 66–76). Florence, KY: Routledge.

Chapter 15
The Psychometric Properties of the Individual-Oriented Achievement Motivation Scale-Short Form (IOAMS-SF): By Structural Equation Modelling (SEM) and Item Response Theory (IRT)

Wing-Yip Chui and Man-Tak Leung

Abstract The Individual-Oriented Achievement Motivation Scale (IOAMS; Yang and Yu in Social- and individual-oriented achievement motives: conceptualization and measurement, 1988) is a reliable and valid measurement tool assessing an individual's individual-oriented achievement motivation (IOAM). IOAM exhibits a functionally automatized (hence still intrinsic) desire via which the process of achievement-related behaviours, standards of excellence, and evaluation of performance or outcome are perceived and determined by an individual oneself. The IOAMS (Yang and Yu 1988) is a reliable and valid measurement tool assessing an individual's IOAM. Chang et al. (J Psychol Chin Soc 1(2):39–63, 2000) found that IOAMS consisted of a sole single-order factor using varimax rotation method. Chang's et al. research was conducted in Singapore, there may be cultural differences between Singaporean and Hong Kong's contexts. Furthermore, varimax rotation method is for exploratory purpose for investigating the factorial structure of the IOAMS. Since the current study targeted at Hong Kong individuals, the present study addressed the issue of cultural difference. Furthermore, in the current study, a confirmatory approach was employed to examine the factorial structure of IOAMS. Hence, the IOAMS was reexamined in Hong Kong context. With confirmatory factor analysis and item response theory, the 30-item IOAMS was condensed to become a 12-item IOAMS-Short Form (IOAMS-SF).

W.-Y. Chui (✉)
Department of Psychology and Assessment Research Centre of The Education,
University of Hong Kong, Hong Kong, SAR, China
e-mail: francischui.fc@gmail.com

M.-T. Leung
Department of Counselling and Psychology, Hong Kong Shue Yan University,
Hong Kong, SAR, China
e-mail: mtleung@hkshyu.edu

M.-T. Leung and L.-M. Tan (eds.), *Applied Psychology Readings*,
DOI 10.1007/978-981-10-2796-3_15

Keywords IOAM · Achievement motivation · Confirmatory factor analysis (CFA) · Item response theory (IRT)

15.1 Introduction

15.1.1 Individual-Oriented Achievement Motivation (IOAM)

IOAM exhibits a functionally automatized (hence still intrinsic) desire via which the process of achievement-related behaviours, standards of excellence, and evaluation of performance or outcome are perceived and determined by an individual oneself (Yang and Yu 1988). Some conceptualized IOAM as the orientation from socialization within individualistic cultures (Yang and Yu 1988; Abd-El-Fattah and Patrick 2011). On the other hand, some theorized that IOAM would be highly associated with intrinsic motivation stated by the self-determination theory (Deci and Ryan 1985; Ryan and Deci 2000). Whenever an individual is intrinsically motivated to achieve, the standard of the individual performances is defined by the individual his/herself, and achievement would be deemed as an individual endeavour (Abd-El-Fattah and Patrick 2011). Hence, the individual's sense of achievement could then be internalized.

15.1.2 Self-Determination Theory

SDT is a theory conceptualizing human motivation which upholds the imperative three fundamental psychological needs: (1) autonomy, (2) competence, (3) relatedness to understand an individual's optimal functioning (Ryan and Deci 2000). According to SDT, in order to attain a sense of well-being, an individual should fulfil the aforementioned three psychological needs, respectively. The need for competence refers to an individual's need to interact with the environment effectively. It is an individual's subjective perception of competence rather than an externally validated achievement (Guay et al. 2003). In accordance with SDT, whenever an individual perceives autonomy while achieving, the individual would experience the sense of competence and the individual's well-being could be attained (Guay et al. 2003). The need for autonomy means that an individual is able to experience and demonstrate freedom to deliberate, maintain, and regulate the individual's behaviours (Guay et al. 2003). Either is the sense of autonomy perceived by the individual rather than is the autonomy be granted by any other hierarchies. Hence, in the current study, the terms perceived competence and perceived autonomy will be employed instead of the fulfilments of the needs for competence and autonomy.

Perceived autonomy has been operationalised via motivational processes (Connell and Wellborn 1991; Deci and Ryan 1985). IOAM is an example of the aforesaid operationalised self-regulatory styles of motivation process. As Deci and Ryan (1985) espoused, there would be different sorts of motivation, representing various levels of autonomy. Intrinsic motivation (e.g. IOAM) refers to the highest level of autonomy. It means that an individual would engage in an activity for the individual's own purpose and experience the joy and satisfaction due to participation (Deci 1975; Lepper et al. 1973). On the other hand, extrinsic motivation would be related to comparatively lower degree of autonomy (Deci and Ryan 1985) which includes different subcategorical self-regulatory styles. In the ascending order of degree of autonomy, the first type of self-regulation would be external regulation (Guay et al. 2003) which would illustrate that an individual's behaviours would be regulated through environmental means, such as reinforcements and punishments. Then, there would be introjected regulation which refers to those who behave with their partially internalized motivation. The third one would be identified regulation which refers to behaviours that are performed by choice because an individual perceives them as critical. So far as SDT, on one hand, individuals behaving with intrinsic motivation or identified regulation would totally or partially fulfil their perceived autonomies, respectively. On the other hand, individuals behaving with introjected or external regulation would not fulfil their autonomy. In consequence, those who behave with introjected and external regulation would have difficulties with attaining their optimal functioning and well-being.

15.1.3 The Individual-Oriented Achievement Motivation Scale (IOAMS)

The IOAMS was devised by Yang and Yu (1988) measuring achievement values, achievement goal, achievement-related behaviours, and outcome evaluation of an individual. IOAMS consists of 30-Likert scale items, ranging from "1" (totally not true) to "6" (totally true). Chang et al. (2000) found that IOAMS consisted of a sole single-order factor using varimax rotation method. Chang's et al. research was conducted in Singapore, there may be cultural differences between Singaporean and Hong Kong's contexts. Furthermore, varimax rotation method is for exploratory purpose investigating the factorial structure of the IOAMS. Since the current study targeted Hong Kong individuals, the present study addressed the issue of cultural differences. Furthermore, in the current study, confirmatory approach was employed to examine the factorial structure of IOAMS. Hence, the IOAMS was reexamined in Hong Kong context.

15.2 The Current Study

The current study aimed at investigating the psychometric properties of the IOAMS in Hong Kong context using confirmatory factor analysis (CFA). With item response theory, the 30-item IOAMS was condensed to become a 12-item IOAMS-Short Form (IOAMS-SF) which would be more parsimonious. Descriptive statistics were analyzed using SPSS 22.0; CFA was investigated utilizing LISREL 9.2; the item parameter statistics and IRT were examined utilizing IRTPRO 2.1.

15.2.1 Hypotheses

There were three hypotheses:

1. Because of cultural differences between Singapore and Hong Kong, the factorial structure of the IOAMS found in Singapore may be inapplicable in Hong Kong.
2. Since there are 30 items comprising the IOAMS, it was hypothesized the presence of second-order factors.
3. Since there are 30 items, it was hypothesized to eliminate the redundant items, i.e. to condense the IOASM for parsimony.

15.3 Methods

15.3.1 Participants

The IOAMS was done on the paper-and-pencil basis. Participants were recruited ($N = 412$) under the criteria of being (1) Hong Kong Chinese, and (2) students by purposive snowballing. There were 155 males (37.56 %) while there were 257 females (62.44 %). The mean age was 21.06 years old and SD for age was 2.02.

15.3.2 Rationale for Analyses

The current studies include four studies. Study 1 would aim at exploring the reliability and factorial structure of the IOAMS using Cronbach's alpha coefficient and the two-stage least squares (TSLS) methods, respectively, by SPSS 22.0 as well as LISREL 9.2 (Hong and Chen 2014; Mitra et al. 2014). Considering the t values of the factor loadings of all the items, the authors would classify the maximum factor loading of every single item to that particular corresponding factor for further confirmatory factor analysis.

In study 2, based on the TSLS factor loading result, the entire IOSMS would undergo a confirmatory factor analysis (CFA). The model fitness of a CFA model would be appropriate given that comparative fitness index (CFI) $\geq$ .90, goodness-of-fit index (GFI) $\geq$ .90, and standard root mean error of approximation (RMSEA) $\leq$ .080 (Bentler 1990; Byrne 1998; Kline 2010).

Study 3 would target at condensing the IOSMS to become a short form using item response theory (IRT). There are three primary assumptions underlying IRT (Bjorner et al. 2003; Brown 2006; Cook et al. 2007): (1) A unidimensional trait denoted by θ, (2) Local independence of the items, and (3) The response of an individual to an item can be modelled by mathematical item response function (IRF). Thus, in studies 1 and 2 CFA must have been conducted to validate the assumption of unidimensionality. Local independence (LI) is also the assumption of CFA (Lazarsfeld and Henry 1968). If the CFA models were validated, local independence assumption would also be validated. IRF would be presented by item parameters (Chui et al. 2016).

According to IRT, item information function (IIF) is imperative to describing and evaluating an assessment (Hambleton and Swaminathan 1985). IIF highlights the contribution of each item to the total assessment information and the consequences of selecting a particular item independently from other items in the assessment independently from other items in the assessment (de Ayala 2009). In accordance with the IIFs, the items with relatively high IIFs were retained whereas other items with relatively low IIFs were eliminated (Toland 2014; Chui and Leung 2016). Furthermore, the total IIF of every single subscale would be investigated. TIF is the summated area under each IIF of the same subscale. Thus, each item would contribute independently unique information to the TIF and is independent of other items. Besides, the expected standard error of estimate (SEE) would be examined. SEE would measure the amount of uncertainty about an individual's IRT score (de Ayala 2009). According to Toland (2014), a satisfying assessment would exhibit the TIF $\approx$ 4.00 and the SEE $\approx$ .5.

Since IOAMS is a polytomous scale, study 3 would investigate the IIF by adopting graded response model (GRM; Samejima 1969). Study 4 would aim at validating the IOAMS-SF CFA model to confirm the psychometric properties by considering the model fitness.

15.3.3 Measures

The IOAMS (Yang and Yu 1988) would be employed. IOAMS consists of 30-Likert scale items, ranging from "1" (totally not true) to "6" (totally true). Chang et al. (2000) found that IOAMS consisted of a sole single-order factor using varimax rotation method.

Study 1—Exploratory factor analysis on the IOAMS by the two-stage least squares (TSLS) method

Before the investigation of the reliability and factorial structure of the IOAM, the skewness and kurtoses of all the items had been examined using SPSS 22.0. The results are illustrated by Table 15.1.

The skewnesses of all the items fall between −2 and 2 while the kurtoses of all the items fall between −7 and 7 (George and Mallery 2010) so that CFA would be applicable (Kline 2010 FI). The reliability, Cronbach's alpha, of the IOAMS was .93 which was larger than the threshold of .60 (Evers 2001) which demonstrated an excellent reliability.

Table 15.1 The descriptive statistics of the IOAM

Item	Means	SD	Skewness	Kurtosis
IOAM 1	4.51	.985	−.501	−.043
IOAM 2	4.42	.939	−.489	.367
IOAM 3	4.07	1.140	−.361	−.202
IOAM 4	4.49	1.002	−.657	.442
IOAM 5	4.38	1.038	−.388	−.222
IOAM 6	4.24	1.081	−.433	.018
IOAM 7	4.32	1.030	−.458	−.098
IOAM 8	4.08	1.036	−.166	−.462
IOAM 9	4.42	1.066	−.536	.113
IOAM 10	4.13	1.156	−.524	.135
IOAM 11	4.27	1.026	−.458	.184
IOAM 12	4.02	1.085	−.347	−.121
IOAM 13	4.46	1.007	−.476	.115
IOAM 14	4.52	.968	−.281	−.468
IOAM 15	4.31	1.065	−.506	.075
IOAM 16	4.08	1.171	−.440	−.200
IOAM 17	4.08	1.025	−.211	−.247
IOAM 18	4.37	1.028	−.244	−.357
IOAM 19	4.05	1.091	−.244	−.106
IOAM 20	4.26	1.045	−.561	.230
IOAM 21	3.99	1.095	−.231	−.329
IOAM 22	3.82	1.169	−.358	−.253
IOAM 23	4.34	1.036	−.656	.726
IOAM 24	4.33	1.015	−.492	.372
IOAM 25	4.21	1.126	−.284	−.427
IOAM 26	3.85	1.173	−.246	−.407
IOAM 27	3.87	1.085	−.121	−.307
IOAM 28	4.26	1.012	−.519	.402
IOAM 29	4.13	1.007	−.423	.216
IOAM 30	4.12	1.197	−.660	.114

* $p < .05$; ** $p < .01$; *** $p < .001$

The TSLS result indicated that the IOAMS had four factors. The maximum factor loadings of all the items on all the factors are illustrated by Table 15.2.

Study 2—Confirmatory factor analysis (CFA) of the IAOMS

The CFA result revealed that the second-order IOAMS model (one single higher order and four lower order factors) did not demonstrate appropriate model fitness to the data: $\chi^2(df = 401) = 1280.42$, $p < .00$, CFI = .81, GFI = .82, RMSEA = .073. In the current study, the authors suspected that some items of the IOAMS were contaminated with some noises. In such a scenario, the IOAMS was analyzed on the item-by-item basis utilizing item response theory (IRT).

Table 15.2 The reference variable factor loadings estimated by two-stage least squares method

Item	Factor 1	Factor2	Factor 3	Factor 4	Uniqueness
IOAM 2	.281**				.625
IOAM 5	.304***				.704
IOAM 6	.314***				.772
IOAM 7	.296***				.732
IOAM 11	.836***				.301
IOAM 12	.486***				.535
IOAM 1		.354***			.715
IOAM 8		.264**			.727
IOAM 9		.495***			.655
IOAM 10		.390***			.612
IOAM 13		.342***			.645
IOAM 14		.494***			.563
IOAM 19		.338***			.557
IOAM 4			.423***		.571
IOAM 15			.504***		.643
IOAM 16			.399***		.618
IOAM 17			.333***		.671
IOAM 18			.776***		.399
IOAM 20			.247**		.713
IOAM 21			.244**		.646
IOAM 22			.290**		.696
IOAM 23			.720***		.482
IOAM 24			.387***		.685
IOAM 25			.356***		.725
IOAM 28			.290**		.709
IOAM 29			.354***		.693
IOAM 30			.290**		.673
IOAM 3				.363***	.586
IOAM 26				.887***	.214
IOAM 27				.538**	.578

Study 3—Item response theory (IRT) of the IAOMS

Unidimensionality is an assumption underlying IRT (Bjorner et al. 2003; Brown 2006; Cook et al. 2007). Unidimensionality could be validated by confirmatory factor analysis (CFA, Cook et al. 2009; Sacco et al. 2011). Thus, before IRT was adopted, CFA had been conducted to ensure that every single subscale was measuring one dimension exclusively. Statistically speaking, every single subscale was hypothesized to be a single factor model. The goodness-of-fit indices of every single subscale of the IOAMS are illustrated by Table 15.3.

All of the above validated models were first-order single factor models. In conclusion, the results indicated the unidimensional characteristics of each subscale per se.

Study 3 investigated the IIF by adopting GRM (Samejima 1969).The goodness-of-fit statistics of the four subscales are illustrated by Table 15.4 while the item parameters are illustrated by Table 15.5 for the factor 1 subscale; Table 15.6 for the factor 2 subscale; Table 15.7 for the factor 3 subscale; and Table 15.8 for the factor 4 subscale correspondingly.

As mentioned above, the IIF of all items were investigated. The item information curve (IFC) of every single item of the factor 1, factor 2, factor 3 and factor 4 subscales are depicted by Figs. 15.1, 15.2, 15.3 and 15.4 correspondingly.

15.3.4 Item Selection

In accordance with the IIFs, the items with relatively high IIFs were retained whereas other items with relatively low IIFs were eliminated (Toland 2014; Chui and Leung 2016). Thus, as for the factor 1 subscale, items 1, 11 and 12 were retained; referring to the factor 2 subscale, items 1, 14 and 19 were retained; with regard to the factor 3 subscale, items 4, 15 and 23 were retained; concerning the factor 4 subscale, items 3, 26 and 27 were retained. The remaining items of the four subscales were all eliminated. The subscales exhibited the TIF $\approx$ 4.00 and the SEE $\approx$ .5. Please refer to Figs. 15.5, 15.6, 15.7 and 15.8. Hence, the IOAMS was suggested to be condensed from 30 items to 12 items to become a short form.

Study 4—Validation of the IOAMS-SF

The Cronbach alphas, composite reliabilities and marginal reliabilities (ρ; Fornell and Larcker 1981; de Ayala 2009; Raykov 2009) of the variables of the selected items were examined and listed in Table 15.9.

Generally speaking, the subscales were found to demonstrate appropriate reliability with Cronbach's alpha greater than .60 (Evers 2001). The overall internal consistency was .87. Moreover, the validity of the Individual-Oriented Achievement Motivation Scale-Short Form (IAOMS-SF) was investigated by CFA. The validated model is depicted by Fig. 15.9.

Table 15.3 Goodness-of-fit indices of all the subscales of the IOAM

Model	χ^2	*df*	χ^2/df	RMSEA	NNFI	CFI	SRMR	GFI	−2ln(L)	AIC	BIC
Factor 1	27.14	8	3.39	.076	.94	.97	.036	.98	2026.28	2052.28	2104.55
Factor 2	28.74	13	2.21	.054	.96	.97	.034	.98	2523.35	2553.35	2613.67
Factor 3	239.59	76	3.15	.007	.88	.90	.053	.92	5042.70	5100.70	5217.31
Factor 4	.00	.00	.00	.000	1.00	1.00	.000	1.00	1215.89	1227.89	1252.02

Table 15.4 The table of the likelihood-based values and goodness-of-fit statistics

Subscale	−2log likelihood	Akaike information criterion (AIC)	Bayesian information criterion (BIC)
Factor 1	6421.62	6493.62	6638.38
Factor 2	7599.13	7679.13	7839.97
Factor 3	14,995.82	15,163.82	15,501.59
Factor 4	3416.47	3452.47	3524.84

Table 15.5 Graded model item parameter statistics of subscale 1

Item	a	b_1	b_2	b_3	b_4	b_5	χ^2	d/f	p value
IOAM2	1.66	−4.01	−2.85	−1.47	0.00	1.87	33.01	39	0.7393
IOAM5	1.25	−5.42	−2.97	−1.51	0.05	1.91	45.63	49	0.6116
IOAM6	1.14	−4.61	−2.71	−1.42	0.32	2.21	65.42	51	0.0841
IOAM7	1.15	−5.82	−2.89	−1.56	0.10	2.26	66.53	47	0.0317
IOAM11	2.83	−2.80	−1.96	−0.97	0.18	1.56	36.08	36	0.4661
IOAM12	2.05	−2.87	−1.86	−0.68	0.43	1.98	50.33	43	0.2056

Table 15.6 Graded model item parameter statistics of subscale 2

Item	a	b_1	b_2	b_3	b_4	b_5	χ^2	d/f	p value
IOAM1	1.56	−2.72	−1.58	−0.21	1.60	–	55.78	47	0.1777
IOAM8	1.17	−5.72	−2.74	−1.01	0.56	2.60	97.58	54	0.0003
IOAM9	1.36	−4.02	−2.87	−1.45	−0.12	1.69	65.23	48	0.0494
IOAM10	1.17	−3.48	−2.50	−1.16	0.34	2.29	80.44	58	0.0272
IOAM13	1.50	−4.73	−2.62	−1.61	−0.06	1.63	72.94	47	0.0090
IOAM14	1.71	−3.08	−1.43	−0.14	1.44	–	57.22	41	0.0474
IOAM19	1.88	−3.04	−1.95	−0.78	0.51	1.88	75.20	46	0.0042

Table 15.7 Graded model item parameter statistics of subscale 3

Item	a	b_1	b_2	b_3	b_4	b_5	χ^2	d/f	p value
IOAM4	2.24	−3.40	−2.15	−1.35	−0.17	1.38	71.22	65	0.2780
IOAM15	1.69	−3.50	−2.33	−1.22	0.07	1.73	102.89	78	0.0310
IOAM16	1.53	−3.19	−1.96	−0.92	0.34	1.96	121.68	89	0.0122
IOAM17	1.61	−4.05	−2.22	−0.90	0.51	2.16	80.58	79	0.4304
IOAM18	1.23	−4.84	−3.50	−1.37	0.10	1.86	74.52	79	0.6225
IOAM20	1.62	−3.47	−2.35	−1.16	0.14	1.99	106.74	81	0.0292
IOAM21	1.49	−3.62	−2.08	−0.73	0.57	2.25	99.02	84	0.1255
IOAM22	1.30	−3.07	−1.87	−0.59	0.80	2.77	93.27	93	0.4734
IOAM23	1.63	−3.32	−2.38	−1.42	0.12	1.79	81.89	76	0.3013
IOAM24	1.52	−3.70	−2.61	−1.42	0.15	1.85	90.62	78	0.1552
IOAM25	1.21	−4.95	−2.42	−1.15	0.35	1.96	94.75	92	0.4007
IOAM28	1.40	−3.75	−2.69	−1.30	0.27	2.21	94.36	79	0.1143
IOAM29	1.55	−3.68	−2.31	−1.13	0.48	2.29	124.53	80	0.0011
IOAM30	1.32	−3.19	−1.98	−1.24	0.30	2.15	111.45	88	0.0464

Table 15.8 Graded model item parameter statistics of subscale 4

Item	a	b_1	b_2	b_3	b_4	b_5	χ^2	d/f	p value
IOAM3	1.43	−3.39	−2.14	−0.82	0.42	2.11	39.95	32	0.1575
IOAM26	2.70	−2.34	−1.31	−0.37	0.56	1.84	29.02	23	0.1790
IOAM27	2.77	−2.67	−1.54	−0.39	0.62	1.87	22.99	23	0.4630

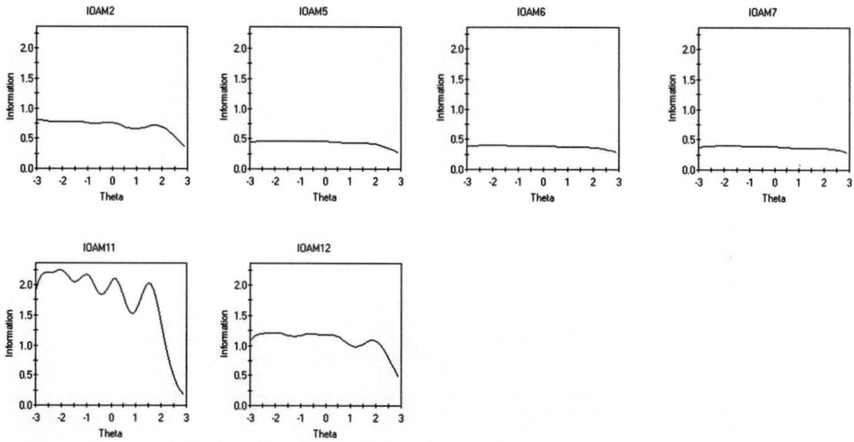

Fig. 15.1 The IFC of factor 1 of the IOAM

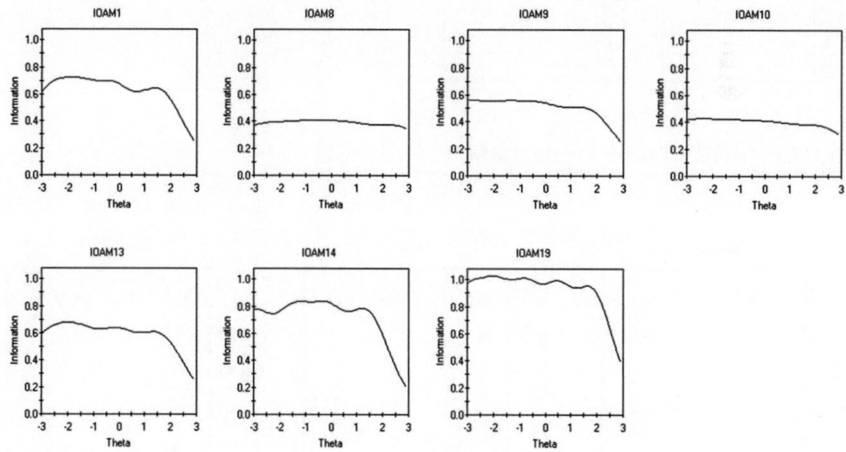

Fig. 15.2 The IFC of factor 2 of the IOAM

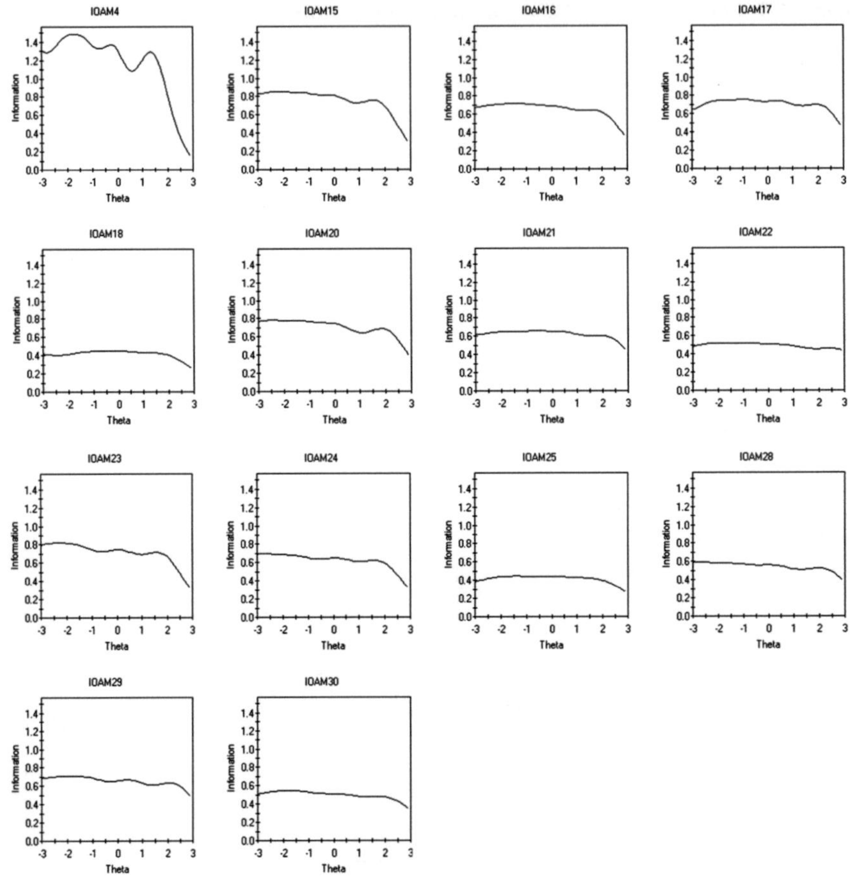

Fig. 15.3 The IFC of factor 3 of the IOAM

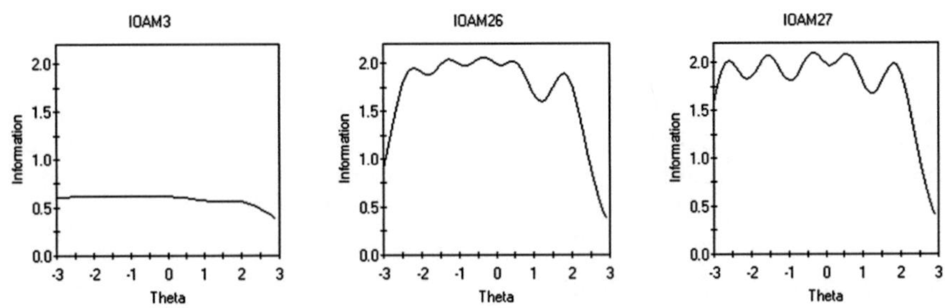

Fig. 15.4 The IFC of factor 4 of the IOAM

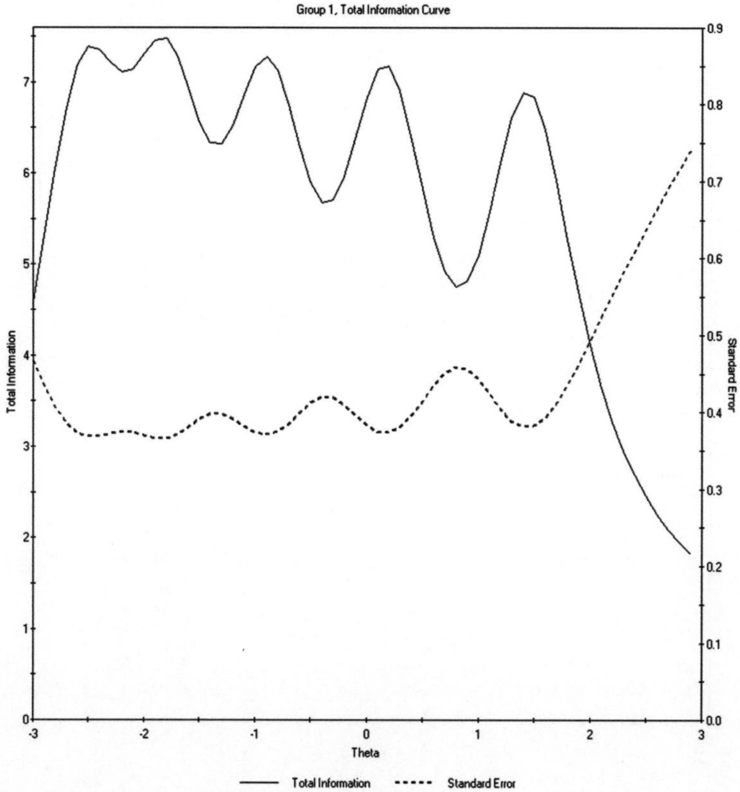

Fig. 15.5 The ITC of factor 1 of the condensed IOAM

The model demonstrated sufficient fit: $\chi^2(df = 48) = 156.09$, $p = .00$, CFI = .94, GFI = .94, RMSEA = .074. To sum up, the indices suggested that the IAOMS-SF would be a valid measurement in assessing an individual's IOAM. The CFA result indicated that the error term of items 14 and 19 significantly and positively covaried ($\theta_\varepsilon = .25$, $p < .001$). Moreover, the error term of items 26 and 27 also significantly and positively covaried ($\theta_\varepsilon = .29, p < .001$).

15.4 General Discussion

The aforementioned CFA model of the IAOMS demonstrated a two-order factor structures with a single higher order and four lower order factors. The result indicated that the four first-order factors would belong to an identical dimension of IOAM. In accordance with the face validity of the items of the second-order factors, the subscales were entitled "persistence", "self-reflection", "inherent values"

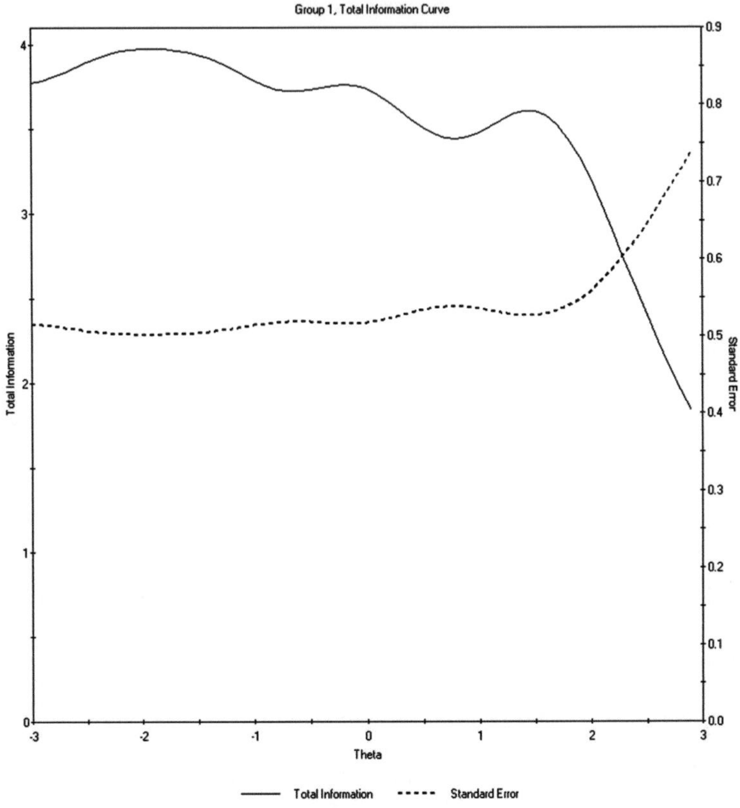

Fig. 15.6 The ITC of factor 2 of the condensed IOAM

and "achievement awareness" correspondingly. The items of the "persistence" subscale describe an individual's resilience and perseverance in goal achievement upon encountering difficulties. The items of the "self-reflection" subscale narrate an individual's willingness and capacity to self-reflect on the underlying motivation to achieve, particularly with respect to education. The items of the "inherent values" assess an individual's intrinsic motivation to succeed. Furthermore, the items of the "achievement awareness" measure an individual's self-perception of the individual self-perceived sense of achievement. This subscale was conceptualized to be associated with an individual's metacognition, i.e. an individual is aware of the individual's own mental state. In the currently studied construct, achievement awareness refers to an individual's awareness of the individual's mental state about success and achievement.

The current study was very different from the previous studies (e.g. Chang et al. 2000 IOAM 2; Abd-El-Fattah and Patrick 2011) as the current study validated the presence of the second-order latent factors and further differentiated the

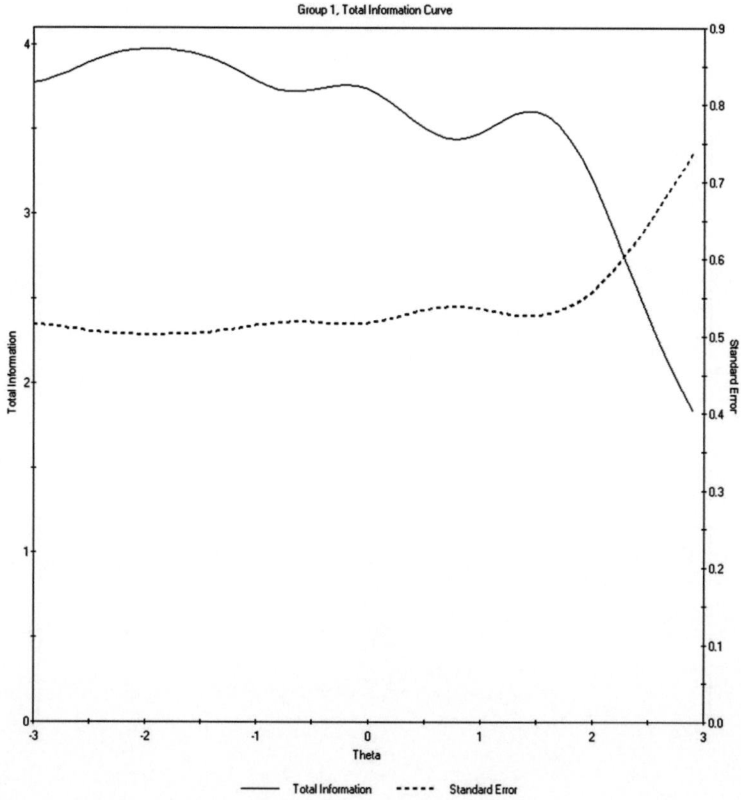

Fig. 15.7 The ITC of factor 3 of the condensed IOAM

entire IAOMS into four different subscales. Despite the four different subdimensions the subscale measuring, they examine the identical construct IOAM as illustrated by the CFA model (please see Fig. 15.5).

The four second-order latent factors echo SDT. As mentioned above, the factor of "persistence" was defined as an individual's resilience and perseverance in goal achievement upon encountering difficulties. According to Ryan and Deci (2000), an individual who has fulfilled the three psychological needs, namely, autonomy, competence and relatedness, would become frustration tolerant and resilient in hard times. The individual would then be intrinsically motivated to pursue the individual's goals regardless of hindrances. The second factor of "self-reflection" embodies an imperative element in lives, the meaning of success, or even the meaning of life (Yalom and Leszcz 2005). Although this factor tends to be existential, not SDT-oriented, an individual will not maintain the individual's intrinsic motivation if the individual recognizes the individual's endeavours meaningless to him/her (Ryan and Deci 2000). Hence, although meaning of achievement is remarkably personal, it is also critical to an individual's intrinsic motivation.

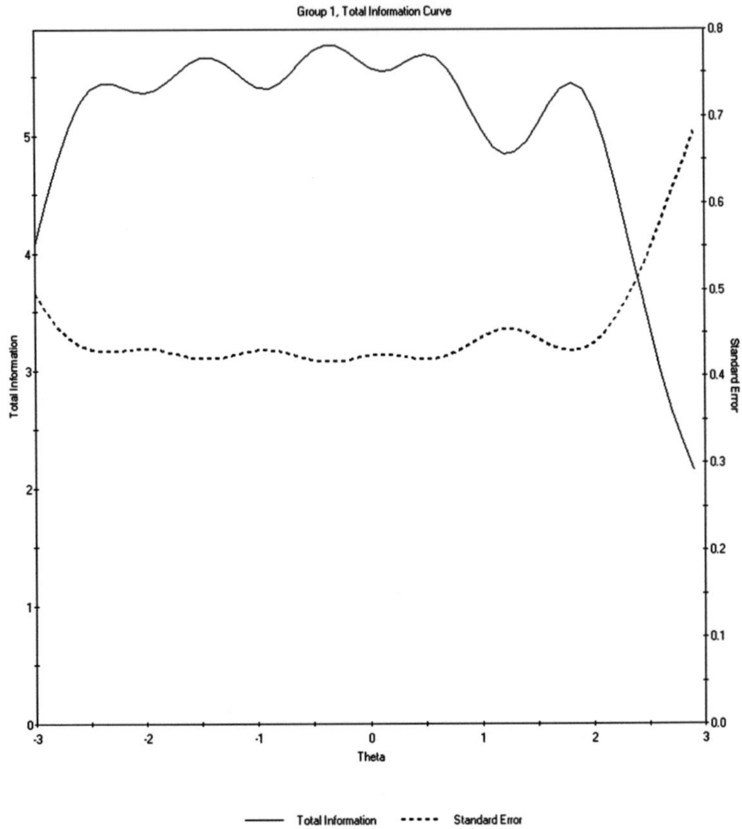

Fig. 15.8 The ITC of factor 4 of the condensed IOAM

Table 15.9 The internal consistencies (α) and composite reliabilities (ρ) of the four subscales

Subscale	Cronbach α	Composite reliability ρ
Persistence	.75	.72
Self-reflection	.68	.63
Inherent values	.68	.68
Achievement awareness	.76	.65
Overall	.87	

The third factor of "inherent values" indicates an individual's intrinsic motivation to achieve, especially in education contexts. Either does it echo with SDT. The fourth factor of "achievement awareness", as mentioned above, is highly associated with metacognition. Metacognition, such as planning and monitoring, were found to be conducive to goal achievement motivation (Zepeda et al. 2015). Therefore, IOAM-SF is capable of assessing a range of areas, not limited to SDT, such as meaning of success, self-reflective capacity and metacognitive level.

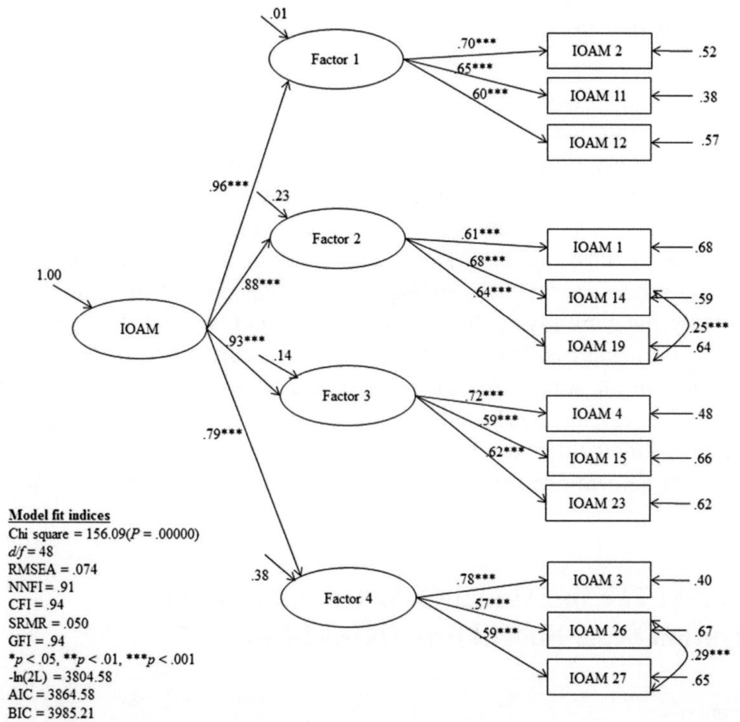

Fig. 15.9 The CFA of the IOAM-SF

Notwithstanding the satisfying reliability and validity of the IOAMS, it comprises 30 items. The IOAMS was found fairly lengthy with items repeating similar ideas. With IRT and IIFs, the original 30-item version was condensed into a 12-item version which would be more parsimonious.

15.5 Conclusion and Implications

The current study validated the IOAMS-SF and further differentiated the entire IAOMS into four different subscales. The IOAMS-SF is capable of assessing a range of areas, not limited to SDT, such as meaning of success, self-reflective capacity and metacognitive level. The IOAMS-SF is found to be a reliable and valid tool assessing an individual's "persistence", "self-reflection", "inherent values" and "achievement awareness" under the mere construct of IOAM. For parsimony, the original 30-item version was condensed into a 12-item short form. It can be applied to measuring individual's IOAM, particularly in education context. Integrating the IOAMS-SF with other scales or inventories, researches on achievement motivation can be facilitated in the future.

15.6 Limitations

Several limitations should be taken into account when evaluating the current study. First, the data collected in the current study were on the basis of self-report which was void of observations of behaviours. The sampling size ($N = 412$) suggested that the potential-biased errors were present and generalization to other samples might be limited. The current study was fundamentally a cross-sectional survey in Hong Kong Chinese culture. The research design was not a longitudinal study investigating the causal effects among the variables. Hence, the causal relationships among the currently studied variables might not be valid. Further interpretations must be made carefully and modestly in the current study. In the future, a causal model of the studied phenomenon should be established which could more elaborately portray the mechanism for devising further therapeutic interventions. Furthermore, empirical researches should be conducted to investigate the effectiveness of the aforementioned interventions in terms of their impacts on the IOAM.

Appendix: The Individual-Oriented Achievement Motivation Scale-Short Form (IOAM-SF)

Persistence

1. While working, I always keep on trying until I am satisfied.
2. I am willing to constantly working hard in order to reach personal success.
3. I usually examine my own performance in an examination, when I do not have the test results, in order to improve myself.

Self-reflection

1. No matter how difficult the task is, I would try my best to do it, if I think it is worthwhile to do.
2. No matter what other people might think, I will try my best to do what I consider valuable.
3. To attain high level of education is glorification of my ancestors but for my own knowledge and interests.

Inherent values

1. I usually think whether my present performance has reached my own standards.
2. I get satisfaction from completing jobs; the reward that comes with it is secondary to me.
3. I usually follow my own studying methods in order to obtain better marks.

Success awareness

1. Even if no one were around, I would still complete whatever I started.
2. I am very clear about how much effort to put in a job in order to reach my goals.
3. After finishing a job, I can usually judge what my performance might be.

References

Abd-El-Fattah, S. M., & Patrick, R. R. (2011). The relationship among achievement motivation orientations, achievement goals and academic achievement and interest: A multiple mediation analysis. *Australian Journal of Educational and Developmental Psychology, 11*, 91–110.

Bentler, P. M. (1990). Comparative fit indexes in structural equation models. *Psychological Bulletin, 107*, 238–246.

Bjorner, J. B., Kosinski, M., & Ware, J. E., Jr. (2003). Calibration of an item pool for assessing the burden of headaches: An application of item response theory to the headache impact test (HIT). *Quality of Life Research, 12*, 913–933.

Brown, T. A. (2006). *Confirmatory factor analysis for applied research*. New York: The Guilford Press.

Byrne, B. M. (1998). *Structural equation modeling with LISREL, PRELIS, and SIMPLIS: Basic concepts, applications and programming*. New York: Lawrence Erlbaum Associates.

Chang, W. N. C., Wong, W. K., & Teo, G. (2000). The socially oriented and individually oriented achievement motivation of Singaporean Chinese students. *Journal of Psychology in Chinese Societies, 1*(2), 39–63.

Chui, W. Y., & Leung, M. T. (2016). Adult attachment internal working model of self and other in Chinese culture: Measured by the Attachment Style Questionnaire-Short Form (ASQ-SF) by confirmatory factor analysis (CFA) and item response theory (IRT). *Personality and Individual Differences, 96*, 55–64.

Chui, W. Y., Lee, S. K., & Tsang, C. K. (2016). Father involvement in Hong Kong: By multitrait–multimethod model and item response theory (IRT). *Personality and Individual Differences, 98*, 333–344.

Connell, J. P., & Wellborn, J. G. (1991). Competence, autonomy, and relatedness: A motivational analysis of self-system processes. In M. R. Gunnar & L. A. Sroufe (Eds.), *Self processes in development: Minnesota symposium on child psychology* (Vol. 23, pp. 43–77). Hillsdale, NJ: Erlbaum.

Cook, K. F., Kallen, M. A., & Amtamann, D. (2009). Having a fit: Impact of number of items and distribution of data on traditional assessing IRT's unidimensionality assumption. *Quality of Life Research, 18*, 447–460.

Cook, K. F., Teal, C. R., Bjorner, J. B., Cella, D., Chang, C. H., Crane, P. K., et al. (2007). IRT health outcomes data analysis project: An overview and summary. *Quality of Life Research, 16*(Suppl 1), 121–132.

De Ayala, R. J. (2009). *The theory and practice of item response theory*. New York: Guilford.

Deci, E. L. (1975). *Intrinsic motivation*. New York: Plenum Press.

Deci, E. L., & Ryan, R. M. (1985). *Intrinsic motivation and self-determination in human behavior*. New York: Plenum Press.

Evers, A. (2001). Improving test quality in the Netherlands: Results of 18 years of test ratings. *International Journal of Testing, 1*(2), 137–153.

Fornell, C., & Larcker, D. F. (1981). Evaluating structural equation models with unobservable variables and measurement error. *Journal of Marketing Research, 18*, 39–50.

George, D., & Mallery, M. (2010). *SPSS for windows step by step: A simple guide and reference, 17.0 update* (10th ed.). Boston: Pearson.

Guay, F., Senécal, C., Gautheir, L., & Fernet, C. (2003). Predicting career indecision: A self-determination theory perspective. *Journal of Counselling Psychology, 50*(2), 165–177.

Hambleton, R. K., & Swaminathan, H. (1985). *Item response theory: Principles and applications* (Vol. 7). USA: Springer.

Hong, J., & Chen, C. (2014). The role of the built environment on perceived safety from crime and walking: Examining direct and indirect impacts. *Transportation, 41*, 1171–1185.

Kline, R. B. (2010). *Principles and practice of structural equation modeling* (3rd ed.). New York: Guilford Press.

Lazarsfeld, P. F., & Henry, N. W. (1968). *Latent structure analysis*. Boston: Houghton Mill.

Lepper, M. R., Greene, D., & Nisbett, R. E. (1973). Undermining children's intrinsic interest with extrinsic reward: A test of the overjustification hypothesis. *Journal of Personality and Social Psychology, 28*, 129–137.

Mitra, A., Bang, J. T., & Wunnava, P. V. (2014). Financial liberalization and the selection of emigrants: A cross-national analysis. *Empirical Economics, 47*, 199–226.

Raykov, T. (2009). Evaluation of scale reliability for unidimensional measures using latent variable modelling. *Measurement and Evaluation in Counseling and Development, 42*(3), 223–232.

Ryan, R. M., & Deci, E. L. (2000). Self-determination theory and the facilitation of intrinsic motivation, social development, and well-being. *American Psychologist, 55*, 68–78.

Sacco, P., Torres, L. R., Cunningham-Williams, R. M., Woods, C., & Unick, G. J. (2011). Differential item functioning of pathological gambling criteria: An examination of gender, race/ethnicity and age. *Journal of Gambling Study, 27*, 317–330.

Samejima, F. (1969). *Estimation of latent ability using a response pattern of graded scores*. Psychometrika Monograph, No. 17. Richmond, VA: Psychometric Society.

Toland, M. D. (2014). Practical guide to conducting an item response theory analysis. *Journal of Early Adolescence, 34*(1), 120–151.

Yalom, I. D., & Leszcz, M. (2005). *The theory and practice of group psychotherapy*. New York: Basic Books.

Yang, K. S., & Yu, A. B. (1988). *Social- and individual-oriented achievement motives: Conceptualization and measurement.* Paper presented at the symposium on Chinese personality and social psychology for the XXIVth international congress of psychology. Sydney, Australia.

Zepeda, C. D., Richey, J. E., Ronevich, P., & Nokes-Malach, T. J. (2015). Direct instruction o metacognition benefits adolescent science learning, transfer, and motivation: An in vivo study. *Journal of Educational Psychology, 107*(4), 954–970.

MIX
Papier aus verantwortungsvollen Quellen
Paper from responsible sources
FSC® C105338

If you have any concerns about our products,
you can contact us on
ProductSafety@springernature.com

In case Publisher is established outside the EU,
the EU authorized representative is:
Springer Nature Customer Service Center GmbH
Europaplatz 3, 69115 Heidelberg, Germany

Printed by Libri Plureos GmbH
in Hamburg, Germany